DATE DUE

The Body Electric

American History and Culture

GENERAL EDITORS
Neil Foley, Kevin Gaines, Martha Hodes, and Scott Sandage

The
Body Electric

*How Strange Machines Built
the Modern American*

Carolyn Thomas de la Peña

NEW YORK UNIVERSITY PRESS
New York and London

NEW YORK UNIVERSITY PRESS
New York and London

Library of Congress Cataloging-in-Publication Data
Peña, Carolyn Thomas de la.
The body electric : how strange machines built the modern American /
Carolyn Thomas de la Peña
p. ; cm. — (American history and culture)
Includes bibliographical references and index.
ISBN 0-8147-1953-8 (cloth : alk. paper)
1. Quacks and quackery—United States—History—19th century.
2. Quacks and quackery—United States—History—20th century.
3. Medical instruments and apparatus—United States—History—
19th century.   4. Medical instruments and apparatus—United States—
History—20th century.   5. Electrotherapeutics—United States—History—
19th century.   6. Electrotherapeutics—United States—History—
20th century.
    [DNLM: 1. Electric Stimulation Therapy—history.   2. Exercise
Therapy—history.   3. History of Medicine, 19th Cent.   4. History of
Medicine, 20th Cent.   WB 495 P397b 2003]   I. Title.   II. American
history and culture (New York University Press)
R730.P39   2003
615.8'56—dc21   2002155358

Acknowledgment is made for permission to quote from the previously
published materials.

Portions of chapter 2 have previously appeared in
"Dudley Allen Sargent & Gustav Zander: Health Machines and the
Energized Male Body," Research in the Philosophy of Technology
(Summer 2002).
"Recharging at the Fordyce: Confronting Machine and Nature in the
Modern Bath," Technology and Culture 40 (October 1999).
Portions of chapter 4 have previously appeared in
"Reading Electric Belts: Sex, Technology, and the Modern Male
Body," Journal of Design History 14, no. 4 (2001).

10 9 8 7 6 5 4 3 2 1

Contents

Acknowledgments

I could not have written this without Elizabeth Ihrig, the librarian at the Bakken Library and Museum of Electricity in Life in Minneapolis. It was Elizabeth who, while I was there on a visiting research fellowship in 1999, suggested that I might want to take a look at a couple of uncataloged boxes of electrotherapy "ephemera." The brochures and business records that I found in those boxes first convinced me that I could tell this story, in spite of the few published secondary sources on the subject. I would like to also thank David Rhees, executive director of the Bakken for his early support of my work on popular electrotherapy, and the Bakken staff for serving as an enthusiastic and critical first audience for this work.

Jan Todd served as a skillful guide through the Todd-McLean Physical Culture Collection at the University of Texas at Austin. It was my good fortune to have close at hand this rich collection of books, pamphlets, magazines, and business records detailing the history of physical training. I also benefited from the time and materials provided by several research fellowships. I spent a wonderful month in the summer of 1998 enjoying the intellectual and botanical riches of the Huntington Library in Pasadena, California. My thanks to the Huntington trustees for the Fletcher Jones Foundation Fellowship that allowed me to put all of my energies into this project during that critical time.

I am also indebted to William Baxter and the staff of the Dibner Library at the Smithsonian for their assistance during a 1999 visiting research fellowship. I completed much of my work on electrotherapy and radium in the Dibner's beautiful reading room.

Additionally, the Helfand Fellowship from the New York Academy of Medicine provided financial support for the last stages of research. My two weeks at the academy yielded several treasures and allowed me to present my work on electric belts for the first time.

I would also like to thank the overworked archivists at the American Medical Association who doggedly unearthed box after box from the Historical Health Fraud Collection (HHFC). The HHFC is a rich source of materials on alternative medical practices of the past century; it is unfortunate that the fees to see these documents make it prohibitive for those without institutional funding to use them. I hope my work leads others to request improved access to the association's documents.

Finally, thank you to the University of Texas for its support through multiple travel and research fellowships, particularly for the year of funding through the Continuing Fellowship program in 1998.

Archivists provided the textual resources essential for this project; my mentors, friends, and family provided the emotional ones. Thank you to my dissertation committee for critical comments that made this book a better one than I could write. In particular, I would like to thank Jan Todd for an encyclopedic knowledge of physical culture that she brought to the first two chapters of this project. It is Jeff Meikle, however, to whom I owe the biggest debt of gratitude. Jeff has always encouraged me to believe that this project was doable, fundable, and finishable. His wide-ranging knowledge about American modernism and technology gave me direction throughout and helped me place my story within a larger cultural framework. And his inimitable editing skills repeatedly found and solved problems conceptual and grammatical. I could not have asked for a more committed, knowledgeable, and supportive mentor.

I am fortunate to have among my friends some of the best American Studies minds on the planet. Joel Dinerstein and Siva Vaidyanathan are two of them; their early support convinced me that I would survive graduate school and complete this project. Kim Hewitt helped brew my ideas through countless conversations about medicine, the body, and our shifting cultural perceptions of the normal. Without Christina Cogdell, I might be thinking about this project right now, but it is doubtful that I would be doing it with a Ph.D. in hand. Thanks to our year of laptop battleship in Austin coffeehouses, we managed to finish dissertations, land jobs in the sunny state, and rethink some of the assumptions of American modernism. Thank you also to Maureen Reed. Her intelligence, incomparable organizational skills, and unfaltering support have continually pushed me to create things better than I thought possible.

I thank my colleagues in American Studies at UC Davis, who are fine teachers, admirable scholars, and generous editors. Thank you particularly to Kay Clare Allen for providing inspiration; to my research assistant Erin McClelland for meticulous work and ample good cheer; and to Sarah Projansky, Vicki Mayer, Joanne Barker, Lara Downes, and Sophie Volpp for unlimited encouragement through the revision process. I am also grateful to Kent Ono, friend and mentor, for commenting on a draft when he had absolutely no time to do it.

My final debts are to my family, past and present. Thank you to my Mimi, Gertrude Vade Bon Coeur. Though she did not live to see this project completed, she gave me the gumption to do it. Thank you to my father, Gary Thomas, for teaching me that learning requires the courage to disagree. Thank you to my mother- and father-in-law, Ardith and Joe de la Peña, for being so proud of my work that it is impossible to fail. Thank you especially to my mother, Catherine Vade Bon Coeur, who has always helped me dream big dreams that somehow come true. And finally, to David de la Peña, master editor and right brain to my left; thank you for immeasurably improving my life and my work. I dedicate this to you, and to our daughter, Sofia. May we always have the energy to create a world of our own design.

Preface

Few of us think twice about building our bodies with machines. Yet almost all of us have spent a good deal of money and time pursuing fitness with technological devices. Perhaps we've bought into the electric belts pitched on infomercials at 3:00 A.M., hooked electrodes to our stomachs and waited for the "six pack" to emerge. Perhaps it was a massager on sale at the mall, one that promised to "reinvigorate" us fully after a ten-minute treatment. Some of us have brought machines for building muscle into our homes. And many of us frequent private gyms where nearly every element of our workout—from StairMaster warm-ups to Cybex lifts to treadmill cooldowns—are choreographed with machines.

Where did these machines come from, and how have they become common tools for our body-shaping projects? What does their ubiquity tell us about the relationship between technology, energy, and the body in modern American culture? These are questions that have driven the explorations in this book. The answers have been found by looking at history, to the particular reasons that Americans once embraced "energetic" technologies, to the products they created and consumed, and to the implications of our dependence on technology to achieve physical health. They reveal that climbing the StairMaster is not merely a way of burning fat; it is also a way of teaching ourselves about the proper relationship between technology and the body. By exploring the values and beliefs at the heart of technofitness habits, we uncover how our bodies interpret technologies in our lives.

Though we rarely think about the lessons our bodies teach our minds, they are, in fact, the most intimate means by which we negotiate the technologies of daily life. We may debate the merits of state-funded birth control, spending on biotech research, and the hospital-industrial complex. It is our bodies, however, that consume the pacemakers, the X rays, and the Viagras that such institutions produce. When we allow a technology intimate entry into our bodies, we become, *on some level*, complicit in the culture that technology represents. Our motivations may be personal, our exposure fleeting, but in the moment of contact we are changed. Should the contact be disappointing, we may be more critical of the technological system it represents. Should it be pleasing, the system may find in us an ally. This is not to say that wearing a pacemaker makes one a supporter of biotech research, microprocessor technology, or managed care—though all are contact points of the experience. It is to say, however, that having this technology in one's body—viewing scars of insertion and experiencing the surge of random regulating shocks—forges a connection that renders a foreign technology temporarily organic; it reminds us, as Donna Haraway has argued, that "the machine is us."[1] Regardless of whether we pay attention to these points of contact, through them our bodies consume lessons about the properties and potentials of technologies. By surrounding or entering our bodies for the express purpose of improving them, technologies become cooperative agents rather than foreign invaders, and grow resistant to critique. Rarely do we debate, dissect, or dismiss the meanings they embed.

I became interested in the ways in which our bodies contextualize new technologies while researching Twilight Sleep, the first method of pain relief widely used in childbirth in this country. Much has been written on the procedure and women's attempts to persuade American physicians to adopt it in the early twentieth century.[2] What particularly intrigued me, however, was the reasoning many gave for advocating its use: its attendant drugs, scopolamine and morphine, were necessary to render bodies natural. To arrive at this conclusion, women, primarily of the middle and upper classes, compared themselves to Native American women, whom they believed experienced painless childbirth.[3] By casting these women as "natural" because of their premodern lifestyle and by arguing, mistakenly, that they experienced little, if any, labor pain, American women were able to conclude that "natural" birth should be pain free. Only modern habits, many reasoned, produced pain. As a result of this correlation, they were able to argue that drugs were "natural" because drugs returned the body to its intended state.

The Twilight Sleep story suggests that our bodies often set the context for understanding new technologies. I began to research current body technologies to see if they had an equivalent to scopolamine and morphine, technologies that because of their desirable ability to lessen pain and remove memory after labor, were regarded as "natural" or "normal" despite their actual composition. I found health machines, electricity, and radium. Each of these technologies, by which I mean materials or substances created or discovered through modern innovations, was defined as "natural" using reasoning similar to that used by Twilight Sleep's advocates, although without the explicit connection to Native Americans. Each appeared as a solution to a physical problem that was particularly pressing due to larger cultural concerns. For health machines, the problem was that human energy was inefficiently "blocked" in the system. For electricity, the problem was that human energy was of an insufficient supply to meet the demands of modern life. For radium, the problem was that human energy was inadequate because it could not continually regenerate itself. Just as the technologies of Twilight Sleep were regarded as natural and welcomed as necessary because they relieved "unnatural" pain, so too were technologies that promised to relieve the "unnatural" lethargy endemic to late-nineteenth and early-twentieth-century life. In both cases, it seemed that the body could be brought closer to its ideal state by "ingesting" modern technology.

This project has four primary objectives. First, it seeks to further develop a theory offered by historian John Kasson. In his *Amusing the Million*, a history of Coney Island's early-twentieth-century amusement parks, Kasson argues that the parks' rides domesticated frightening new technologies for a generation of Americans who confronted unprecedented industrial and urban change.[4] By focusing on the rides, technological products that people voluntarily put in contact with their bodies, Kasson discovered a rich space within which individuals interpreted the nature of new technologies.[5] My search for materials that had a similar effect uncovered hundreds of technological products marketed to consumers between 1870 and 1935 with the explicit promise of physical benefit: once they were attached, inserted, or ingested, improved energy and health would follow. Many of these objects, such as exercise machines and electric belts, appeared in forms typically associated with urban life and industrial production. As a result, they allowed consuming bodies to bridge the gap between dangerous and restorative energies. These devices functioned in a manner similar to Kasson's rides but on a more intimate level and with a more explicit connection between physical power and technological prowess.

A second goal of the project was to craft a narrative that put bodies at its center. In the past decade, a growing number of scholars have theorized connections between humans and machines. Lead by Donna Haraway, they have used the cyborg as a rhetorical and metaphorical tool for understanding how, in the broadest sense, science and technology have impacted our "lives, subjectivities, and concepts."[6] In spite of this groundbreaking work, we have yet to fully understand the ways in which individuals have shaped and been shaped by human-machine contact. By expanding our inquiry into the history of this interaction, we uncover the complex and varied motivations that have driven producers and consumers to willingly intertwine the fates of humans and machines.

A close study of these individual stories accomplishes several objectives. Most important, it reveals that people embraced physical technologies because they hoped to gain something in return. There was no technological imperative at work. Technologies have not emerged out of thin air, nor have they been created and consumed out of an abstract human desire to become more machine-like. Instead, they have been accepted, and rejected, based on their ability to create culturally determined "ideal" bodies at particular moments in time.

Further, as David Nye has recently documented in *Consuming Power*, the twentieth century has been one of phenomenal increases in American energy consumption, increases that on a per capita basis far exceed those of any other similarly developed nation. His study looks at the changing institutional and cultural climates around energy production and consumption; here I reveal that there is also a more intimate story to tell. Exploring the body allows us to theorize that we consume more energy because we once believed that industrial and physical energies were interchangeable. By expanding the production of our productive energies, we expanded the possibilities of our physical selves.

We can also use these experiences to better understand the cultural relevance of neurasthenia. Those who write about the disease often cite S. Weir Mitchell and George Beard, stressing their doomsday predictions about physical decline that trapped women in traditional gender roles at a time of cultural change. The story of technological devices, however, challenges this theory by affirming more recent scholarship: males, not females, actually made up the majority of neurasthenics.[7] Further, the devices' popularity suggests that people did not passively accept as a truism experts' speculative correlations between modern life and ill health. On the contrary, many bought gadgets expressly to fight "neurasthenic" decline, contradicting the advice of elite physicians. Experts may have written treatises about conserving energy to fight neurasthenia, but individuals often chose to augment—or forgo—conservation in favor of expansion by means of electric belts and radium waters. By exploring what bodies did instead of what experts advised, neurasthenia's story of decline emerges as one of many possible interpretations available to those who sought to understand the new relationship between energy, modernity, and the body. This approach supports recent work that challenges theories of technological determinism. Forgotten sites of techno-body contact like Health Lift studios and storefront I-ON-A-CO treatment centers, once reconstructed, remind us that individuals have actively used their bodies to accept certain technologies and reject others. The appeal of the promise a technology makes to consumers is as important as any innate momentum it may possess.

A discussion of energy enhancers blurs the line between regular and irregular medicine. Much effort has been expended by physicians and academics over the past century to carefully distinguish between the theories of regular, or licensed, medical practitioners and those of unlicensed "quacks."[8] The distinction, however, is much more relevant with the aid of hindsight. During the late nineteenth century and early twentieth, few Americans granted licensed physicians exclusive domain over medical treatments. Instead, most people conceived of medicine as a smorgasbord of possible panaceas, some from licensed doctors in their offices and some from quacks selling from carts on street corners. Lax standards in medical licensing meant that there was often little distinction between the efficacy of a regular or a quack cure; a patient chose between the two based on the seriousness of the illness, the proximity and cost of a treatment, and the resonance of its promises with what he or she wanted to hear. The fact that we now know that electric belts do not cure most physiological ailments does not mean that they were unimportant as curative devices. They, along with radium waters and health machines, were products in which people invested and believed. Understanding the power of "medicine" at the turn of the twentieth century, as today, means accepting that "bad" science can make "good" cures.

Finally, it would please me if this project proves the cultural relevance of Spiderman. It is easy, but incorrect, to assume that once these gadgets fell from favor in the 1940s, our hopes of technologically powered bodies disappeared. Admittedly, there was no longer a direct stream of consumer products linking physical fantasies to technology purchases. By the

1950s, science and medicine had proven the fallacy of energy-absorption theories: machines could improve cardiovascular health and skeletal strength; electric "acupressure" could relieve pain when used precisely; radium could, under expert supervision, fight disease. These things could not, however, "power" the body. This does not mean that our belief in technopowered bodies disappeared. Once we uncover the promises of machine, belt, and water promoters, a clear connection emerges between them and the superheroes who were a standard part of most twentieth-century American childhoods. There are striking similarities between Spiderman, an average guy who, after a bite from a radioactive spider, gains paranormal abilities, and Vigoradium water drinkers; or between Flash Gordon, a man who wields physical power through lightning bolts, and wearers of the German Electric Belt. Certainly connections can be made between our current electric exercisers and the I-ON-A-CO "horse collar." Even our vision for cyber bodies has been built on this earlier era in which bodies could reach their ultimate potential only by connecting to technologies. What one generation embraced as reality has become another generation's fantasy. The power of the underlying mythology is not necessarily weakened in the exchange.

The Body Electric

Introduction

Everything, of course, depends on what we define as normal.
— Joseph B. DeLee

In 1923, Henry Gaylord Wilshire, well-known California socialist, socialite, and real estate tycoon, left sunny Los Angeles in search of renewed energy, eternal youth, and a second fortune. It was a risky venture but not his first; Wilshire loved to take chances. Land speculation, one of his most profitable ventures, had already paid off big, as evidenced by Wilshire Boulevard, Southern California's "miracle mile" of high-priced leases and elegant shopping. To the surprise of many, Wilshire left it behind to pursue the path of technological "invigoration." He moved to Oregon, putting his fortune, his reputation, and his remaining years into the I-ON-A-CO company, the leading producer of electric belts.

Little attention has been paid to Wilshire's electric belt business. Other than one article written two decades ago, the I-ON-A-CO has not been mentioned beyond an occasional paragraph in medical fraud reports. Yet Wilshire's promise of extended youth and vigor by means of electricity resonated with his time; hundreds of thousands of the belts were sold over a ten-year span. The American Medical Association's collection on historical health fraud reflects the immense public interest in Wilshire's product; it contains multiple folders documenting the successful I-ON-A-CO marketing campaign. The AMA's intensive efforts to label individuals like Wilshire as quacks and their supporters as misguided have largely succeeded; as of yet, no one has taken seriously Americans' eighty-year enthusiasm for technological energy enhancers.

In the hundred years between 1850 and 1950, Americans became the leading energy consumers on the planet, expending our physical

1

resources on energy exploration, our mental resources on energy exploitation, and our monetary resources on energy acquisition.[1] Research in the history of technology has revealed much about the great "energy" inventors of our time. Recent scholarship has uncovered the complex combination of self-promotion and ingenuity that drove Edison and Ford.[2] What remains less understood are the average American's reasons for embracing the technologies that fascinated experts.

Between the end of the Civil War and the beginning of World War II, a significant number of Americans purchased technologies sold explicitly to improve their bodies. We may assume, using historical accounts of Americans' celebratory attitudes toward technologies, that in doing so they were simply adding another layer of mechanization onto their daily lives. Once we connect this popular enthusiasm for physical gadgets to the cooperative relationship between technology and the body marketed by manufacturers, however, an experience distinct from riding a streetcar or turning on a light emerges.

There is ample evidence to document Americans' fascination with power during the late Victorian and early modern eras. Icons like the great Corliss engine of 1876, the electric amusements of Coney Island, and the glimmering "great white ways" have been evoked repeatedly to express technological enthusiasm. Energy sources have convincingly been described as tourist attractions, spaces where Americans gathered to witness firsthand the power of steam engines, the beauty of electric displays, and the showmanship of radium. Yet it is incorrect to posit that Americans worshiped new sources of power only because of their ability to perform work and inspire awe. In reality, many Americans imagined a cooperative relationship between such "dynamos" and their own bodies. Scientific and pseudoscientific medical theories suggest that individuals actively experimented with ways to increase their internal energy by putting it in contact with external energies. Few have taken these attempts seriously; contemporary Americans did. Over an eighty-year period, numerous fortunes were made and lost as popular medicine sought to make good on an implicit promise of an age of "limitless" energy.

A unique combination of pseudoscientific theories of health and Americans' rudimentary understandings of energy created an age in which industrial energies seemed capable of curing the physical limitations and ill health that plagued Victorian bodies. Licensed and "quack" physicians alike pushed machines, electricity, and radium as ultimate energy cures, veritable "fountains of youth" for their eras, substances that would infuse the body with energy and push out disease and death. The "work" of these technologies was twofold. First, they domesticated frightening new forms of energy. One could easily fear an industrial engine twenty times the size of man that whizzed and rumbled at a deafening level. It was harder, however, to sustain that fear if it greatly resembled the engine that powered a muscle-building machine one had used that morning.

Second, these technologies physically carried the body into the modern era. In all likelihood, this was not something that users of energy enhancers consciously noted. One did not strap on an electric belt and imagine the body transported from the Victorian environments of horse-drawn carriages to the modern environments of streetcar systems. Yet on an intuitive level, exposure to energy-enhancing products did allow people to see themselves as part of the modern project. By directly transferring energy from external, unlimited "dynamos" to internal circulatory and muscular systems, mechanical, electric, and radioactive technologies promised to bring the body along on the road to rapid modernization. They fostered a world in which unbridled technological optimism and industrial plenty seemed necessary components for individuals' full physical development.

Technological devices alone did not link energy acquisition to physical health. Throughout the nineteenth century, Americans gradually moved away from viewing the body as a set entity determined by God and toward viewing it as raw material malleable under man's direction. Two popular pseudosciences emerged by 1850 that successfully challenged ideas about the body's immutability. The first, phrenology, gained American converts in the early 1820s. Its promoters stressed that the brain was not, in fact, a single entity. Rather, it was made up of thirty-seven "organs" that one needed to develop equally for physical and mental health. The conception had two important implications for later energy theorists: it recast the body as a system of individual parts, each of which had to be "toned" to create a healthy whole, and it established a precedent for regarding the body as infinitely improvable. Phrenological experts such as Orson Fowler argued that one's shortcomings need not be permanent. Each of the brain's organs controlled an aspect of the personality. To become friendlier, for example, one need simply exercise that "organ." By the late nineteenth century, even if one did not agree with phrenology's findings, the idea that the body could be altered by applied energy was an acceptable proposition.

If phrenology established that the body should be altered, mesmerism made energy enhancement the most effective way of doing so. Another nineteenth-century pseudoscience, mesmerism purportedly healed bodies by redirecting blocked internal energy. Out of the hands of a skilled mesmerist, followers believed, energy traveled from practitioner to patient, resulting in increased vitality. If mesmerists never won over a majority of physicians and scientists to their cause, they did capture an American popular audience. Over a period of fifty years, itinerant mesmerists wandered the country's rural areas, introducing two generations to the idea that the body's energy could be manipulated through external force for improved health.

By the late nineteenth century, it was possible to believe that external energies could alter the physical body. To understand why individuals may have wanted to alter their bodies with those energies, however, we have to explore changing attitudes about energy itself. Although it had once seemed plentiful on the "new" continent and in its inhabitants, energy seemed rapidly diminishing in both as the new century approached. In the external physical environment, this gave rise to energy conservation movements, such as the national parks system. In the internal physical environment, it encouraged attempts to shore up physical energy, most notably through neurasthenia treatments. Both conservation and neurasthenia "treatments" were attempts to halt energy dissipation, but only the external approach could be taken with any assurance of success. One could erect a barrier around open spaces and decree by law that the resources within be permanently preserved. The body proved a more challenging terrain to police.

First diagnosed by physician George Miller Beard, neurasthenia entered the conservation dialogue by defining the body as a system continually diminishing in energetic strength. The body's energy, Beard argued, was finite. Every individual was born with an allotted amount of energy to perform daily tasks. Once that supply had been used, no more could be added. According to Beard, this fixed-energy system had served individuals well in premodern conditions. When people traveled by foot or horseback, labored near their homes, and engaged in simple social activities, their energy was never dangerously depleted. However, once individuals sought higher education and exposed themselves to the strains of modern city life, their bodies demanded increased amounts of energy from the same limited reserve. As a result, the mere process of navigating a day could leave the modern city dweller critically exhausted. The result was an epidemic of "wasting" diseases such as consumption, fatigue, excessive nervousness, impotence, and heart palpitations. For experts like Beard, the solution lay in establishing a system of energy conservation. Without it, they predicted that men and women would face a physical demise similar to the planetary "heat death" postulated by physicists.

Many health experts, licensed and unlicensed, refused to see neurasthenia's symptoms as a harbinger of demise. If a barrier could not be erected around the body to preserve energy from within, they reasoned, perhaps the body's own barrier could be relaxed to absorb energy from without. These efforts to redefine the body as an energy-absorbing organism have been overlooked. By relying upon Beard's written theories of limited energy resources instead of his actual attempts to facilitate limitless energy absorption, we have often interpreted the modernist body narrative to be primarily about decline.[3] Yet as much as Beard emphasized conservation, encouraging women, for example, not to engage in advanced study because brain work drained from the body energy that could be better used for reproduction, he was not content merely to sit back and watch the body destroy itself. His writings and speaking engagements may have stressed the taxations of modern life and urged audiences to conserve their own energies in self-defense, but his practice sought to use the very resources that depleted the body to infuse it with infinitely renewable energy. In fact, a mere ten years after citing electricity as among the "modern stresses" that caused the disease, Beard began working with it to treat neurasthenia. What actually emerged from his neurasthenic paradigm was something far from a fatalistic view of a modern body in precipitous decline.

Most individuals who developed energy-enhancing products demonstrated what Tim Armstrong has called modernism's "desire to *intervene* in the body; to render it part of modernity by techniques which may be biological, mechanical, or behavioral."[4] These entrepreneurs recognized that modern energy was indeed more powerful than human energy. Like Beard, they believed that mechanized factories and electrified cityscapes increased the amount of energy human bodies needed to expend merely to survive in modern society. Yet instead of fearing those energy sources as agents for human displacement, these businessmen actively sought to harness them for use within the body itself, an attempt made possible by their amateur status. Few of them had formal training in medicine and physiology to call upon while creating their products. Even fewer had more than a layman's understanding of mechanics, electricity, or chemistry. As a result, they were not restricted to what experts deemed possible. Their products offered a kind of informal modern homeopathy: by using machines, electricity, and radium to infuse bodies with small doses of "modernity" over time, many provided patients with resistance to "diseases" they believed it caused.

Those who, in 1900, regarded energy-enhancing products as a menace to public health were far outnumbered by those who purchased them. In doing so, they reflected the cultural moment, one in which it was easy to believe the "inaccuracies and exaggerations," as one reporter called them, broadcast by creators of technological cures.[5] Given the sheer speed of technological change, it did not seem so far-fetched to believe that electricity might drive disease from one's veins, or that radium could create an internal fountain of youth. The generation that made decisions about whether to pursue mechanized, electric, or radium cures was the same that would look incredulously upon reports of electricity, the telephone, X rays, and the automobile. There were always the disbelievers, those who doubted that electricity would light private homes; that telephones would replace personal visits; and that the automobile would supplant the horse and buggy. In each of these instances, the technology prevailed. And each time, what had once seemed fantastic had turned out to be fact.

There was little reason to believe that technologically curative products were fraudulent. Users eagerly endorsed each new item that came on the market. Some of their testimonials were undoubtedly created by professional marketers, particularly those that appeared in advertising circulars, yet there were enough well-regarded voices among advocates to counter physicians' attacks of fraud and consumers' occasional doubts. When popular preacher Henry Ward Beecher endorsed the Health Lift machine, people listened. When real-estate mogul Henry Gaylord Wilshire praised the I-ON-A-CO belt, people purchased. And when industrialist Eben Byers touted the Radithor drink as the "fountain of youth," people drank it.

It is easy to assume that these prominent endorsers must have been in on the joke. Or that perhaps they were all, as was Wilshire, motivated at least partially by financial gain. Or perhaps they were merely naïve pawns in the hands of crafty quack promoters. Yet it is not inconceivable that many endorsers said that technological health products worked because they did. Once we expand our definition of cure beyond the strictly scientific and into the psychological, we can imagine that many users did find their health improved by machines, belts, and radium waters. Today, physicians recognize the power of the mind in effecting physical cures. Placebo studies have found people inexplicably helped by sugar pills; the only reason for their recovery, it seems, is that they believed recovery was possible. This may have been the primary curative power behind such pseudomedical products. In some cases, low-level electrical currents may have relieved pain; health machines may have built muscle to overcome fatigue; small amounts of radium may have given consumers, at least at first, the sensation of energy. Yet by and large, the thousands of individuals who purchased these products were cured more by their minds than by their bodies. In an age when technology posed the primary threat to human health, the psychological value of consuming technology to improve health should not be underestimated.[6]

This book explores these issues through the frames of three specific health technologies: muscle-building machines, such as the ones developed by Dudley Allen Sargent at Harvard in the mid to late nineteenth century; electric invigorators, such as electric belts, vibration devices, and "magnetic" collars sold from 1870 to 1930; and radioactive elixirs sold between 1910 and the late 1930s. These technologies, while promising to "energize" the body, actually offered three specific means of revitalization: they could "unblock" energy trapped in the system, "transfer" energy from an external source to the body, or "create" new energy within the body itself. Together, they suggest that Americans increasingly sought health in the productive capacities of modern life.

Health machines were designed primarily to unblock energy that the body already possessed. Using language familiar to those living in an age of neurasthenia with its excessive concern with "waste," machine creators theorized that lifting heavy weights was a means of unplugging stopped-up energy embedded in the system. Energy was not, then, actually added by machines; it was merely pulled to the usable surface. Later, as the properties of electricity were enmeshed within earlier theories of machines, this understanding of technology's effect on the body shifted from "unblocking" to "transferring."

Electricity's dramatic energetic properties were the topic of much speculation: in the age of the first electric injuries and electric executions, few people could ignore the fact that electricity dramatically altered the body upon contact. Electric cuffs, belts, and suppositories were all marketed for this ability, albeit at a safer voltage level: each was sold as a means of expanding energy through physical contact. The final trajectory of energy theories was reached with radium, a substance that seemed able, by altering cellular composition, to turn the body itself into a mechanism for producing continuously renewable energy. It is this trio of approaches that created the foundation for our notion of the technologically improvable body. It also explains why, after radium failed to deliver on the promise of continuous energy, the quest was not abandoned. Because the belief in energy enhancement had been built on three foundations, removing one did not fatally weaken the structure as a whole.

Chapters 1 and 2 explore why individuals once believed that energy had become fatally "blocked" in the body and could be released only by machines. Chapter 1 looks into strategic shifts in nineteenth-century attitudes toward the body that allowed people to believe in machine-generated energy, and how those shifts led to the Health Lift, the first mass-marketed machine in the United States to successfully create a theoretical link between technology and physical health. Today, so entrenched are machines in our fitness regimens that systems like Pilates can differentiate themselves merely by offering "fitness without machines."[7] Yet machines were not always such natural physical allies. Entrepreneurs like George Windship and David Butler sought that relationship by promoting the regulated mechanical motions of their health machines as uniquely capable of releasing physical energy.

Chapter 2 directs attention to the process by which these theories influenced a wider circle of Americans, and how, in doing so, they domesticated new technologies and quantified "strong" bodies. Here I explore Dudley Allen Sargent's machine-training program at Harvard College and Gustav Zander's equipment used at popular health resorts. Machines created a new visual definition for the fit male body as a result of Sargent's routine whereby each muscle had to be fully developed in order to achieve perfect health. By defining the body as a machine that could "leak" energy if not strengthened in each muscular component, Sargent made non-mechanically trained bodies, meaning those without access to public or home gymnasiums, inferior. In the days of Theodore Roosevelt's public warnings of an impending "race suicide," this was probably a comforting thought to many young men of the middle and upper classes because it allowed them to distinguish themselves from encroaching "inferiors" by using quantifiable measurements of strength and mass. I also explore how machines domesticated modernity for those with the means to take "spa" vacations. Many American resorts installed complete sets of Zander equipment between 1910 and 1925 as a way to attract customers.

The combination of natural motion and mechanical process advertised and experienced in Zander machines allowed users, primarily members of the nation's business class, to believe that machines did more than harness human energy to efficiently produce products; they also harnessed mechanical energy to produce efficient humans.

The third and fourth chapters explore how technological health devices, between 1880 and 1930, promised to transfer energy from external sources into the body. The advent of electricity allowed individuals to improve upon earlier ideas of "unblocking" energy with machines. Electricity seemed uniquely capable of going beyond merely redirecting the body's energy. As anyone who came into contact with it could attest, electricity infused the body with a palpable force. As a result, many saw electric health aids as capable of driving power directly into the nerves and muscles, leaving the body with more reserve force as a result.

Chapter 3 looks at the unintended cooperative relationship between "quacks," or unlicensed medical practitioners, and regular physicians who contributed to a popular cult of electric devices. Here I argue that although unlicensed practitioners have often been cited as the primary purveyors, licensed physicians were actually the first to advocate use of electric devices. They were the first to ignore scientific evidence about electricity's limits, instead anointing it as, in the words of Galvani, the "life force itself." By the time the American Medical Association's health fraud division cracked down on tales of fantastic electric therapies, it was too late; irregular practitioners had captivated a popular audience. I explore three particular pseudoscientific electric products, the electric belt, the electric oxygenator, and the I-ON-A-CO magnetic collar, arguing that each sold, in spite of its questionable medical value, by curing illnesses physical and cultural during a rapidly electrifying age.

Chapter 4 is a case study of the relationship between electric technology and changing definitions of sexuality. I explore electric belts and vibration devices aimed at male consumers and argue that these sold by offering men two cures for contemporary sexual confusion: (1) a way to overcome Victorian fears that masturbation caused irreversible physical decline, and (2) a way to believe, in the face of women's increasing sexual demands, that the male body remained sexually superior.

The fifth chapter explores radium, a substance that seemed capable of creating energy by causing a cellular change that rendered the body infinitely able to renew its own energy supply. Between 1900 and 1940, scientists, quacks, and consumers alike struggled to turn radium into an energetic fountain of youth. By promoting a mythology of energy "continuously created," radium's advocates argued that with the element's discovery, they had at last found the ultimate physical rejuvenator. Whereas machines had promised to unblock energy and build muscles, and electricity had promised to transfer energy and temporarily power the body, radium, it seemed, could permanently modernize the body through cellular renewal. In the end, the use of radium revealed the risks of putting one's physical future into the hands of technology. Many users found out too late that product claims were indeed too good to be true. After several well-known people died from radium poisoning in their pursuit of "super health," the uncritical campaign to wed technology and the body ceased. But its promises still echo.

The conclusion looks at the aftermath of this first wave of techno-physical enthusiasm, including the end of practical experiments with technology transfer in the 1940s; a lingering spirit of techno-body enthusiasm in the myths of Marvel Comics and fantasies of television; and our current enthusiasm for cyber bodies.

It is tempting to generalize and say that these devices impacted the lives of all Americans. Certainly they were seen by a cross-section of the general public. One's class, race, and, in some cases, gender made little difference in how familiar one would have been with the products or claims; basic literacy was the only requirement necessary to read the advertisements placed in local and national papers, handed out on street corners, and delivered door to door by salespeople in large and small towns. Yet class, race, and gender did play a role in determining whether one would actually have access to the products themselves. Four distinct groups of people used these devices during their roughly fifty years of popularity. The first included the products' designers and promoters, individuals whose simultaneous roles as professionals and entrepreneurs placed them solidly within the middle class.[8] Their understanding of science varied; some, like Dudley Allen Sargent and William Hammer, had advanced degrees and were considered experts in their fields. Others, like Henry Gaylord Wilshire and Thomas Edison, Jr., were more versed in self-promotion than in scientific theory. Yet all were outside the realm of experts; because of their working-class backgrounds, their lack of scientific knowledge, or their penchant for hyperbole, none of these promoters, who often declared they used the devices they sold, was fully accepted as a scientific or medical expert. The other three user groups comprised upper-class, middle-class, and working-class consumers.

Access to money, status, and "regular" medicine made one a member of the "upper class" among device consumers. These individuals, like other consumers, had access to electric and radium devices. Unlike other consumers, however, they also had access to health machines in elite universities like Harvard and in the privacy of their own homes. Unlike owning an electric belt or water dispenser, ownership or restricted access to health machines, which sold for as much as three hundred dollars in the late nineteenth century and were decorated with fancy ironwork suitable for parlor display, marked one's upper-class status.

Middle-class Americans appear to have been the most likely to sample each device. Health Lifts, although cost prohibitive for home use, were available at YMCAs and health clubs in urban centers, where most members were white-collar workers. Existing records reveal that many who purchased or considered purchasing memberships were teachers, clerks, and preachers, members of solid middle-class professions.[9] Further, the rhetoric of marketing material frequently evoked long work hours, stressful lives, and minimal physical strength as reasons for using a device, all "problems" associated with the turn-of-the-century white-collar class.

Each of these products also had some following among members of the working class. YMCA membership was within reach of blue-collar laborers, as was the cost of radium water dispensers. Visits to spas, where Zander machines and radium baths were located, were not. It is electric belts, however, with their low prices and affordable installment options that were most attractive to the working class. It is also likely that their expressly prescriptive advertisements appealed to persons unable to afford regular medical treatment. Physicians reportedly found men who could not afford "proper" food, housing, and medical care in possession of an electric belt.

Gender also determined who consumed these products. Product use tended to be aligned with gender conventions of the late nineteenth and early twentieth centuries. Thus, when promoters made explicit promises that products would transfer or generate energy, they were making those promises mainly to men. At a time when notions of "separate spheres" still dominated, it made sense that men would be encouraged to merge their bodies with technology in order to continually increase their physical strength and that women would be instructed to use technology to gain energy sufficient to perform domestic tasks. It was acceptable to promote a Health Lift for men and women because it merely advocated unblocking the natural energy one held within. Once energy technologies could actually promise to deposit additional energy, to make one's body more powerful than it was "naturally," courting female consumers would have contradicted gender roles that defined women as caregivers in the domestic sphere.[10] Such standards made active, vital energy primarily a male terrain.

Products that were marketed to women, such as the Electropoise "oxygenating" electric ankle cuff, were typically pitched to restore depleted bodies; advertisements often showed women wearing the device while striking a "consumptive" pose on overstuffed Victorian furniture. The gendered iconography in early advertisements is striking. Whereas male bodies are typically displayed in revealing, muscular, energized poses to sell products, female bodies are rarely shown at all. When they do appear, they tend to be either fully clothed and either of average strength or obviously weakened. This is not to say that women did not use the products I discuss here; certainly they did use Health Lifts, and they are likely to have used other products, even if they were not the intended consumers.[11] In fact, recent scholarship has shown that women did go against the advice of experts when it came to technological devices, often taking pleasure in their transgressive actions.[12] Yet the dominant narrative of "energy enhancement" was told on the bodies of men until the 1920s. Only then, possibly coinciding with women's increased social equality, did products like the I-ON-A-CO and radium water begin to offer genderless visions of limitless energy.

The men and women in this story are predominantly white. Yet this is not a narrative of relevance only to Anglo-American history. The whiteness of brochure images, the device inventors' oft-told parables of immigrant laborers defeated by techno-powered "Americans," and the Eurocentric rhetoric of companies like Pulvermachers of London, in Cincinnati, and German Electric, in Brooklyn, appeared in response to the challenge to whiteness posed by turn-of-the century immigration and African-American emancipation. It was this cultural shift that gave rise to fears of decreasing "potency" and "power" in white males.[13] Without the perceived threat of nonwhite bodies, the cultural space necessary for energy devices to succeed would not have existed. As a result, this work, like any on turn-of-the-century bodies, is inherently a discussion of race and nation.

This project is the first to place changing ideas about fitness and gender in dialogue with the popular culture of technology. It is possible to make this connection only now, with the benefit of critical work on masculinity and technology that has been done over the past decade.[14] And although much of this work has helped us understand the connection between bodies, technological change, and energy enhancement, it has remained primarily focused on experts: the doctors, scientists, engineers, and industrial theorists who formally applied technologies to the body. These individuals undoubtedly had a tremendous impact on how laymen and laywomen understood physical capacity and on the environments in which nonexpert bodies worked. What the focus does not do, however, is reveal the individual energy enthusiasms that brought bodies into desired contact with machines.

Elites did not always successfully define the limits and applications of modern energies. The deregulation of the medical industry, the proliferation of "popular science," the convenience and privacy of mail order, and the proximity of door-to-door salespeople created a climate in which individuals were more likely to learn about scientific theories from circulars than from textbooks. Further, even if Americans did learn much about new technologies from official sources, such mental lessons were not likely to have been more powerful than those learned on the body directly. Hooking on electric belts, climbing into machines, and ingesting radium-laced water allowed bodies to absorb technological promise without interference from rational minds. We cannot underestimate the lessons that materials teach our bodies about the world we live in, even when the lessons directly contradict the best expertise of our time.

This is not to say that the popular spin Americans gave to energy theories were correct or more important than the theories developed by scientists and strategists. It is to say that until we combine the theories of experts with the physical experience of laypersons, we will not create a complete picture of how modern energies reshaped modern bodies. In a world where science and fantasy met in the marketplace, there could be no strict divide between "pure" and "popular" technologies. By reanimating the energy dialogue with the popular, the pseudoscientific, and the fantastic, we gain a glimpse of a world of unlimited technological potential that once stood.

A century ago, people postulated that ultimate physical freedom would somehow be realized in technological advances. Today's discussions about cyberculture and the "escape" it allows from physical restraints and decay are not far off from conjecture a century ago about the I-ON-A-CO's electric fountain of youth. We are part of a coping strategy for American technological innovation created by individuals who sought to prove that although modern energy production might exact a physical price, the benefits far outweigh the risks. We are left with a complex vision of technology's ultimate physical promise, one that combines Hiroshima's images of radioactive destruction with Spiderman's radioactively enhanced "superpowers," and stark images of the electric chair with the electric-belt recharger. Like George Beard, we continue to fear the ultimate physical costs that technology may one day demand from our bodies, yet we enthusiastically pursue the physical enhancements that only technology can provide. It is in this space between fear and fantasy that the story of the energized body emerged and continues to be told.

1

The Machine-Built Body

We believe that the Lift produces physical perfection; that physical perfection begets mental vigor, which, in turn, by appropriate tuitions begets moral power; that this combination makes the perfect man.

—J. C. Zachos, MD, "The Butler Health Lift: Its Reasons and Its Facts," 1871

Every man longs to keep his body dynamized with vibrant energy.
—Advertisement, Vig-Row Health Riding Machine, 1932

In 1871, Henry Ward Beecher wrote a letter to the editor about a recent cure he had found for nervous exhaustion. Beecher was not only a well-known preacher, considered by many "the great popular phenomena of the era," he was also widely praised for his athleticism, a trait that made him a prime example of what is typically called "Muscular Christianity."[1] Among his contemporaries, Beecher was often cited as a figure worth emulating, a man of education, religion, and morality who had not fallen victim to what seemed a nearly ubiquitous physical decline among the middle and upper classes.[2] Along with five of his fellow Brooklyn clergymen, he wrote to *The Lift*, a journal published by the Butler Health Lift Company, about what he asserted was a renewed strength and health that had resulted from using its product. Though none of the five men had previously suffered from ill health beyond an occasional bout of fatigue, each had nevertheless "derived great benefit" from several weeks' training at Brooklyn's Health Lift Studio.[3] There, under the tutelage of professional trainers, the six men had followed a systematic exercise routine of weight lifting using dumbbells and specially developed Health Lift machines. Without expending much of their valuable time,

Beecher reported, each had improved his physique and energy level dramatically. The letter, which the journal printed, recommended the Health Lift "to the attention of all persons whose avocations severely tax the brain and to all whose nervous system is run down."[4]

Beecher was one of many to praise the Health Lift in late-nineteenth-century America. Yet his popular image as healthy and rugged, as well as his ability to attract upwards of three thousand parishioners to his Sunday sermons, made his accolades more resonant than most.[5] By publicly endorsing a mechanized health system, Beecher broke with Muscular Christianity's tendency to equate health with outdoorsmanship and organized sports.[6] Regulated machine lifting, Beecher declared, not football or hiking, was the best method to relieve the intellectual stress of modern middle-class life. The message likely was relevant to Beecher's primary audience: farmers, clerks, lawyers, small businessmen, carpenters, and masons, young men squarely placed within the rising middle class. It was these individuals whose lives were becoming less about physical labor and more about management and specialized skills.[7] It was also these individuals who were increasingly suffering from ill health.

Surprisingly little attention has been paid to Health Lifts.[8] One would assume, from the relative silence, that few were sold or that their influence was short-lived. Just the opposite is true. By the late nineteenth century, gyms in cities throughout the country offered Health Lift training. Living near an exercise facility like Beecher's Brooklyn studio was not a prerequisite to using the devices. Advertisements in popular magazines brought the message of machine lifting to urban and rural residents and regularly urged people to consider purchasing a machine of their own and having it shipped to their homes.

We need look no further than our local health club to prove the Lift's lasting impact on American culture. Our own weight machines are updated and bear little outward resemblance to the basic Health Lift, but many of them act in quite similar ways upon our bodies. Quad machines use the same principle of platform weight borne by the lower body; squat machines use a similar, if inverted, motion. If only as examples of early incarnations of these currently ubiquitous machines, Health Lifts have much to teach us about the origins of weight training. Their significance, however, goes beyond historization. They also reveal the ways in which health machines have enabled users to interpret technology as a benevolent force.

There remains an unexplored connection between mechanized power and human potential in the industrial era. Although numerous studies have looked at the way that Americans adapted to the mechanization of modern life, they have not explored the role that exercise machines played in the narrative. Most studies of American mechanization focus on factories and workers. The best of these, including Terry Smith's work on Ford's River Rouge plant, examine how workers' actual bodies interacted with the machines they operated.[9] In Smith's reading of Diego Rivera's mural done for the plant, the job of men is to toil under the weight of machines. Here, bodies are mechanized; arms and legs move in an unchanging rhythm dictated by all-powerful machines. The men's muscular bodies, developed in response to the inhuman pace set by machines, are external symbols of internal human suffering. Technology oppresses these bodies; they have no more power over the machines they run than they will over the products those machines create. Such a reading is perfectly sound; it parallels Rivera's Marxist perspective on the role of laborers in a modern capitalist society. At the same time, one wonders whether this is the only possible interpretation of what it meant for strong bodies to interact with powerful machines. Examining the images in light of contemporary attitudes about mechanized human potential, there is room to posit that the bodies and not the machines may be the real beneficiaries. In an era of obsession with reducing fatigue, bodies that collaborated with mechanized power would have been regarded by many as symbols of vigorous health.

Alone, an institutional lens cannot reveal the effects of machines on American life, for although Americans have always been workers in one sense or another, their motivations for accepting or rejecting machinery in their daily lives are only partially explained by work environments.[10] Regardless of its methodology, research on the restrictions of mechanized workplaces and the oppressive calculations of scientific management can inform us about only the eight to twelve hours a day that someone spent at work. If the pace and repetition set by machines oppressed their human operators, that tells us only part of the relationship between body and machine. On the way to work, during breaks, after work, on weekends and vacations, turn-of-the-century Americans were surrounded by machines. It is certainly conceivable that any detrimental impressions made by industrial machinery could have been reversed by recreational machinery during the off hours. One might forgive the machine-enforced monotony of the widget line (or at least exonerate the machine itself) after a night of machine-generated fun on the streetcars and at Coney

Island. Rural Americans too could witness the positive side of mechanized life by purchasing kitchen gadgets and electric belts from Sears, Roebuck and Co. catalogues. Thanks to mail order, both groups could at least consider Beecher's advice that they install a portable version of the Health Lift in the privacy of their own homes.

We cannot understand the role of machines as producers until we look at the part they played in producing bodies as well as finished goods. In an age of massive industrialization, when the limits of productive energy were redefined almost daily, it was natural to assume that expanding possibilities would affect more than goods. The harder we look, the less we will see of an exclusively adversarial relationship between bodies and machines in the United States between the Civil War and World War II. Industrial machines certainly subjected workers to monotonous factory routines. Mechanical innovations did, in fact, make many trades obsolete. Machine production may have strained the relationship between craftsman and product. Yet at the same time, numerous Americans welcomed machines into their lives, hoping that they might help create an economically *and physically* sound nation.

Antebellum America offered a vast array of strategies to improve physical performance, among them vegetarianism, Fletcherism, boxing, and Boy Scouting. However, the most popular shared space in which physical improvements were pursued was the gymnasium.[11] Organized fitness centers began appearing in urban areas in the 1860s; by 1900, eighty thousand Americans belonged to YMCA gyms and thousands more belonged to the roughly one hundred gyms connected with athletic clubs, hospitals, and military bases.[12] These gymnasiums offered a combination of inexpensive, portable equipment, including parallel bars, heavy clubs, tossing rings, and climbing ladders. Most, even smaller athletic clubs for whom the expense would have been significant, also offered muscle-building machines.[13]

The gyms provided one of the first structured environments in which bodies encountered health machines. Gym members typically came at regular times, developed regular routines, and were advised by trainers who associated machine training with optimum physical health. This interaction was not limited to bodies of privilege. Some facilities, such as private athletic clubs and military bases, restricted membership to those who met entrance requirements: money and enlistment, respectively. YMCAs, however, were accessible to the majority of the urban middle class. These mechanized environments provided the nucleus of organized physical activity for a rapidly expanding "fitness" age. To understand what such environments taught the bodies that inhabited them, we need first to set aside our twenty-first-century perspectives and view them as they were originally encountered. These devices may appear antiquated today, but to their contemporary users, they embodied the best that technology had to offer.

Premachine Fitness: The Acrobatic Athlete

In the early nineteenth century, a strong body came second to a strong character. Within this system, physical health was important, but it was not as conscious a pursuit for most men as were moral strength, religious piety, and cultivated intelligence. Being healthy typically meant moderate eating, moderate exercise, and avoiding disease. This, however, changed dramatically over two generations. By century's end, fitness guru Bernarr Macfadden, a devotee of daily rigorous exercises, proclaimed that "weakness is a crime." In Macfadden's era, a healthy body was not merely a foundation for an accomplished character; it was a visible symbol of one's essential value. Macfadden's journal, *Physical Culture*, enjoyed a wide readership by presenting strong bodies as the single most important ingredient for personal and economic success. These bodies, in *Physical Culture* and in gyms across the country, were increasingly to be achieved through the calculated use of machines.

Before modern physical conditioning initially appeared, the emphasis had been on acrobatic performance rather than pure strength. In the 1820s, German immigrants introduced Americans to gymnastics, or *Turnen*. Designed by Frederick Jahn to strengthen German youth in the wake of the nation's defeat in the Napoleonic Wars, *Turnen* stressed intensive exercises such as running, jumping, tumbling, and parallel bar work.[14] It was not an immediate success. Well after the first schools were established in the Boston area, the system continued to attract primarily German immigrants. Twenty-five years later, however, when the upheavals of the 1848 revolutions brought another, wider wave of German immigrants, many began to pay attention to the young muscular gymnasts in their midst. Americans' interest in the games of ancient Greece, the result of a midcentury revival in Greek architecture and design, further enhanced the esteem accorded gymnastics.[15] By the mid-1850s, Harvard had established a formal gymnastics program. Ten years later, Luther Halsey

Gulick, gym superintendent of the YMCA of Jackson, Michigan, helped establish complete gymnasiums in cities throughout the country.

Although *Turnen* professed to be a system for every young man, it was not something at which the average person could easily excel. Exercises such as the pommel horse, the suspended rings, and the parallel bars helped practitioners improve their strength. Yet these kinds of activities were not easy to master; performing many of the *Turnen* exercises required a combination of upper-body strength, balance, and muscular control. The emphasis on performative strength, along with the frightening heights that accompanied exercises like the parallel bars, showed beginners little sympathy. For a young man who had never developed his biceps and chest muscles, it could take months of hard work to make a respectable showing on an apparatus like the pommel horse. Still, it was difficult to argue with gymnastics' successful results: when men practiced hard enough and long enough, they built muscles and performed impressive physical feats. Yet for those without the inclination toward physical exhaustion, or for those who simply lacked sufficient upper-body strength, *Turnen* seemed more a form of torture than a method for improving physical health.

By the 1830s, individuals like Dio Lewis and Catharine Beecher were beginning to encourage colleagues to prescribe more-well-rounded and less physically stressful exercises to improve their accessibility, particularly to women. By the 1880s, physicians had joined them. In an 1882 talk, Dr. Alfred Worcester promoted the value of exercise for men and women of all shapes and sizes, yet feared that gymnasiums were actually preventing healthy muscular development by encouraging students to develop only those muscles necessary for specific events. "It was the fashion for the would-be gymnast . . . to exercise only his best-developed muscles," he commented. "If a good vaulter, he spent his hour in vaulting; if strong-armed, his exhibitions were on the swings and bar."[16]

Other contemporary exercise systems posed similar problems for critics like Worcester. Calisthenics, which originated in the 1820s and remained popular through the Civil War, appeared in numerous schools and private gymnasiums. Unlike *Turnen*, calisthenics required little skill or muscular strength of the beginner; most maneuvers depended upon simple, repetitive motions, requiring only the ability to lift the legs, raise the arms, and bend at the waist.[17] As a result, calisthenics had no gender bias and did not require practitioners to be physically gifted. What it lacked in drama, it made up for in relative safety. Yet Worcester's criticism could have been well applied to its marches and drills. Calisthenics may not have required the kind of concentrated muscle building of *Turnen*, but it too exercised muscles individually rather than developing the body as a unified muscular system.

In his 1873 exercise guide, *New Gymnastics*, Dio Lewis, a well-known advocate of exercise for men and women, declared that calisthenics did students as much a disservice as did traditional gymnastics. The "numberless schools" using the system had, as a group, failed completely to produce what he called a "muscle culture." The excessive reliance of calisthenics on marching, turning, and walking created students with strong legs but weak chests, arms, and backs.[18] In a problem similar to that diagnosed by Worcester in gymnasts, calisthenics devotees could easily end up strong but only half developed. To Lewis, the burly arms of the pommel-horse performer and the solid calves of the drill sergeant might be impressive when each engaged in their respective "sports," but such attributes were those of dangerously undeveloped athletes.

Dio Lewis was the first to offer a corrective to these "imbalanced" systems by theorizing the body as a machine for development. In 1862, inspired by studying gymnastics in Europe, he published one of the most widely read texts on exercise, *New Gymnastics for Men, Women, and Children*. Lewis devoted the remainder his life to teaching his unique combination of calisthenics, strength drills, and rhythmic dance.[19] His system provided the muscular benefits of gymnastics and military drills but with two fundamental improvements. First, it was a system at which every practitioner could excel. Instead of death-defying feats, his students executed rhythmic dance performances, lifting light weights in time with music that regulated the pace and length of exercise routines. Second, it was also a system that Lewis believed left practitioners stronger in all parts of their bodies by incorporating repetition and adding maneuvers with equipment designed to simultaneously exercise the upper and lower body.

In his best-known exercise treatise, Lewis stressed repeatedly that being fit was more than having strength in one's arms or legs. It could be achieved only by engaging the entire physical structure in balanced movements. "Is the body one single organ," he asked, "which, if exercised, is sure to grow the right way? On the contrary, is it not an exceedingly complicated machine, the symmetrical development of which requires discriminating, studied management?"[20] Lewis believed it was, and designed a system thorough enough, in his opinion, to fine-tune each part. Adaptable for men and women, "new gymnastics" consisted mainly of partner exercises augmented by calisthenics done with light Lewis-designed apparatus.[21] A Lewis session in action looked like playtime with oversized youngsters; for much of the period students tossed rings or bean bags to their partners or rhythmically lifted and turned large hoops. Musical accompaniment assured a steady pace and helped develop coordination.

At the root of Lewis's exercise philosophy was the concept of regulated tension. Exercises in gymnasiums or with dumbbells failed, he reasoned, because of two factors: they were too dangerous, and they did not apply the correct amount of tension to each area of the body. In free gymnastics, or *Turnen*, students could easily strain muscles by exerting too much force at one time, such as in an ill-fated turn on the parallel bars. Dumbbells could also do damage when excessive weights were handled. According to his biographer, Lewis considered heavy weights more damaging than beneficial; if they did not result in pulled muscles, they certainly caused stiffness in overused areas while other muscles remained inactive.[22] When students used tension generated by partner exercises, they regulated the amount of force each exercise applied. Rings, for example, if properly engaged, allowed a user to stretch and build muscles by working against a partner's pushing and pulling. Whether using light dumbbells, wands, or rings, students were taught to gauge the proper resistance required for each body part to become as strong, as Lewis described, as a well-oiled machine.

Lewis was one of the first exercise theorists to regard the body as a machine. He made comparisons between the two, regularly referring to the human machine in passages such as one from *New Gymnastics* on the benefits of warming up before exercise: "No machine can suddenly be put in motion at its highest possible speed, and as suddenly stopped, without risk of destroying it." Yet although Lewis thought of the body as a machine, he did not typically use machines in training.[23] Perhaps his machine metaphor was one of convenience: merely a way of making the myriad parts of the body comprehensible to a general audience more familiar with mechanics than physiology. Still, his philosophy on strengthening makes him arguably one of the first to envision the possibilities of a mechanically trained body, even if he did not explore it himself.

Lewis was the first to declare that the healthy body was one built by exact tension distributed equally over the muscular frame. His reliance on well-regulated, adjustable, and evenly distributed resistance would later be associated with machine-based training systems. Further, unlike previous programs, Lewis's allowed for minute adjustments so that users could strengthen without injury. For example, by using a heavy partner for arm exercises and a light partner for back exercises, one could apply varied force to the body. Lewis also trained his students to equate apparatus with strength building. Thus, although he never advocated using machines exclusively, and, at times, outright discouraged their use, Lewis taught students that bodies required mechanisms to build proper strength. By regarding the body as a machine with complex parts requiring balanced development, Lewis helped initiate a search for equipment that could bring it to its potential.

The Body as Machine: A Metaphor of Power

The idea that the body is a machine stretches at least as far back as Descartes, who in 1637 described humans as God-made animal machines "incomparably better ordered [and] more admirable in [their] movements than any of those which can be invented by men."[24] By the late nineteenth century, both European and American scientists had accepted some version of the analogy. Advances in physiology and anatomy explained the body as a system of interlocking parts, each of which depended on the others for growth and sustainability. The rise of increasingly complex factory systems driven by steam- and electricity-powered motors further strengthened the association. One medical textbook, *The Motive Power of the Human System*, published in 1840, explained at its outset that human and machine power could be compared. "In studying this subject," author H. H. Sherwood wrote, "it will be necessary to examine the different structures of organized bodies, and to understand their mechanism, as the mechanist understands a machine, before we shall be able to ascertain the kind of power by which they are moved."[25]

By the 1880s, physicians were recognizing the comparison's ubiquity. One, in 1884, complained in *Popular Science* about the "somewhat trite" practice of comparing the muscular system to an engine but recognized that such imagery had "pretty clearly formulated the idea as generally accepted."[26] According to its author, J. M. Stillman, the comparison might have as much to do with what scientists did not know as with what they did. "We are in almost complete darkness," he commented, about the processes that took place in a gland, muscle, brain, or nerve. Because scientists could not accurately explain them, they settled for metaphors. It was easier to compare the human muscular system to an engine, in that it was "generally accepted that fuel produces force."[27] During the late nineteenth century, it was common for books on popular health to refer to hearts as "motors" or "pumps" and food as "fuel." Even physical imperfection was described as a mechanical failure. One 1911 article in *Everybody's Magazine* explained disability as having a "flaw in [one's] casting, with a twist in [one's] transmission."[28]

These comparisons stretched beyond the specialized audience of physicians and scientists and readers of a few select magazines. Abundant examples of human-machine analogies appeared in popular turn-of-the-century novels. In Robert Herrick's *Together* (1908), a woman suffering psychological problems wonders if "we are just machines with the need to be oiled now and then." Despite her own comfort with mechanized analogies, she is disturbed by the supplanting of humans by machines. When her nerve doctor promises to cure her through treatments in which he will act as her "temporary dynamo," she can respond only with skepticism.[29] Machine analogies are equally common in Jack London's writings, in which dogs are described as "perfect mechanism[s]" with muscles that stretch "like steel springs."[30]

Such human-machine comparisons were not new, but they did represent a fundamental shift in how individuals viewed their physical frames. Enlightenment philosophers and physicians had speculated that the body might be a rational collection of mechanized parts. Yet their understanding of the body as machine-like was a means to understand the body, not to improve upon it. By 1860, machine analogies were not merely being used to describe complex physiology to a general audience. They also began to reflect a popular belief that machines could improve upon God's given body. We can see this emerging in Henry Ward Beecher's Health Lift endorsement. A generation earlier, Beecher would have accepted the body as predetermined by the creator. In the late nineteenth century, however, Beecher saw no contradiction between simultaneously following God's will and altering his body with man's technology. His efforts to build muscle and his urging that others do the same suggest that for Beecher's contemporaries, bodies were given by God but perfected by man. Once we understand this cultural shift, Herrick's prose does more than prove that people thought bodies and machines similar. It suggests that people had begun to embrace a cooperative relationship between mechanized power and human potential.

The shift is especially important because mechanistic physical metaphors are commonly given as evidence of man's subservience to the machine. Anson Rabinbach rightly asserts that one of the goals of modernity was to harmonize the body with mechanized rhythms.[31] He convincingly argues that this harmonization often exacted a great physical and mental cost from workers as assembly lines sped up and basic human needs like variation were ignored. Still, descriptions of the body as machine are not merely evidence of industrial strategies to increase worker productivity. They also indicate that individuals desired greater control over their bodies, over the way they performed, the way they looked, and the rate at which they decayed, than had any previous generation. For those on and off assembly lines, mechanized physical metaphors could represent a desire to craft bodies into entities *as powerful as* machines. This possibility allows for a cultural context in which machines became agents for physical vigor and weapons against the threat of terminal fatigue.

Empty Buckets: Neurasthenia and Physical Breakdown

Americans had good reasons for turning to mechanical metaphors to describe human energy in the late nineteenth century. Machines were not failing, people were. Neurasthenia, a term coined by George Beard in 1869, gave a name to a set of mysterious ailments plaguing primarily business-class white Americans and Europeans at midcentury.[32] Symptoms varied: some sufferers reported sleeplessness and anxiety; others experienced weariness and despondency. And although Beard believed in a specific neurasthenic etiology, discussions of the illness in mainstream magazines and newspapers suggested that any sign of weakness might indicate impending onset of the disease. There seemed few regions of the body safe from a neurasthenic attack. Headaches, back pain, groin discomfort, and limb atrophy all appeared common symptoms in popular accounts and physicians' reports.[33]

If prospective patients and physicians could not agree on symptoms, they could agree on a culprit. According to Beard, widely regarded as an expert on the illness, the problem was a depletion in "nerve force," which the body possessed in limited amounts. Contemporary reports revealed that nerve force could be depleted by a number of typical daily activities, including education, employment, and exercise. Such endeavors could have a cumulatively dangerous effect, but were commonly regarded as productive: energy expended was at least partially returned in the form of health, wealth, or status. Unproductive, illicit activities, such as masturbation and gambling, however, were regarded as particularly destructive because they merely drained precious force from the body. The result of one or both activity types, Beard explained, was often that "[T]he central nervous system . . . loses somewhat of its solid constituents . . . and as a consequence becomes more or less impoverished in the quantity of its nervous force."[34] Beard's diagnosis reflected his contemporaries' closed-system view of human energy: the body had a limited amount of force or energy that traveled through the nerves and produced productive force. According to Beard, when this energy was spent, the body required almost five times as long as the original spending activity to recover from the strain. Excessive thought, work, physical activity, or ejaculation used energy beyond that which could be easily recovered during a normal period of rest. Physical breakdown, the first stage of neurasthenia, was the all-too-frequent outcome.[35]

Cures for neurasthenics tended to vary depending on gender. Physician S. Weir Mitchell prescribed women a regimen of bed rest of at least a month, no reading, and a milk-heavy diet spoon-fed by a nurse. Physicians treating famous neurasthenics like Theodore Roosevelt and Frederic Remington advised long trips in the West for fresh air and strenuous exercise. Beard himself favored treatment with faradic currents, a procedure he perfected in experiments with Edison on electricity and physical force.[36]

Physicians agreed that sufferers were primarily middle-class workers and women: the latter because of a perceived incompatibility between their intellectual and procreative pursuits; the former because of white-collar stress. Physicians repeatedly emphasized the problem of excessive thought, asserting that people in business, writing, law, and the professions were most precariously weakened. Yet white-collar stress was not merely a profitable notion invented by physicians, though the general malaise of weakness among new professionals did certainly increase the many coffers.

Writers of popular fiction also began to explore the physical and psychological costs of work in which "products" were profits accrued through skillful sales pitches and managerial savvy. Edgar Burroughs's Tarzan novels spoke to the disenchantment of those so employed, a group whose membership, by 1910, consisted of one-fifth of the entire male labor force. As John Kasson reveals, Burroughs's own experiences as a "very minor cog in the machinery" as an office manager and as a door-to-door salesman who "recite[d] my sales talk like a sick parrot" undoubtedly contributed to his own eventual ill health. After working six years without a vacation, Burroughs estimated that he suffered "tortures from headaches" during "fully half my working hours."[37]

Physical depletion among middle-class, white males reached epidemic proportions by 1900. That year alone, the U.S. Surgeon General's index listed more than one hundred studies of muscle fatigue, a number that did not include studies of "nervous exhaustion," "brain exhaustion," and "spinal exhaustion."[38] The state of pervasive weakness created more than a physical change in American culture; it also created a cultural change, as white, middle-class men attempted to build muscle in emulation of new vigorous heroes like Harry Houdini, Eugen Sandow, Bernarr Macfadden, and Teddy Roosevelt, fellow white-collar men who embodied the self-made confidence and physical strength they lacked.[39]

"Neurasthenia" was the word most Americans came to equate with the problem of energy depletion, and it continues to be the focus of most of our studies of nineteenth-century fatigue, but this climate of ill health was originally understood as a physical manifestation of global energy depletion. In 1852, William Thompson, also known as Lord Kelvin, published "On a Universal Tendency in Nature to the Dissipation of Mechanical Energy." His work, combined with Rudolf Clausius's, offered proof for what came to be known in the 1860s as the second law of thermodynamics, a theory that argued that in the material world, energy, once applied to a task, could never be restored to its original quantity. The conversion process did more than turn mechanical energy to heat energy as previously hypothesized; it also diminished the total amount of energy available.[40]

The second law of thermodynamics was particularly distressing, given that it followed the optimistic first law of thermodynamics by only a few years. Suddenly, energy that had appeared constant now appeared to be energy in a state of constant decline.[41] To ascertain the relevance of this for bodily fatigue, one need look only at its underlying perspective on energy. Work, or the use of energy to accomplish a given task, resulted in heat loss. This meant that all mechanical processes resulted in a net loss of total energy available because energy could flow undisturbed in only one direction. Heat energy could become mechanical energy but, once transformed, it could never be restored to its original mass; thus, entropy was always increasing. The result was a dramatic recasting of Newton's self-perpetuating universe. Instead of a world running indefinitely on a re-cyclable energy supply, theorists posited a world tending inevitably to decline. "Heat death" would be its final destination, a point at which energy would continue to exist, but not in a form suitable for human consumption. The universe would lock its energy away in a state of maximum entropy, or an ongoing diminishing available force. There would be no other option, as Herman von Helmholtz put it, but that "all natural processes must cease."[42]

Entropy's discovery in physics did not gain a following equal to neurasthenia's, a fact likely due to neurasthenia's greater salience with the average person. One might occasionally be concerned about universal heat death, but the concern for something thousands of years away was not nearly as immediate as one's current sensation of debilitating fatigue. The law did, however, become a part of popular culture by becoming embedded in neurasthenia's rhetoric. Beard's writings and speeches on energy depletion and terminal fatigue reveal similarities to the law. Whether it was referred to as entropy or an overtaxed system, the idea was clear: modern life demanded more from living systems than they could supply. The growth of cities, the increased attention to time and scheduling, and the quickened pace of transportation demanded that late-nineteenth-century bodies move faster and late-nineteenth-century brains process an ever-increasing amount of information. According to the discourse, there appeared two options available: to find additional energy or to suffer the "heat death" of humanity.

When experts worried about progressive physical decline, they did not worry that every American was approaching physical ruin. On the contrary, many were believed immune to the second law's predictions. Immigrants from rural areas of southern and eastern Europe reportedly suffered far fewer ailments of fatigue than did the American-born middle and upper classes. According to contemporary theories, such people enjoyed better health and plentiful progeny because they avoided the "over-civilization" that frequently followed advanced education and white-collar work. The inevitable consequence of the physical disparity, as argued by Theodore Roosevelt in the early 1900s, was that established Americans of northern European descent who occupied the middle and upper classes were declining in number while new immigrants from "less desirable" regions of Europe were increasing. For people like Roosevelt, the nation's resulting prognosis appeared bleak: physical decline would lead to democratic decline, as members of what he saw as the superior class of individuals slowly died out through "race suicide" and were overtaken by intellectual inferiors with higher birth rates.[43]

For many middle- and upper-class Americans who believed in the threat of race suicide, the best defense lay in combating the loss of middle-class vitality. Throughout the 1870s and 1880s, the middle-class readers of *Popular Science Monthly* became familiar with Kelvin's second law of thermodynamics through his article "The Available Energy of Nature" and through his colleagues' articles "The Physiological Significance of Vital Force" and "The Dissipation of Energy."[44] Few of these authors, including Kelvin, were content merely to forecast the world's doom. Instead they used it as an opportunity to hypothesize alternative energy sources. According to Kelvin, the exhaustion of mechanical energy might lead us to discover future resources in tidal energy, wind, and rain.[45]

Other authors also contested fears of entropy, saying that the supposition "that the sun will finally grow cold" was "inconsistent with the theory of continuous evolution."[46] Because the universe extended indefinitely, these authors suggested, energy might be ever-expanding, albeit in different forms. The search for energy went well beyond scientific journals to reach a popular audience. "The Problem of Increasing Human Energy," by one of the best-known researchers on electric energy, Nikola Tesla, appeared in *The Century Illustrated Magazine*, urging readers to support new research on solar power.[47] These expert recommendations provided numerous places Americans might look to replace diminishing energies. Physical conditioning movements, however, suggest that people increasingly sought a source closer to home.

Muscles became cultural status symbols largely because of the contemporary obsession with halting physical decline. At the heart of the shift was a new understanding of the relationship between muscle and physical power that emerged from advances in circulatory research. Whereas individuals had previously believed that energy was produced in the lungs, mid-nineteenth-century researchers discovered that the body was actually a system of exchanges. The lungs channeled "fuel," which was sent to the blood for "transport" into the "furnace" of muscle fibers.[48] Muscles thus became the core component in turning raw materials into usable energy for the body. Writers commonly used machine analogies to express this relationship, as chemist Justus von Liebig did in a *Harpers* article covering the century's progress in anatomy and physiology up to 1898. Here readers learned that any "general and comprehensive view" of the human organ had to include the "digestive apparatus and lungs as the channels of fuel-supply"; the blood and lymph channels as "the transportation system"; and "muscle cells . . . as the consumption furnaces where fuel is burned and energy transformed and rendered available for the purposes of the organism."[49]

The subtle, mechanized redefinition produced a revolution in the way the body was regarded. If energy was produced in the lungs, one could access only energy brought to the "surface" by an already weakened system. Unlike lungs, however, muscles could be trained and dramatically expanded. Thus, if muscles transformed fuel into energy, the possibility of an expanding energy reserve existed. Such a theory, however, appears in conflict with entropy's law: if the second law of thermodynamics stated that all usable force is constantly diminishing, how could the body become a machine for increasing energy? Muscle advocates did not argue that expanding one's physical size could expand the body's energy indefinitely. They did argue that muscles increased the body's *usable energy*. Just as the second law theorized that energy was not actually disappearing, it was only becoming less usable, physiologists theorized that muscle did not actually increase the total energy in the body; it merely brought that energy to the body's usable "surface," making it at once more accessible and visible.

The result was a two-part improvement in the existent energy system: muscles could both expand energy production and increase the efficiency of energy consumption. As readers of the well-regarded domestic writer Catharine Beecher's *Physiology and Calisthenics for Schools and Families* (1856) learned, muscles did more than produce energy; they also helped ensure that that energy traveled through the circulatory system as efficiently as possible. Only muscle, if used "strongly and quickly," could accelerate circulation by encouraging blood to flow through the body and toward the heart.[50] This, she asserted, explained why it is "that exercise gives new life and nourishment to every part of the body."[51]

By the late 1860s, physician and physiology expert Austin Flint could declare that the "powerful influence of the muscular system on the heart" is a fact so familiar "that it need not be further dwelt upon."[52] Yet, building the body did not merely add energy to one's organs; it also refueled one's mind. If we return to George Beard's neurasthenia diagnoses, strong muscles might help speed up the process of cellular renewal he deemed essential. Rather than wait, as was normally required, for the existing supply of nervous force to be replenished, one could, with sufficient muscular development, create additional nervous force to draw upon in the interim. As early as the 1830s, one physiology text posited that "persons of great muscular firmness are not generally subject to what is called 'nervous excitement.' They are not easily thrown into trepidation; they keep cool and quiet on all occasions."[53] Though published before Beard's thesis, it presented muscle building as a definitive solution to what would later be understood as neurasthenia's ills.[54]

By the 1870s, such studies had advanced from drawing correlations between muscular and mental states to experimenting with ways to maximize muscular mass. Flint's second book, a methodical study measuring the maximum energy output available from each of the body's muscles, enjoyed wide readership. We can assume that muscle measuring had become a pastime for many Gilded-Age Americans, given that *Popular Science Monthly* published a review of Flint's book in its April 1878 issue.[55]

By late in the century, muscle had emerged as a key component in physical and mental health. According to one physician who wrote a series of articles published in the *Boston Medical and Surgical Journal* in the late 1880s, exercises that built muscle were not just about increasing physical size or strength. Instead, they were "much more exercises of the central nervous system of the brain and spinal marrow."[56] Popular enthusiasm for methodical physical conditioning increased as muscles were elevated from attractive aesthetic objects for the few to a means for physical and mental salvation for the many.

If muscular power could bestow salvation, one can imagine long lines formed at the church of *Turnen*. After all, by the late nineteenth century, the system had been around for fifty years and had proven itself capable of developing muscles of ample strength and size. Yet the rise of numerous machine-based treatments during the period of entropy anxiety suggests that such was not the case. For most Americans, gymnastics remained an artisan's craft in the machine age. If much of the anxiety that caused neurasthenia stemmed from rapid industrialization, then tossing rings and touching one's toes left something to be desired as a treatment.

Interestingly, the rise of health machines accompanied the decline in reported neurasthenia sufferers. This, combined with the repeated claims by health machine companies that they alone could cure ailments associated with neurasthenia, suggests that many who used machines did so expressly to fight the disease of energy depletion. What emerged was a variation on the theory of homeopathic treatments whereby the disease is ingested incrementally to effect a cure. If a fundamental part of neurasthenic anxiety was the fear that bodies would not measure up to the world of machines, then it is logical that many sufferers sought relief in mechanized physical training.

Chiosso and Windship: Building Machines for Modern Energy

Although weight training is ubiquitous in the United States today, an American did not invent the first weight-training machine. It was created in 1831 by Captain James Chiosso, a professor of gymnastics at London's University College. Long an advocate of traditional gymnastics, Chiosso had been searching for a way to bring healthful exercise to individuals who were intimidated by organized fitness or who were without access to public facilities. He believed the solution lay in bringing a gymnastics routine to people who would not come to it. Yet he found nothing available to replicate the graduated, controlled motions of calisthenics for the lone home practitioner. One could use dumbbells; these required neither gymnasium nor lengthy instruction.[57] The problem there, Chiosso believed, was a lack of guidance. Stationary weights could easily be misused, causing muscle strain and uneven development. What was required was a system that carefully guided the body through gymnastic movements, making sure that muscles worked neither too much nor too little.

The Polymachinon was Chiosso's answer. After twenty-five years of experimentation, he settled on the right ratio of wooden parts, heavy weights, and metal pulleys. In 1855, he published a Polymachinon pamphlet that served as part catalogue, part instruction guide, and part philosophy lesson. Though there is no direct evidence that Dio Lewis and Chiosso ever met, Chiosso did share Lewis's idea that exercise should stress each part of the body equally. In the publication's introduction he explained that "Bodily exercise, to be of use . . . must be of such a nature as to act gradually on the various complicated sets of motors of the body in every possible way . . . without the chance of their receiving the least strain."[58]

The Polymachinon achieved uniform muscular tension by bringing machine technology to physical fitness. Roughly eight feet high, it appeared to be a cross between a pulpit and an ionic column. To call it a machine seems misleading; there was actually little that looked mechanical about it. Yet it was the first exercise tool to put mechanics at its center. Embedded in the wooden structure were more than twenty compartments, from which protruded metal pulleys with handles for gripping. At the base of the machine, hidden doors concealed a solid base with removable heavy weights. One could stack weights inside the machine to increase tension. The machine thus served as a mediator, regulating the amount of stress on the body as one raised and lowered the various pulleys.

Chiosso's was the first universal machine marketed to build physical strength (fig. 1).[59] Most exercises were done facing the machine, either while sitting in a chair or standing and supporting oneself against it for balance. Even though the Polymachinon's machinery was hidden from view, the source of muscular progress was clear: between exercises, one had to reach into the machine and adjust its weights. Most of the exercises replicated the mundane tasks of daily life. During "general rotation," a typical Chiosso exercise, users hooked one of the lower pulleys over their shoulders, raising and lowering their bodies from the waist as if lifting a package or a small child off the ground. Other exercises were similarly evocative of familiar tasks, such as the "prone and supine movement of the trunk," which users would have found almost identical to the motion involved in rowing. The "downward traction or extension" replicated stair climbing, with the Polymachinon's sides acting as banisters. Were these exercises done in amounts necessary for daily life, they would be unlikely to dramatically increase strength. Yet because the machine had adjustable weights, users could gradually increase resistance. By climbing increasingly elevated stairs and rowing increasingly heavy boats, users could expand muscular strength beyond that required for natural motions. The results would have left few doubting the machine's contribution to their physical gain.

Despite his obvious vested interest in popularizing his system, Chiosso failed to articulate a theory of mechanized training. Instead, he promoted his machine as one part of a gymnastics routine that included traditional exercises like parallel bars and calisthenics. Chiosso stopped well short of developing a complete system of physical development. In his mind, the primary virtue of machines was their ability to bring gymnastics to people who could not meet for group exercise sessions. Chiosso's significant financial investment, exemplified by high-quality pamphlets with more than eighty pages of detailed instructions, did not make the Polymachinon a household name in Europe or abroad.

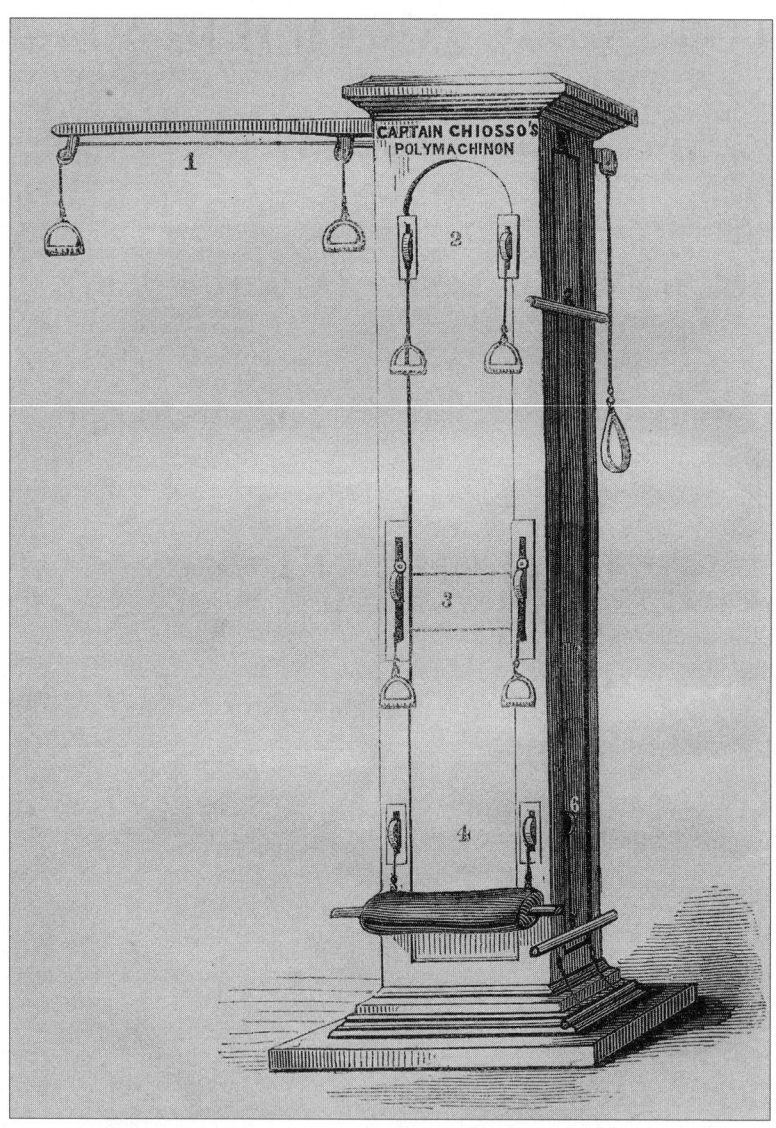

Fig. 1. Chiosso's Polymachinon. Captain Chiosso, *The Gymnastic Poly-machinon: Instructions for Performing a Systematic Series of Exercises on the Gymnastic & Calisthenic Polymachinon* (London: Walton & Maberly, 1885), back page. Todd-McLean Physical Culture Collection, University of Texas at Austin.

Chiosso's failure to gain acclaim from his machine was largely due to timing. The machine preceded by twenty years the widespread interest in entropy and neurasthenia that it might have addressed. Further, because he developed his machine before research on muscular energy emerged in the 1850s, Chiosso could not have known the profit potential in portraying it as uniquely capable of increasing stamina.[60] In the end, he contributed only a prototype awaiting an entrepreneurial American twist.

That twist came from George Windship. From inauspicious beginnings as a "puny" Harvard undergraduate, Windship became, by his late twenties, the "Roxbury Hercules," famous for lifting hundreds of pounds before sold-out audiences along the East Coast.[61] Like many of his contemporaries, Windship began physical training after growing dissatisfied with his small size. Shortly after entering Harvard in 1850, he found *Turnen*-inspired gymnastics and, with monastic dedication, set out to gain as much muscle mass as possible. By his senior year, Windship was able to turn the tables on the Harvard bullies who had previously threatened him. His work on the parallel bars, rings, and horse, as well as with free weights, had made him one of the university's strongest students.

Windship's assessment of his strength changed dramatically when he encountered a street-corner lifting machine in downtown Rochester, New York. Like an organ grinder or street entertainer, the pitchman was more promoter than instructor; he offered the machine as a temporary amusement to passersby. It was the first such device that Windship had seen, but it is likely that he understood it as part of a recent popular interest with feats of strength. Many Americans' first exposure to "strongmen" occurred in the antebellum era, when touring circuses, many imported from Europe, traveled the country showcasing performers capable of lifting immense weights and battling ferocious beasts.[62] By taking a turn on a street-corner machine, regular folks could compare their performance to the stars'.[63]

To gauge their strength, users stood on a platform, bent down, and pulled upward on handles. It was possible for a relatively strong individual to lift well over five hundred pounds this way, for the lifting was done primarily in the legs and the weight need come only inches off the ground. Windship expected his turn on the machine would "make the crowd stare" in amazement. Instead he lifted 420 pounds, no more than average for a man his size.[64] For the first time, Windship's strength had been quantified, and the results were unimpressive. Harvard's gymnastics routine had made him look strong, he reasoned, but had actually left him physically weak. "I found what many other gymnasts will find," he later recalled, "that *main strength*, by which I mean the strength of the truckman and the porter, cannot be acquired in the ordinary exercises of the gymnasium."[65]

In search of "main strength," Windship designed a crude machine to replicate the street-corner lifter. He dug a hole in the ground into which he dropped a large barrel with a rope tied to it. The other end of the rope was tied to a set of handles, and weight was added to the barrel. Windship used the machine religiously, gradually increasing the weight. In little more than a year he was able to lift 700 pounds. Within another two years, he could lift 1,208. By November 1861, he had gone beyond what his hands could lift, and he replaced the handles with leather shoulder straps. On this new apparatus he reached his maximum squat: 2,007 pounds.[66]

Windship was more than a backyard fanatic. He entered medical school and embarked on the New England lecture circuit when he finished. Part performer and part health advocate, Windship packed houses in cities already besieged by antebellum health reformers such as Baltimore, Philadelphia, Cincinnati, and Albany.[67] Some of his appeal probably lay in the curiosity of seeing someone "lift with his hands 929 lbs.," as a circular for a Cambridge lecture advertised.[68] But Windship's philosophy kept the crowd engrossed after his lifting feats were finished. He called his theory "strength is health," meaning that all of the proper eating and light exercise in the world could not make a healthy body if strong muscles were lacking. "Lifting, if properly practiced, was the surest and quickest method of producing harmonious development," he explained in 1860.[69] In both his lectures and in his private clinical practice, Windship became the machine theorist that Chiosso did not, teaching students that only machine-developed muscles could ward off ill health.[70]

Windship's method for proving his strength suggests that for some upper- and middle-class men, machine training was appealing, in part, because of its ability to render their bodies superior to those of the working class. It is telling that when Windship first realized that his gymnastics training had left him unable to demonstrate impressive strength, he characterized it as failing to give him what he called "main strength," or "the strength of the truckman and the porter."[71] This failure to demonstrate working-class strength motivated Windship to deem his machine training successful only when it could grant users strength not equal to but *in excess* of that of laboring men. In fact, he defined his body as "strong" only after it had successfully defeated a laborer's body.

After six weeks of lifting on his home-made machine, Windship invited a "stout gentleman" whom he had regularly seen unloading barrels of whisky to try the apparatus. When the worker was unable to match Windship's lift of roughly 600 pounds, the inventor delighted in the failure. He recalled watching the man as he "tugged until he was so red in the face that apoplexy seemed imminent," finally giving up "dejectedly." Thanks to his his lifting apparatus, Windship noted, it would be only a matter of time before this laborer's reputation as "one of 'the strongest men about'" would fade from view.[72]

Through their access to a machine's precise exercise of muscles not normally used even in the most strenuous of daily labors, men from the middle and upper class, the very "depleted" bodies described by Burroughs, could prove themselves superior *in spite of* the fact that their bodies were no longer employed in manual labor. By determining that the ultimate "good" produced by men should be massive muscle as opposed to productive labor, machine developers like Windship could bring about the physical defeat of the *performatively superior* bodies of immigrants, African-Americans, Native Americans, and the Anglo working class. Regardless of how many sacks of flour or barrels of whisky a man could haul, without access to a machine's specialized harnesses and pulleys, he would remain "undeveloped," unable to perform the feats of power deemed essential for Windship's masculine vision of "harmonious development."[73]

David P. Butler: When Only Cannon Balls Will Do

As Windship's popularity grew, so did the number of machines on the market that replicated his lifting feats. These became known, generically, as "health lifts."[74] By the 1870s, the term "health lift" had become so common that even simple rubber bands, to be placed under the heels and pulled upward with the hands, were sold by that name.[75] The devices, however, had not yet become popular for gymnasium or home use. Arguably, the thousands who came to see Windship's performances appreciated his feats of strength but may have lacked the motivation to develop their own "main strength" in his image. To capture a popular audience, the health lift had to be placed in the context of late-nineteenth-century energy concerns. Lifting weights had to become both something that average men and women could add to the routine of their day and something that gave them the exceptional strength necessary for physical health in an "entropic" age.

David Butler, like Windship before him, began as an unhealthy Bostonian. Like many midcentury Americans, he had pursued various doctors' cures to no avail. Self-described as having suffered in youth from "moribund debility," and having been "given up by physicians to die," Butler took matters into his own hands by beginning weight training in the late 1850s.[76] Soon he was developing his own machines to increase the weight loads. By 1867, he had opened a gymnasium in Boston and patented two lifting machines. Three years later, he was manufacturing models of his Health Lift for sale to gymnasiums and home users. By 1871, he was publishing the Health Lift newspaper and running a successful franchise operation, selling his methods and equipment to individuals interested in opening their own Health Lift studios across the country, such as the one Beecher's friends had visited that same year.[77]

We can credit entrepreneurial skills and advertising savvy for some of Butler's sales success. Yet while Butler spent more money than his predecessors on pushing his product, he also distinguished himself by more than sales skills. Butler succeeded where both Chiosso and Windship had not because he placed machine technology within the context of entropy and physical decline. Chiosso had developed a machine fifty years before Windship, one that was very similar in sophistication and use. Yet Chiosso had not explained how his mechanical training system differed from regular gymnastics. Further, his machine was bulky, expensive, and decidedly not in tune with most ornate Victorian home decor. If machines were an imitation of gymnastics, many likely reasoned, why not save money and space by going to a gymnasium? Windship addressed the specific benefits of machines with more precision, but he too failed to sell audiences on why the cumbersome devices were essential for health. His focus remained fixed on his own lifting abilities. Such excessive showmanship may have kept many from following in his footsteps. If one were not driven to lift thousands of pounds, Windship's method might have seemed like excessive energy expended for limited gain.

David Butler's program was based on his theory that machine technology could "unblock" energy that was currently in the body but unavailable for productive use. He disseminated this theory widely through his self-published newspaper and books, one of which went through six editions in three years.[78] His ideas about physical enhancement offered a counterpoint to the decline of "neurasthenia," a disease codified in Beard's *American Nervousness* only one year after Butler's first publication. Human energy, Butler argued, was sufficient to accomplish all of the tasks necessary in modern life. All one needed to do was uncover a hidden energy reserve. Unlike Beard, who blamed modern "energies" for physical decline, Butler insisted that modern energies were in fact the solution to all problems of physical weakness. By their literally embracing the technology of his machines, he promised users bodies as vigorous as the pace of modern life.

Insufficient energy was not to blame for unhealthy bodies, Butler told readers; *insufficient access* to the energy one possessed was. Americans were not necessarily weak but simply had not yet found a system that exploited their energy reserves. According to Dr. J. C. Zachos, a former army surgeon who collaborated with Butler on many of his instruction books, Butler believed that the body reserved a healthy amount of "vital force," which it kept "stored away, as it were, in the healthy organs."[79] The problem was that without what Butler termed "appropriate stimulus," the energy remained dormant.

Zachos established Butler's system as a "middleman" between vital force and the body. In his theory, vital force was an unpredictable agent. Often it remained locked in one region of the body, away from the muscles that required it to perform work. The machine regulated this relationship. As one raised the weight on the machine, Zachos reported, an enormous amount of vital energy was unlocked and sent directly to the muscles doing the heavy lifting. By applying a significant amount of force to the body at one particular time, such action concentrated "all the [body's] strength in one unitary and powerful effort, which [was] slowly but surely communicated to the largest number of muscles possible."[80] This created energy diffusion; as released energy traveled toward the working muscle, it was simultaneously absorbed into the neighboring muscle, and that muscle's neighboring muscle, and so forth until the entire body was energized with the previously dormant force. This was what Zachos called the Health Lift's "secret": it was able to "awake a torpid Liver or a tired Brain by distributing to them the latent energy that had remained unused in other parts."[81] The theory took the basic ideas from recent muscular and circulation research and applied them to mechanized exercise. Just when scientists were realizing that muscles created healthy hearts and circulatory systems, Zachos asserted that only machine lifting could build muscles to their maximum capacity. It was an equation that rendered the Health Lift synonymous with overall physical health.

Zachos's theories reflected those of contemporary physiology: circulation and muscular systems were beginning to be decoded, but physical energy continued to mystify. Although ideas about "vital fluid" and "flow" abounded in popular and scientific journals, these terms remained curiously undefined. Butler filled the void by arguing that energy traveled in a linear fashion: once it filled one muscle, it then traveled to the next and so on. His description is similar to that of an electric shock where energy is produced by weight friction and then transferred through "touch" between muscles. The connection was no accident. Zachos described the sensation of using the machine in terms of electricity: when lifted, "it has the effect of a galvanic shock to the whole system."[82]

It is probable that Zachos chose his electric analogy to cover up what he did not know. Electricity in the 1880s was still a mysterious force to most Americans, who had little contact with it in their daily lives. Yet few who read the numerous stories of electrocution in the popular press would have doubted its power. By presenting the Health Lift as a similar technology, Zachos could suggest that it, too, was a modern energetic element, one that undoubtedly worked even if it was not completely understood.[83] In fact, the very imprecision of the Health Lift's instructions may have ensured its success; by offering vaguely defined cures, it became a perfect remedy for a vaguely defined disease. Many described neurasthenia as a "general weakness" that left sufferers with a variety of symptoms including hysteria, fatigue, headaches, and impotence. Such symptoms left no one region to blame for the disease.[84] Similarly, Butler's machine made it unnecessary to pinpoint the area of the body affected by weakness. It made no difference whether it was a weakened liver or a wearied mind or an atrophied arm; the Health Lift promised to deliver sufficient strength to the entire system.

The crux of Butler's sales pitch, however, was not a cure for neurasthenia. He was far more interested in promoting "cooperative mechanization," a theory of his own design. In their writings, both Butler and Zachos stressed that cooperation was essential between one's exercise method and the body's natural movements. This informed their critique of popular therapies, including Dio Lewis's light gymnastics and the heavy gymnastics that had preceded it.[85] Those who read Butler's promotional materials learned that most of the leading systems of exercise in the late nineteenth century worked against the cooperative relationship between muscles. "They proceed too much in the analytic method of exercising one organ," explained Zachos. Using this reasoning, he asserted that exercise systems that compartmentalized muscular work could not condition the weak muscles most in need of vital force. For example, doing Lewis's exercises with the arms might also bring energy to the wrist; yet following Zachos's theory of energy transfer, it would not be enough to cure a torpid liver. In his words, such systems were akin to "trying to batter down a wall with bullets, when only cannon balls will do."[86] Without a significant force, such as the four or five hundred pounds borne by most Health Lift users, the body's strong muscles would fail to push energy into their weaker neighbors, leaving fatigue behind.

The theory of cooperative action created an exercise regimen well suited to its cultural moment. According to Butler, the system mirrored the way that Americans lived. "Excessive action is the bane of the American people," he declared in his popular *Lifting Cure*. Exercises involving numerous repetitions and strenuous movements like the Lewis system might be fine for the Germans and Swedes who, he believed, still lived lives "characterized by a lack, rather than an excess of activity."[87] American fitness, however, had to counter the frenetic pace of modern life with its increasingly populated cities and highly organized production systems. For Butler, this meant an exercise system must increase strength while conserving energy. Only such cooperative conservation would release "reserved organic power" when needed and "secure vigorous health and long life."[88]

In Butler's opinion, machines alone accomplished that twofold task. As a result, his system relied first and foremost on machine technology. Butler's main treatise, "The Lifting Cure," published in 1868, inextricably linked the machine to human health. In a section subtitled "Man a Machine," he argued that mechanical action was the fundamental law of the universe. Everything stemmed from mechanical action, including "the laws of vitality, electricity and chemical action."[89] By virtue of its being part of the system of life, the human body was a machine, and a nearly perfect one at that because of its superior organization. When the body stopped functioning correctly, Butler theorized, it must be treated as any mechanical system would be treated: with a thorough examination of its parts, or organs.[90] Butler found medicine old-fashioned. In all probability, he shocked readers in an age of pills and quick-fix potions by explaining that medicines had no inherent value.[91] They allowed users to feel better, relieving symptoms, but left the damaged system unrepaired. Only treating the action of the organs themselves would guarantee health. Like a steam engine, the body could be cured only by "obedience to the fundamental law of mechanical action."[92]

Butler's machine analogy fit an age that commonly referred to "the human engine" and "the heart pump." Butler described bodies as machines in much the same way as did physicians: to help people who were more familiar with machines than with internal organs to envision physiological function. Certainly he did use a familiar trope when he explained that the body, like a steam engine, required all parts to be working to function properly for "perfect action."[93] John Leavitt, who trained Health Lift users in one of Butler's exercise facilities, described the body's physiology in of one his exercise manuals as so similar to machines that "in mechanics, the steam, its regular alternation, the fire-box, steam-chest, driving-wheels of the Locomotive, might have been formed from seeing down through the breath, stomach, lungs, arms, and legs of man."[94]

Yet Butler's comparisons of body and machine were more than convenient analogies; they stemmed from his belief in cooperative action between the two. By connecting the body to a machine and accomplishing a series of regulated movements, users could increase usable physical force. This was the revolutionary element in Butler's system. Because the system established a cooperative relationship between mechanical and physical forces, Zachos could declare it natural to look to a machine to recalibrate the body. "[I]f by mechanical exercises the action of the organs can be regulated," he postulated, "and their latent power as effectively developed, the gain must be incalculable."[95] A century before medical science would catch up with his proposal, Zachos articulated a vision of the machine-regulated body as the apex of physical health.[96]

Butler manufactured several Health Lift models.[97] Varying in appearance, all worked under the same principle. His basic wooden machine functioned much like Windship's (fig. 2). It consisted of a raised platform standing above weights of differing amounts. To use it, one stepped up on a stool, walked onto the platform, and took hold of the handles of a pole that supported weights underneath. To lift impressive weight loads, users stood over the rod, grasped the handles in both hands, bent their knees, and lifted upward. After the weight cleared the floor ever so slightly, it was carefully lowered and the exercise was repeated three or four times

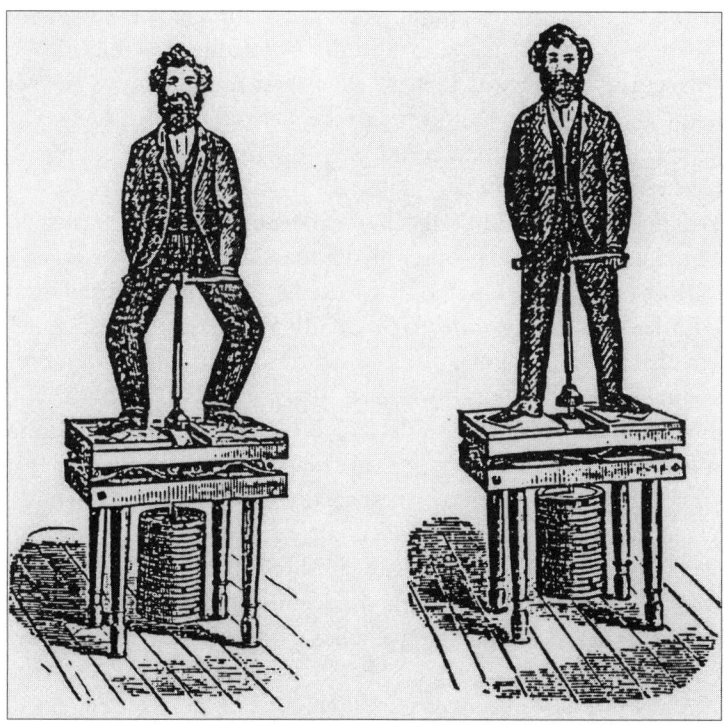

Fig. 2. Butler's standard Health Lift. Lewis Janes, *Health Exercise: The Rationale and Practice of the Lifting-Cure or Health Lift*, 6th ed. (1871).

with five minutes rest between each attempt. Butler's higher-priced model, the standard iron machine, differed in design but not function: it had a built-in step for ascending and a chair for resting during breaks.

It would have been difficult for users not to notice that Butler's exercises connected their bodies to machines. Unlike Chiosso's Polymachinon, the Health Lift's operating mechanism was in plain view.[98] Its tightly coiled springs separated the top and bottom layers of the platform, and additional springs on the base of each supporting leg provided a slight rocking motion when one ascended the device. Heavy iron weights were stacked below the platform as a reminder that this was a machine, not a breakfast table. Butler and his associates often discussed the springs in promotional materials, describing them as the heart of the machine's effectiveness. By dividing the force of lifted weight between the body, pulling up, and the springs, pulling down, the force was evenly dispersed over the whole body. The "natural order" of lifting was thus allowed to take place; the weight was lightest when first raised and, as the springs reached full extension on a lower surface, became heavier. Only with the visible springs as mediators, could one "obtain complete co-operation" between weight and body.[99]

Even if the Health Lift's mechanical features escaped one's notice, plenty of guides would have provided a machine context for users' exercises. Most promotional materials stressed that the mechanized exercises made Butler studios more effective than others. Further, Butler's machines were neither cheap nor portable; a standard iron machine cost more than three hundred dollars and weighed seven hundred pounds without weights.[100] As a result, few readers of Butler's advertisements followed the suggestion that they purchase his machines for home use. Instead, most interacted with machines in specially designed studios where they witnessed firsthand the importance of machines in effecting Butler's "cure." Further, all Butler studios were directed by a group of personal trainers schooled in the Butler method and familiar with Butler's own promotional materials, including Zachos's book. Their interactions with students would therefore have emphasized that the machines were at the heart of any physical improvements they saw.

Butler actively sought to connect his Health Lift to industrial machines. The introduction to "The Lifting Cure" describes how Butler's machines cure the body by creating a protective "iron brace of muscles." This was not the only time he associated machines with armor; throughout the pamphlet he referred to protective muscles shaped by lifting. His use here of the term *iron*, however, is significant. Butler would have been aware of iron's vogue in the Gilded Age. Periodicals, newspapers, and traveling medicine shows offered iron bitters, iron solutions, and iron pills to cure a variety of ailments. Many were specifically marketed as "nerve tonics" and "strengtheners" for young and old. Clearly such panaceas found a receptive audience; as early as 1860 a major text on medicinal drugs listed more than eighty forms of iron for therapeutic uses.[101]

The fact that this iron vogue coincided with the primary period of American industrialization suggests that Butler desired customers to connect his machine to industrial power.[102] "Iron bracing" would have evoked, for consumers familiar with advances in structural engineering, a vivid connection between Health Lifts and modern architecture. Known as the "cast iron age" in American architecture, the 1850s through 1880s saw iron-casting adopted for commercial buildings as a strong, less-expensive support system than wood or masonry. Health Lift users thus "built" themselves out of the same material that built their towering urban structures, perhaps imagining them equally suited to bear the load of modernity.[103]

Butler strengthened this connection by marketing his most profitable apparatus as an "iron machine." He even suggested that his machines possessed power superior to iron's, as they produced a force on the body equivalent to "the trip hammer that crushes tons of iron at a blow, or cracks a single nut by adjustment."[104]

To Butler, there was no reason that machines should revolutionize industry and not the body as well:

Why should not machinery be adapted to this high purpose? This is preeminently the age of invention and discovery. Intelligent labor was never so honorable. Brain labor is fast superseding physical drudgery. By the invention and use of machinery, the civilized world is fast being revolutionized and reconstructed. Every thing is being done better and more profitably by machinery than ever before. Productive energy is increasing with the speed and capacity of mechanical action. But commerce, agriculture, and manufactures must not monopolize the use of machinery: we propose to apply it directly to the culture of man, physically and mentally.[105]

If machines could not be applied to man's body, according to Butler, the bountiful energy that industry produced would be physically irretrievable. If machines allowed us to produce, trade, and consume in ever-increasing quantities without correspondingly increasing our productive capacities, we would be left behind physically, relics of a simpler time before mechanized enhancements. Butler's perspective rendered physical improvement programs like gymnastics antiquated. Throwing a hoop to a partner twenty times or doing fifty toe touches became akin to pounding out widgets by hand: time consuming, fatiguing, and premodern. Butler's argument, though preceding Frederick Winslow Taylor's theories on industrial efficiency by some thirty years, suggests that efficiency was a concern in both industrial and physical production. Even if gymnastics had been an appropriate way to build the body, which Butler's cooperative training theory denied, there was simply no time to waste on extraneous movements in the modern age: "Men cannot afford to occupy hours in securing exercise through the usual forms of manual labor or the old systems of gymnastics," Butler advised, "when better exercise can be obtained in ten or fifteen minutes, two or three times a week, by the use of machinery."[106]

This joining of human possibility with mechanical principles makes Butler one of the first to promote what would later be called the cyborg. By actively envisioning a cooperative relationship between users and his lifts, Butler became more than an inventor and trainer. He became a prophet for a new era in which human bodies should be linked to machines. Butler believed that one could not gain maximum energy until he or she reached a "feeling of oneness with the apparatus at an exercise, as if it were a part or prolongation or added sense of the body itself. The general rapport of the mechanism" was to be "like that of the rider with his horse."[107] This advice would have dramatically shifted the perspective of Butler's followers: the base was not merely a platform to stand on but an extension of the feet; levers were not metal bars but strengthened segments of users' arms. The effect went beyond blurring the distinctions between the animate and the inanimate. Because users believed that embracing an intimate relationship with machines extended their bodies' power exponentially, they had reason to eagerly anticipate further mechanization in their lives. At a time when the machine age was running full-speed ahead, dynamos taking center stage at expositions, the Brooklyn Bridge changing the dimensions of engineering capacity, and skyscrapers breaking through urban skylines, the Health Lift demonstrated the power of technology to improve human life on an intimate scale.

Butler enjoyed influence with people of power on both coasts throughout the 1870s. He was particularly successful in New York City, where, within several years of writing "The Lifting Cure," he opened four Health Lift studios on Broadway. At the same time, he oversaw rooms in Brooklyn, San Francisco, and Providence, all the while continuing to run the original studio on Boston's west side.[108] By 1871, he had enough studios and members to offer subscriptions to multiple sites, allowing clients to use Butler facilities as they traveled between urban centers. It is difficult to determine just how many Americans came into contact with the machines, given the variety of sales to private buyers and gymnasium operators and the use of Health Lifts in several YMCAs.[109] One must also factor in the success of imitation Health Lifts, which according to Harvard's physical fitness director, by the late nineteenth century had sprung "up in parlors and offices and schools everywhere."[110] None of these provided an explanation of how they worked to rival Butler's, but persons who had read Health Lift manuals would have recognized the body-machine connection the machines facilitated. Often lighter and more portable, the knockoffs took Butler's cooperative mechanization beyond lifting rooms and into the private homes of the well-to-do.[111] It is safe to assume that tens of thousands used original and imitation lifts in homes and training centers nationwide.

Butler primarily spoke of his clients as "men" in promotional materials. In reality, men and women were both featured in Health Lift advertisements for Butler's version and its progeny. This was not merely "equal-opportunity" advertising. Women did have access to Health Lift machines, at home if they had the means to purchase one, and in public gymnasiums if they did not. They could also use them at one of Butler's two studios that had women supervisors and special women's sessions.

Yet Butler's rhetorical emphasis on men reveals the impact that machines had on the gendering of physical culture programs. Whereas earlier fitness promoters like Dio Lewis had encouraged women to adopt their programs, Butler tended to include women as an afterthought, if at all. There are two explanations for this change. First, by promoting his products as tools for "depositing strength" into the body, Butler entered into an energetic space not zoned for women. Like most nineteenth-century activities, fitness was constrained by gender conventions. It was fine for women to improve posture, coordination, and general vitality with ring tosses and calisthenics. It was even acceptable to pursue the same ends with heavy weights and Health Lifts. But, arguably, as machines became increasingly theorized as *agents for* transforming the body into a productive force, they began to pose a threat to accepted ideas about female power. Butler, after all, never distinguished female from male potential energy; in his system, all bodies were equal storehouses for untapped energetic potential waiting to be "unblocked." Had women been too actively encouraged to tap into this reserve, they might have physically outgrown their culturally prescribed positions as the mental and physical inferiors of men.

One cannot say whether Butler consciously sought to exclude female consumers; his insistence, however, that the device worked by applying "the invention and use of machinery" to the physical and mental "culture of man" and that as a consequence of using his machine "all the elements of a perfect manhood are increased" shaped a space more comfortably

male than female.[112] By maintaining that he was bringing the outside productive world of invention, discovery, and labor into the body, Butler created a system of energy that mirrored the convention of separate spheres.
His theories were the beginning of what would become an increasingly
masculine world of energy enhancement, one where bodies might be
"revolutionized" and "reconstructed," but would rarely escape the confines of gender.

Existing evidence makes it easier to know the gender than the class of
Butler's clientele. His promotional use of Henry Ward Beecher suggests
his primary target was the middle class. Yet we also know that Butler
counted among his clients the well-to-do. This is clear from his home
equipment, which offered ornate, iron Health Lifts suitable for parlor display for amounts well out of reach of the middle class.[113] Additionally,
Butler's list of clients reads as a who's who of East Coast male professionals. Among those listed as "references" in *The Lift*, a promotional
journal sent to current and prospective users of Butler's rooms, were doctors, lawyers, bank presidents, military officers, corporate presidents,
publishers, clergymen, and editors such as Horace Greeley of the *New
York Tribune*.[114] The status of such individuals reveals much about who
used the machines.

Butler would have valued endorsements from people with whom other
prospective clients could identify. Advertising concerning upper-class and
famous patrons would have appealed to his largely middle-class clients,
who imagined themselves upwardly mobile. At the same time, Butler
made Health Lifts available to the working class. Yet as with women, Butler limited their facilities, offering "low rate" memberships in only two
Butler centers.[115] That Butler's target audience was the white-collar class
is evident in Beecher's *Lift* endorsements to people "whose avocations severely tax the brain" and Greeley's expressed hope that the device would
appeal to "thousands of our sedentary workers with brain and quill."[116]

Butler told readers that his machines were the only way urban professionals could regain their health. In articles like "Our Danger," he credited "active business men and capitalists" for shrewdly making money yet
chastised them for being "fatally reckless and extravagant in the use of
their own life force." Why gain property, he asked, if one did not have the
vitality to enjoy it? Look to the "hundreds of your friends and neighbors
. . . who have made their mark among you as able preachers, lawyers,
men of business"; they could testify that the machine had doubled and
tripled their strength.[117] By marketing his machines as facilitators of

white-collar recuperations, Butler tapped a market already primed by neurasthenia's panic. His targets were the men who came into close contact with what Zachos called the "productive energies" of machines, through riding to work on streetcars, using switchboards and calculators at work, and experimenting with gadgets like radio kits at home. These were the individuals who would have realized that Zachos and Butler turned accepted ideas about the effects of mechanized life upside down. Not only could the Health Lift add energy to the body enervated by the pace of modern urban life, it could use the very mechanism that threatened men's obsolescence to ensure their success.

Butler's reign over the fitness world was temporary. His crafted mosaic of entropy rhetoric and neurasthenic concerns, of Chiosso-inspired mechanics and Windship-like self-promotion, held the public's attention for little more than a decade. New machines displaced his Health Lift, many offering features that the Health Lift had not. Pulley systems promised to work arms, legs, and chests. Home exercise systems appeared that allowed users to convert walls into universal sets. In all, they allowed a greater variety in both exercise and interpretation. Windship's death in his early forties dealt a further blow to Health Lift promoters; many concluded that the massive weights he had lifted had contributed to his stroke. Increasingly, new companies produced and marketed their health machines by stressing that they *were not* Health Lifts. One 1886 advertisement for a home gymnasium trumpeted: "The principles embodied in its use are, that by its use it is nearly impossible to overdo, as the system is not called upon to exert any sudden efforts, as in the health lift."[118]

Butler's philosophy of mechanized cooperation, however, retained its influence. Many advertisements for similar products continued to promote Butler's ideas, including mechanized balance and maximum energy, if simultaneously decrying his method. Others appeared, offering a systematic approach, one that promised safe lifting and varied muscle work but that continued Butler's focus on machine energy. All pursued the promise he first made: only machines could power modern bodies by reaching into their reserves and bringing to the surface "an actual deposit of organic strength."[119]

2

Measuring Mechanical Strength

I developed manhood.

—Dudley Allen Sargent

Every man who has not gone through such a course, no matter how
healthy or strong he may be by nature, is still an undeveloped man.

—Advertisement for Sandow's Physical Development for Men

In 1869, Dudley Allen Sargent laced up his boxing gloves,
climbed into the ring, and set out to prove his manhood. He had already
been hired by the president of Bowdoin College to be its new gymnasium
director. The president, however, was not the one whom Sargent needed
to impress. Although, at only nineteen, he may have proven himself intelligent and experienced enough to win over the school's head administra-
tor, it was the students who would have the final say. They had selected
the strongest and quickest of their peers to put Sargent to the ultimate test:
ten rounds of boxing. To the students crowded around the ring, Sargent
demonstrated his strength and agility by making short work of his chal-
lenger.[1] The bout settled the question of whether he was qualified to teach.

The initiation emphasizes the dramatic difference between the physical
training of Sargent's early career in the 1860s and the one that he would
help create by its end in the early twentieth century. Along with individuals like Swedish inventor Gustav Zander, Sargent was influential in
changing the definition of "strong" men from those who won boxing
matches to those who possessed machine-balanced physiques. Sargent
made a career out of augmenting boxing rings, and the high bars and
standard rings of traditional gymnasiums, with sleek weight machines of
his own design. Under his tutelage at Bowdoin, later at Harvard, or indirectly at one of the many institutions that adopted the "Sargent system,"

students learned that real, energy-enhancing strength could be built only with the help of machines. Unlike Health Lifts, which limited users to prescribed motions, Sargent's and Zander's machine-training routines targeted specific muscles with their movements and established a means to build and measure muscle strength. In so doing, they created a physical assembly line that produced strength and dependency on the machine.[2]

Sargent's inventions made their middle- and upper-class users a compelling, three-part offer: redemption from physical obsolescence; integration into a mechanized modern world; and possession of calculable "balanced" physiques.

Turning to Machines: Sargent's Early Life

Little about Dudley Allen Sargent's early experience suggested he would, in the words of one historian, exert "a greater influence on the development of physical training . . . than any other."[3] He first became interested in fitness in the 1850s through a school hygiene program in the small town of Belfast, Maine. In the early 1860s, he came across Thomas W. Higginson's "Gymnastics" in the *Atlantic Monthly*, an article he deemed to be important enough to save and study.[4] Soon after, he organized his own boxing and gymnastic club.

Like many midcentury athletes, Sargent equated strength with the ability to attract a crowd.[5] As a teenager he organized "Sargent's Combination," a group of Belfast gymnasts that toured neighboring towns.[6] At the age of eighteen, Sargent joined a variety show that had come through town, reasoning that his own skills were at least as good as those of the featured tumblers. On the road, he alternated between performing with various circuses and training at gymnasiums to build strength. By 1869, Sargent was tired of circus life and what he called "the inevitable company of loafers."[7] Seeking to further his education and pursue his gymnastics interests, he took a job as director of gymnastics at Bowdoin College.[8]

It was at Bowdoin that Sargent began theorizing about muscular strength. He had ample time to think, for few students ever entered the decaying former dining hall that then served as the school's gymnasium. The equipment, like that in most gymnasiums, had not been improved since the early nineteenth century: its high bars, rings, and pommel horse reflected an emphasis on *Turnen's* upper-body athleticism.[9] The only machines were heavy pulley weights and one rowing device. With the exception of the latter, the equipment was usable only by students with either advanced gymnastic skills or of significant upper-body strength. According to Sargent, most students thought the equipment was merely "a form of torture."[10]

Ironically, Sargent discovered that machines were necessary only after he eliminated them. With little budgetary and college support, he first built a program the cheapest way possible, with Indian clubs (similar to juggling pins) and dumbbells. The lighter weights did allow more students to begin training, but Sargent found that many saw them as "an admission of weakness," perhaps because of their frequent use in women's gymnastics.[11] Moreover, Sargent deemed them unsatisfactory in training anything other than the upper body.

With the money from his first raise, Sargent bought adjustable machines to augment the lighter equipment. These, he hoped, would be heavy enough to challenge weak and strong students alike. Sargent also modified the heavy pulley system himself, adding a higher level of pulleys that made lifting lighter amounts possible. He based his design upon experiments he had conducted in Belfast: by introducing a system of adjustable iron bars attached to a cord, Sargent had discovered that weaker children could gradually build the upper-body strength needed for his gymnastics feats. What had worked in Belfast worked at Bowdoin; after installing several of these "developing appliances," Sargent saw results that "seemed magical."[12] Students who had believed themselves weak now came to the gymnasium to try his building machines. According to Sargent's own accounts, class enrollments tripled. By 1872, his success had convinced the faculty to make gymnastic development, which meant machine training, compulsory for all students.[13]

Bowdoin gave Sargent two important resources: a college degree and a philosophy of mechanized human development. Sargent earned the first by taking classes part-time; the second by observing his students over years of teaching. In "The Limit of Human Development," his junior oration speech, Sargent lauded the balanced men he had built with Bowdoin's machines: "Perfection of man on earth, whatever may be his condition hereafter, comes not from the surpassing development of his highest faculties, but in the harmonious and equal development of all."[14]

By stressing equal development, in mind and body, Sargent moved away from his earlier interest in physical feats of strength. He began to realize, as had Windship before him, that his own training as a teenager, although physically impressive, was incomplete. Years of practice had left him able to swing from the trapeze and entertain a crowd, but had left him "overtrained" and depleted internally. "I had learned how to work and develop my muscles," he recalled, "but I had not learned how to conserve my energy."[15] During his Bowdoin years, Sargent had a chance to rethink the purpose of muscular development from a student's perspective. Future leaders needed bodies that built maximum energy for physical and mental tasks.

William Blaikie, one of Sargent's supporters and friends, first articulated Sargent's new philosophy. An alumnus of Harvard's rowing team and a New York attorney, Blaikie enjoyed influence among Harvard administrators and New York professionals. His book *How to Get Strong and Stay So*, published in 1879, proclaimed Sargent the creator of a new machine system. Blaikie's description of the properly developed body sheds light upon Sargent's reappraisal of the machine. Sargent would never credit Blaikie for his new approach to physical fitness, but his biographer did document the close pace with which he followed Blaikie's recommendations.[16]

For Blaikie, the Health Lift and heavy lifting in general were improper physical applications of machine technology. They created "work of the grade suited to a truck-horse," he told readers, at once rejecting claims that the lift trained muscles equally and equating lift-trained bodies with genetically inferior stock. Blaikie drew such conclusions from his own Health Lift training: eventually he could lift one thousand pounds but found his back stiff and his inner-thigh and upper-back muscles "abnormally" developed. In Blaikie's assessment, Butler had overlooked the latent potential of machine-based training: a perfectly contoured, symmetrically developed muscular physique. It was this, not brute strength, that distinguished the scientifically fit body from its laboring counterpart. In the controlled, supervised environment of the studio, the body could be strengthened without the detrimental effects of manual labor. "Scarcely any work in a farm makes one quick of foot," Blaikie explained, citing the reason that farmers often suffered from ill health. "All the long day, while some of the muscles do the work . . . the rest are untaxed, and remain actually weak."[17] Athletes suffered equally from this imbalance-induced weakness, asserted Blaikie; through illustrations of "poorly developed athletes," he made his point (fig. 3). The subjects' deficiencies are

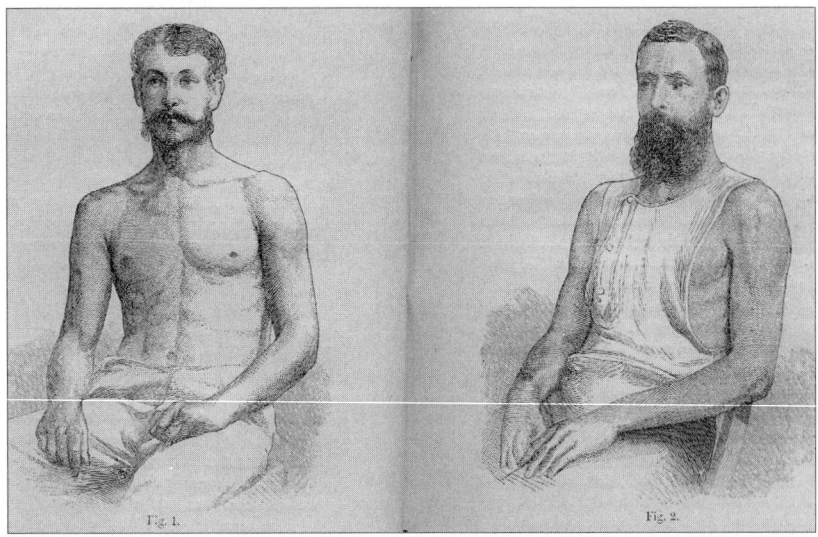

Fig. 3. Blaikie's illustration of the half-built athlete. William Blaikie, *How to Get Strong and How to Stay So* (New York: Harper & Brothers, 1879), 36.

not readily apparent to us today, but Blaikie saw bodies not yet perfected and drastically out of proportion with excessive shoulders, sunken chests, and weak legs.

Blaikie's musings challenged American paragons of masculine strength. To Blaikie's eyes, the yeoman farmer, symbol of vigorous national health since Jefferson's time, and the athlete, a hero of strength since ancient Greece, were proven weak through the very accomplishments that once validated their strength. By insisting that the strength and energy came from balance, not performance, Blaikie promoted a new ideal that could be achieved only by new systems of training. This established an elite group, the only one with access to the facilities, machines, and instructors necessary for proper energetic strength.

For Blaikie, earlier machine systems like Butler's had left users as weak as the unfortunate laborers and athletes. By failing to take advantage of machine precision, the systems had neglected the adjustable resistance required to fully develop all muscles. He proposed, alternatively, Sargent's light pulley system, which he knew from the Bowdoin experiments. Blaikie familiarized readers with Sargent's approach, giving a detailed description of the machine and a full-page illustration in his text. Only this kind of graduated weight training system, Blaikie argued, could relieve a "clogging," or "lack of complete action," in the body's energy.[18]

As part of a broader industrial standardization after the Civil War, Blaikie's emphasis on balance corresponded with the precursors to Progressivism, such as the U.S. Sanitary Movement. By the 1870s, many Americans no longer marveled at the brute force of machines, as Windship had praised the Lift for "crushing a ton of iron in a single blow." As technology developed, more subtlety was expected. Trains needed not merely to run but to run on time and over standardized tracks; factories needed not merely to produce but to produce cheaply with efficient labor. The refinement and systematization of machines was impacting the fabric of daily life, and with the help of Blaikie and Sargent, so too would it be brought to bear on the body itself.

Harvard and the Hemenway: Building a System of Machine Energy

Harvard's regents hired Dudley Allen Sargent as the school's first director of physical education in 1879, a position he held for more than forty years. Prior to his arrival, Harvard's Hemenway gymnasium had been, like Bowdoin's, ignored.[19] With only a few old-fashioned rowing machines, a generic health lift, and several older pulley weights, it was, primarily, a place for gymnasts and boxers to practice.[20] Harvard gave Sargent relative freedom and ample resources to develop his ideal mechanized fitness system. The Hemenway's renovations had cost $110,000, nearly double the cost of other university gymnasiums. Its running track, rowing room, fencing room, baseball cage, and tennis courts made it one of the most impressive in the world.[21] Harvard spared no expense in developing a fitness program to build students' health and athletes' performance.

Sargent used Harvard's financial resources to create and build advanced versions of the machines he had first used at Bowdoin.[22] In addition to standard gymnastics equipment such as parallel bars, the pommel horse, and Indian clubs, he installed thirty-six new machines manufactured by the Narragansett Machine Company according to his own specifications. Sargent's minute attention to muscular detail is evident in the machines he created. In addition to back, abdominal, chest, arm, and leg machines, Sargent built machines specifically to strengthen necks and fingers, as well as those targeted at body deficiencies. One such machine purported to correct "any erratic twist or turn in one or both feet."[23]

A total of fifty-six machines lined the walls, commanding attention from all who entered the Hemenway. Much of the regular gymnastics equipment was hung from the ceiling, so even users who did not work with Sargent's machines directly hovered over them as they trained.

In arrangement and quantity, the Hemenway's equipment was visually striking. The machines, however, also invited a sense of physical intimacy with their users. The collection included both standing and sitting machines. Sargent's devices for lower body work, as well as those for head and finger strength, required individuals to sit on or inside them. According to one user, the machine for building calf muscles felt much like a comfortable "arm-chair," in which one sat and pushed a foot weight up and down.[24] Sargent also mechanized traditional gymnasium offerings: counterweighted parallel bars made lifting one's weight easier and spring boards on iron pedestals pivoted in their sockets for increased bounce. He drew attention to these improvements, saying that although "all the old-style apparatus has been added," it had been "with improvements in form, structure, and arrangement."[25] The innovations allowed students to feel themselves part of a mechanized environment. Enhancements such as parallel bars shaped to students' hands and ladder-rungs polished for easier gripping meant an environment reflective of machine-age design and ergonomics a generation before such theories came into vogue.[26]

Sargent's goal was not to give students a comfortable and modern method of exercise. It was to produce the healthiest bodies possible. His means to that end were his machines. His theories are best illustrated by exploring in detail three units of the Hemenway apparatus: the chest pulley, the abdominal pulley, and the Inomotor. Sargent's most popular machine was his basic chest pulley. Not only did the Hemenway have more of them than any other, they were also the machine most frequently imitated.

Peck and Snyder, one of the best-known sporting-goods manufacturers in the 1880s, carried several examples of pulley machines. Professor D. L. Dowd's home exerciser and its list of muscular exercises were clearly imitations of Sargent's system.[27] The Narragansett Machine Company marketed pulley weights so similar to Sargent's that he sued the firm, despite having promised Harvard that he would not patent his devices.[28] The basic pulley weight was a modified version of those he had encountered at Bowdoin. By dividing the block weights into iron bars and attaching

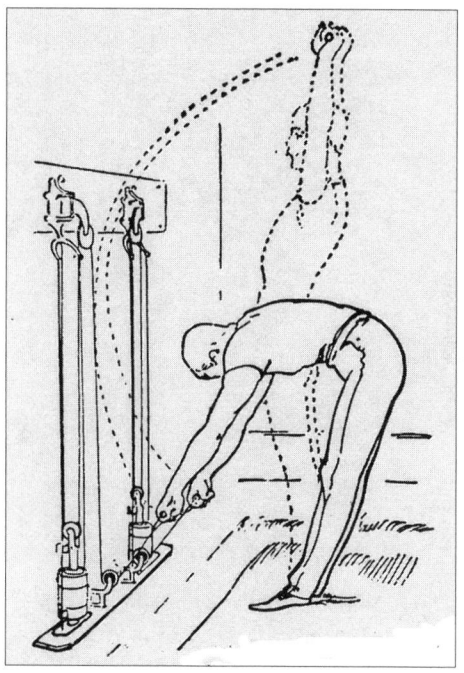

Fig. 4. Sargent's "chopping wood" pulley exercise. Narragansett Machine Company (catalogue, 1887), 33.

the bars to the pulley in desired increments, Sargent created a weight system that, as he put it, was "adjustable to the strength of the strong and to the weakness of the weak."[29] As he did for all of his machines, Sargent developed specific exercises for the pulley weight. Rather than completely new movements, he prescribed mimicry of movements from everyday life. These allowed students to "work" by "chopping," moving the arms over the head and down, or "sawing," moving the weight front to back (fig. 4). They could even engage in "swimming" by pulling their arms in circular motions.[30]

Sargent had noticed at Bowdoin that the students who had the strongest arms or legs were often those who engaged in regular labor, such as that of blacksmiths and lumberjacks. He identified labor as the source of strength, but it is significant that Sargent did not simply send his students out to chop wood. Following in the footsteps of Windship, Butler, and Blaikie, Sargent argued that manual labor led to overdeveloped, inferior muscles. A laborer would be unlikely to saw, row, swim, and chop all in an afternoon as would be required for even muscular development.

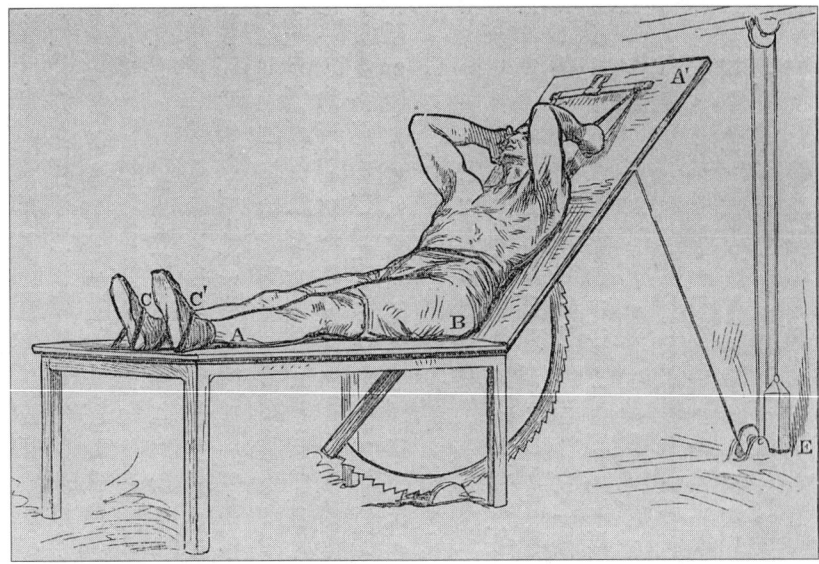

Fig. 5. Sargent's stomach pulley machine. William Blaikie, *How to Get Strong and How to Stay So* (New York: Harper & Brothers, 1879), 225.

Moreover, his pulley system could mimic these natural movements more efficiently by providing them all in the same place. For Sargent, pulley weights created many light "jobs" that could be done in a short time, and thus were the best means for "giving one an all round [*sic*] development of the whole muscular system."[31]

With balanced development as his goal, Sargent needed machines that allowed students to work underutilized muscles. Accordingly, he fashioned a series of involved pulley systems that could fortify each part of the body. His abdominal pulley shows how his basic pulley principle could be adapted for different movements (fig. 5). A standard chest pulley system was not well suited to abdominal training, unless one understood that the resistance could be transferred to another device, in this case a hinged table that required stomach muscles to do the lifting. Machines like the abdominal exerciser distanced working bodies from trained bodies. The chest pulley machines would have developed muscle that looked visually similar to those developed through daily labors, given that the motions of pulling a weight and pulling a barrel are quite similar. Abdominal muscles, however, were not intensely exercised in labor. "Sculpted" abdominals, then, were muscles effectively removed from productive labor and, because one needed machines to develop them, achievable only by those who had access to and time for machine training.

For young men at Harvard, machines offered a route to superior strength that conserved nerve force, a distinction between Sargent's system and its predecessors. According to one journalist, most gyms actually hurt users because they required "too great [an] expenditure of nerve-power in the effort to keep the muscles up to their highest tension."[32] In other words, people tended to leave training with less energy than they brought. Sargent's system seemed to allow even the weakest students to develop strong muscles while preserving their delicate health, thanks to new machines like the abdominal pulley.

Sargent's Inomotor best reflects his belief in the compatibility of machine technology, physical health, and energy conservation. Patented in 1899, the Inomotor was both a vehicle and exercise machine, and a reflection of twenty years of active experimentation (fig. 6). The device, which never enjoyed popular success, looked highly unusual, like a vehicle's chassis without its protective metal exterior. The user manipulated a combination of levers and a sliding seat so as to do two tasks at once: move the vehicle forward and exercise arms, legs, and torso. In principle,

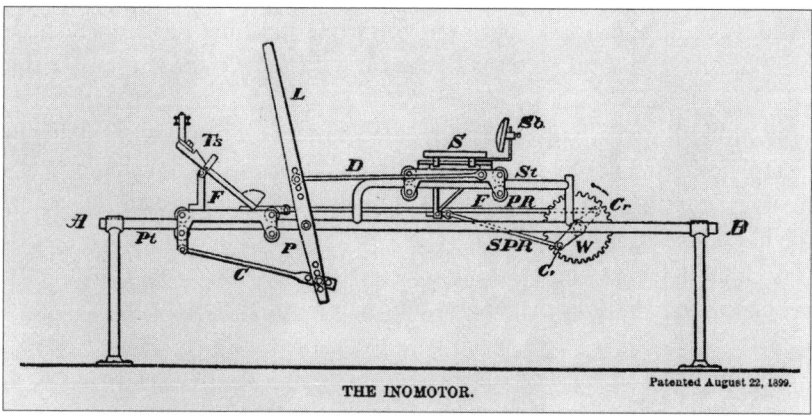

THE INOMOTOR.   Patented August 22, 1899.

Fig. 6. Sargent's failed Inomotor. D. A. Sargent, "The Inomotor: A Fundamental Mechanism for a New System of Motor Vehicles, Testing Apparatus and Developing Appliances," *American Physical Education Review* 5 (December 1900): 319.

it worked like an exercise cycle: a series of user movements turned the gears of the machine. The Inomotor, however, offered something unique: when the optional wheels were attached, it actually moved.

Unfortunately, Sargent sketched more than he wrote about the Inomotor. Though he never articulated how the machine fit into his system of pulley devices, Sargent's intentions are legible in a proposal to modernize the Hemenway in the early 1900s. His idea, which was rejected by Harvard's administration, was to place the Inomotor at the center of a new, dynamic training program.[33] The gymnasium's interior would be gutted, its fencing rooms and batting cages demolished to make room for a wide track. On it, students would propel their way to health. Sargent's vision would allow the machines to reach their fullest potential: not only would they build operators' muscles through resistance to the levers and pedals, they would also allow students to enjoy a tangible return on their energy investment.

Harvard's administrators perceived the scheme as misguided. Yet Sargent's sketches and limited writings on the machine's function suggest that he was actually trying to take mechanized muscle building to a higher level of energy production. For although Sargent believed that pulley weights developed the body's muscles equally, he was ambivalent about the strength students thereby acquired. Students needed cardiovascular exercise to get their pulmonary and circulatory systems flowing over an extended period of time. This was impossible with pulley weights. Regardless of how fast students went from one machine to another, there were inevitable pauses between devices and during weight setting. On the other hand, cardiovascular exercise alone could not ensure balance, because, like all unmechanized activity, it expanded some muscles while neglecting others. The key seemed to be to find a way to use machines to actually pump the body as a whole, building balanced muscle and speeding the heart simultaneously.[34]

In his single essay on the Inomotor's efficacy, Sargent first clarifies the problem with previous machine training by using the analogy of

a factory that has been accustomed to work only a few of its machines at one time, and has an engine adapted to that purpose. If all the machinery were started up at once, the boiler could not generate enough steam to supply each machine with its requisite power, consequently permitting little effective work to be accomplished by any one of them. The remedy for the factory is to build a larger engine, or to generate more steam. In the case of an individual, the remedy is to invigorate the heart and lungs and, if possible, provide more nerve power.[35]

Sargent acknowledged that students could be well-trained at his system of individual machines, yet still lack the overall "boiler" or heart-pumping capacity to work each of the machines at the same time. This was a theoretical problem because no student could actually work all "machines," or muscles, at once. The Inomotor provided an actual solution to the theoretical problem: a cardiovascular apparatus that Sargent believed could actually give more "nerve power" to the body by invigorating the heart and lungs.[36] When students "drove" the Inomotor, they expended their available energy to move its pedals and levers and send it into motion. Unlike stationary machines that merely provided resistance to expended energy, the Inomotor returned energy back into the driver.[37] As the vehicle raced faster and faster, force theoretically reentered the student's body, a unique by-product of the human-machine interaction.

This concern with energetic force was not unique to muscle building. "Force" was at the forefront of American intellectual and business life in the Gilded Age, thanks to the embrace of British psychologist Herbert Spencer. Spencer's theory of social Darwinism attempted to apply biological evolutionary theory to social and psychological concerns. An advocate of big business and small government, Spencer was a hero to a generation of emerging capitalists eager to use biology to justify their great personal wealth. At the heart his theory, however, was an exaltation of force. In *Principles of Psychology*, he argued that his purpose was to interpret "life, mind, and society in terms of matter, motion, and force." All social systems, including ethics, morality, and status, were actually produced by a universal force. For Spencer, this energy was the engine that drove evolution. At the heart of all life, all change, and all organization was a "persistence of force" driven by nature and impervious to human machinations.[38]

Although life was being driven by force, individuals were not entitled to sit back and wait for universal energies to reveal a perfect society. Spencer envisioned an ideal world in which universal force was met with individual resistance. As a result, desirable traits were inherited and improved upon as generations moved closer and closer to social perfection. This Lamarckian worldview provided Spencer, and those who heard his lectures, with a new energetic model of society. Instead of merely evolving along a predetermined course, individuals could add to their hereditary inheritance by exercising particular thoughts, feelings, and emotions over a lifetime.[39] With a proper regimen of "fitness," individuals could thus improve national health by passing on their improved traits to the next generation.

Spencer's language intersects in several places with that of health theorists like Sargent, Butler, and later, Gustav Zander. His use of the terms *force, exercise,* and *resistance,* as well as his emphasis on man's innate muscle sense rhetorically connected weight training to directed evolution.[40] This is not to argue that Sargent's machine-training system shared social Darwinism's goals, though Spencer's ideas circulated in the United States in the 1880s when Sargent was developing his theories. The cultural context out of which weight machines emerged, however, was one in which the "universe of force" was depicted as a coconspirator in attempts to justify class distinction and disparate wealth.[41] Middle- and upper-class Americans, to whom both Spencer and Sargent directed their attention, could interpret their own force-built bodies as further justification for their position at the top of Spencer's capitalist-evolutionary ladder.

Ultimately, Sargent did not have a chance to develop the Inomotor's program of force expansion. Although several stationary devices were placed in the Hemenway, the Inomotor gymnasium never materialized. Nonetheless, the Inomotor leaves little doubt that Sargent conceived a relationship between human and machine force. It was one he shared with far more students than just the number who sought out the Hemenway's offerings. Although he was never able to make training mandatory for students, Sargent did persuade Harvard's administration to require all athletes and scholarship holders to go to the Hemenway, meet Sargent, get a physical examination, and be shown an exercise regimen. Those students would not actually have to do the exercises they were given, but they had to be taken through the exercises, ensuring that all interacted with Sargent and his machines. Further, each entering freshman had to visit the gymnasium at least once, a meeting Sargent used to deliver "specifications of the movements and apparatus which he may best use."[42] Even if each freshman entered the Hemenway only once, at least 250 a year received a personal introduction to Sargent's machines.[43] Individual accounts of students' experiences with the machines are scarce, but there is evidence that students chose machines over traditional equipment. Participation in gymnastics exhibitions decreased dramatically after Sargent arrived, in spite of his own skill as a gymnastics teacher.[44] The shift suggests that many transferred their interest from *Turnen* to machines. Additionally, President Charles Eliot publicly endorsed Sargent's system for even the least athletic students, citing its "greater service to weak, undeveloped persons than to those already strong" and its training of athletes through "moderate and symmetrical muscular development."[45]

For some students, the Hemenway's equipment became an integral part of their lives. One alumnus reported in 1919 that as students in the 1880s, he and his friends had "exercise[d] there almost daily." They recalled that Sargent had measured their strength, "showed us where we were weak and assigned us to practice on his development apparatus."[46] Popular articles support this account of frequent Hemenway exercise; an 1889 article declared that "at present the average student, with no thought of training for any contest, devotes an hour or so a day to exercise in the gymnasium, or to whatever may be his chosen game."[47]

It is noteworthy here that Sargent's students at Bowdoin and Harvard were all men. Sargent would later be renowned for opening his Cambridge institute for women in 1881.[48] Like Butler, Sargent believed that both men and women should use his machines, and his summer institutes regularly trained women in how to administer the Sargent system. During Sargent's formative years, when he developed his theories of mechanized physical development, however, his students remained primarily male. Throughout his career, men constituted the majority of his students, and his most extensive collections of machinery were consistently made available only to men.[49]

Sargent's work with the men at Bowdoin and Harvard had important implications. It provided those who would join the white-collar industrial class with firsthand evidence of a symbiotic relationship between machines and health. Sargent's repeated emphasis that muscular balance meant physical health further suggested that only machines facilitated complete development. These conscious and unconscious lessons likely facilitated an association between mechanized systems and human progress. By handing each Harvard student a card that calculated his weaknesses and directing him to the machine whose use would fix them, Sargent taught him to think of his body as a system of imperfect parts best repaired by machines.

Measuring Mechanized Progress: Sargent's Anthropometric System

Upon their matriculation at Harvard, young men found their bodies fully qualified by Sargent—a process involving some forty calculations in all.[50] On the basis of these measurements, each student received a chart detailing which body parts were average, above average, and below average. Sargent then provided a prescriptive training regimen of machine exercises. Ideally, an examination in six months would show that the student had moved closer to the average and had "remed[ied] defects." Should that not be the case, a revised training schedule would be attempted.[51]

Sargent employed a variety of devices to measure each student's strengths and weaknesses. For example, he clocked students to see how fast they could run and measured muscles with tape to check development.[52] He also used tools such as calipers to measure abdomens and chests. Yet these appliances measured only what one could see. To perform internal measurements, Sargent used three machines: the spirometer, the manometer, and the dynamometer.[53] Each required the user to exert force upon an apparatus to produce a strength reading. The spirometer was a modified bucket-and-straw apparatus; users took in as much air as possible and exhaled into the mouthpiece, giving a reading of lung capacity in water displaced. The manometer worked in a similar fashion, except that the user blew with one quick blast into the mouthpiece and the pressure applied through the process appeared on the top dial.

If the number of illustrations in his publications is any indicator, dynamometers were among Sargent's favorite machines. They appeared in numerous guises; the back dynamometer, the hand dynamometer, and the chest dynamometer were the most common. With the back apparatus, muscle strength was measured as a student stood on one side of the machine while pulling up on the other. As with Butler's earlier Health Lift, the user bent slightly at the knees and then straightened his back to raise the "weight."

The chest dynamometer afforded an equally close connection between user and apparatus. The user held handles on both sides and pushed each hand toward the other. The result could be read in kilograms of force on the display dial. The hand machine worked similarly; the user pressed his fingers toward one another, forcing the machine's metal exterior to bend.[54]

Of the myriad sensations one would have experienced using these machines, one of the most startling would have been the translation of strength into data via machines. Whereas other physical educators had developed their own measurement systems, Sargent's was the first to chart physical power by mechanized means.[55] Sargent referred to these measuring techniques as anthropometry. The word, coined in the eighteenth century, had been popularly used for several decades by the time Sargent began his Harvard experiments.[56] Studies of anthropometry tend to focus primarily on the ways it was manipulated in the nineteenth century to "prove" Anglo superiority.[57] Anthropometry, although scientific when rigorously applied, had a chameleonlike character; it could easily be used to prove whatever a researcher set out to find. It lent itself to racist applications; findings often "proved" the inferiority of certain groups based on prejudice masquerading as science.[58] Because of this association, Sargent's system has been largely ignored, though he was arguably the best known anthropometrist of his time.[59]

By virtue of his long-held position at Harvard, his summer school program that enrolled thousands, his popular writings, and his role as a founder of the American Social Science Association, Sargent defined anthropometry for an educated American audience.[60] His work offers an important corrective to definitions of anthropometry as an exclusively racially determinist endeavor. Sargent did propagate a rigid standard of the "ideal" body and trained bodies that were almost exclusively white, but he did not exclude nonwhites from learning his methods or applying them to achieve "ideal" physiques.[61] Booker T. Washington, in fact, was one of Sargent's summer institute students.[62]

Sargent's anthropometric studies were part of a late-nineteenth-century flood of efficiency experiments. Taylorism is one of the best known; its promoters sought to measure the exact movements of industrial workers to determine the path of least resistance in manufacturing.[63] Scholars have focused on the American Frederick Winslow Taylor, arguing, rightly, that his theories successfully distanced workers from their products, replacing craftsmanship with speed.[64] Yet Taylor's project was part of a general climate of efficiency of the time. Many of the projects were designed to speed up industrial production; others were undertaken to understand the body's processes and extract the most energy from them possible. One historian has called their combined efforts an attempt to develop "a new calculus of fatigue."[65] Studies emerged in calorie counting or "scientific eating," researching how to receive the maximum "energy" from food.[66] By the late 1890s, researchers in France, Germany, and Italy were developing ways to best measure and utilize physical energies. Much of this took the form of breaking down bodily processes, internal and external, into their constituent elements.[67] The most famous of these researchers, Eadweard Muybridge, published a series of body-in-motion studies in the late 1870s.[68]

Unlike most of his contemporaries, Sargent was more interested in examining body measurements than in observing bodies at work. He viewed machine-derived measurements as accurate gauges of strengths and weaknesses. His detailed calculations are illustrated by his anthropometric chart for Eugen Sandow, an Austrian strongman famous in America (fig. 7). The chart, which included Sargent's standard forty measurements, shows Sargent's goal of "perfect symmetry" realized.[69] Sandow is far to the right of the middle line, meaning his measurements are largely 90 percent greater than those of other individuals. Further, when connected, the individual measurements follow an almost perfect line reaching from the top of the chart to the bottom, excluding deviations in knee, shoulder, and elbow strength. For Sargent, the strongman's symmetry proved the possibility of physical perfection. Sandow was widely recognized as having "a machined figure" that could "be admired, imitated, and industrially reproduced."[70] He courted this image of replicatable perfection by offering charts of himself in his books and showing readers how they might measure their own bodies in comparison. Further, he offered his own machine-training system as an aid to such replication. Sandow's machine, a modified pulley-weight developer, was so associated with the performer that Marcel Duchamp, in his sculpture *The Bride Stripped Bare by Her Bachelors, Even (The Large Glass)*, included a pulley machine he called a "Sandow" in order to create what Linda Henderson has called an "ideal human-machine analogy."[71]

When Sargent emerged from his 1893 measuring session with Sandow, declaring him "the most wonderful specimen of man I have ever seen," he confirmed a new alliance between the popular world of strength performance and the scientific pursuit of muscle building.[72] It is tempting to portray Sargent's mechanized system at Harvard as something distinct from the world of working-class strength amusements. Certainly the future professionals measuring and building their bodies with machines under Sargent's tutelage were learning a definition of strength that differed from the feats of "strongman" performers.[73] "Sargentized" bodies were neither those capable of doing immense work, such as Windship's

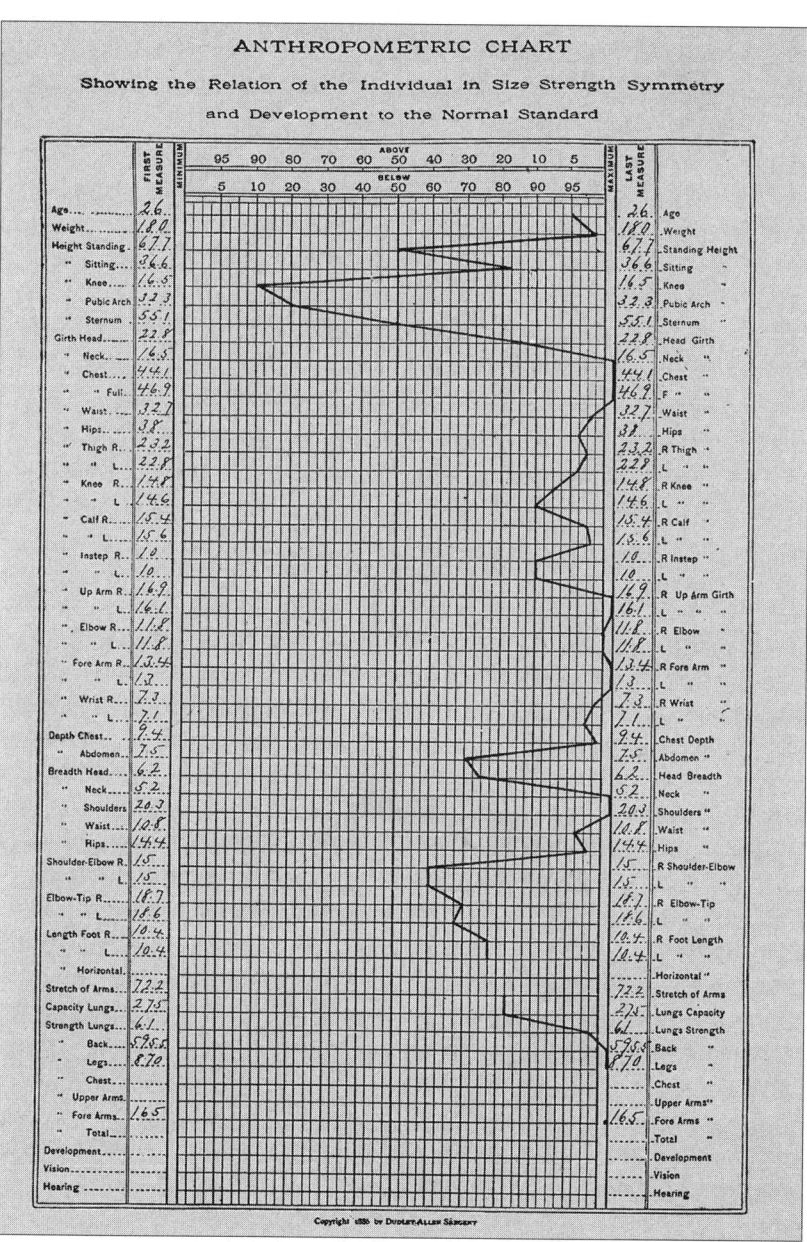

Fig. 7. Sargent's anthropometric chart for Eugen Sandow. G. Mercer Adam, ed., *Sandow's System of Physical Training* (New York: J. Selvin Tait & Sons, 1894), 241.

mythologized "laborer," nor those capable of phenomenal feats of strength, such as popular nineteenth-century circus performers like Sampson and Atilla. Yet Sandow's popularity with professional muscle strategists like Sargent and with the general public in search of a good show attests the cross-class appeal of scientific strength.

Throughout the second half of the nineteenth century, traveling gymnastic shows like "Sargent's Combination," circus shows with resident strongmen, and boxing bouts attracted audiences in urban centers and small towns. The skill level of performers ranged from Sargent's amateur Belfast gymnasts to practiced promoters like Atilla or John L. Sullivan, but the product they offered was similar: a chance to watch men display their muscles by lifting weights, mastering parallel bars, straddling the pommel horse, or knocking out opponents.

These men represented a world apart from Sargent's systematized Hemenway training. They did not develop theories of muscle building or design specialized machines, and they privileged localized muscle strength over "balance." For popular strongmen performers, the goal was to gain fame, pack houses, and make money. To do so, they put on a show with their excessively strong arms, backs, and legs. This was the world Sandow entered as a traveling circus performer in the 1880s early in his career when, trained by the master self-promoter "Professor Louis Attila," he took to the stage to lift weights of more than one thousand pounds, break chains with his arms, and bend iron bars with his bare hands.[74]

By the time he met Sargent in 1893, Sandow had become more than a strongman. Throughout the 1890s, in shows at the Casino in New York and the Tremont Theater in Boston, and with Florenz Ziegfeld's performers in Chicago, he presented a body that consciously combined working-class popular strength with upper-class systematized training. In his writings on muscular development and in his interviews, Sandow presented himself as an educated, gentleman strongman who embodied the best of brute strength and scientific erudition. Sargent remarked in his notes on Sandow's measurements that his "behavior under the tests was admirable" and described him as "a perfect gentleman" who possessed "considerable knowledge of anatomy, and can call the muscles by their proper names."[75] It is telling that in a session ostensibly devoted to muscle measurement, Sargent would spend much time thinking about Sandow's station as a proper gentleman. He had made no such remarks when measuring the working-class boxing champion John L. Sullivan months earlier.

In Sandow, Sargent had found what John Kasson refers to as the "messiah" of fitness: a man who possessed unequaled physical strength *and* understood his body as a complex system to be trained by machines. The public's overwhelming embrace of Sandow, and in particular its fascination with the extraordinary development of each muscle in his body, and his abdominal muscles in particular, reveals that the emphasis on "balance" coming out of Sargent's mechanized muscle-building program was not merely an upper-class fixation. Suggestively, part of the attraction of watching Sandow perform was that it allowed working-class audiences to connect their own strength-training strategies with the scientific rigor of emergent mechanized systems like Sargent's. Devices such as the popular modified health lifts and dumbbells sold by Sears, Roebuck and Co. and street-corner lifting machines bore similarities to the platform lifts and iron weights mastered nightly in Sandow's performances. As a result, Sandow's shows throughout the 1890s may have affirmed the value of working-class performative strength. At the same time, Sargent's pronouncements of Sandow's muscular balance, "gentlemanly" status, and superior anatomic knowledge, which ran in urban newspapers simultaneously with Sandow's performances, as well as Sandow's own connection to Harvard (he spoke at the Hemenway where a cast of his physique was installed as an inspiration to students) placed him squarely within the rarefied world of machine training seeping out of the Hemenway and YMCAs across the country.[76] Exploring Sandow's connection to Sargent allows us to reinterpret Sandow's body as a site where separate definitions of working- and upper-class strength merged to create the perfect modern man.[77]

During his fifty years in physical education, Sargent influenced strength training far beyond the confines of the Hemenway. At Harvard and in summer training sessions, Sargent trained roughly three thousand students from one thousand institutions who went on to shape fitness programs across the nation. Sargent counted among his summer students Booker T. Washington and prominent women like Dr. Helen Putnam of Vassar and Dr. Carolyn Ladd of Bryn Mawr; many used their training to begin similar systems at major universities.[78] Edward Hartwell brought the Sargent method to Johns Hopkins; William Anderson, to Yale; and R. Tait McKenzie, to the University of Pennsylvania.[79] Luther Gulick, who guided YMCA training in the late nineteenth century, was also a Sargent student. Gulick's YMCAs bought Sargent's developing machines and adopted his measurement system, allowing thousands of men and women across the country to build bodies and gauge progress with Sargent machines.[80] Sargent also reached a wide popular audience through articles in *Scribner's Magazine*. With titles like "The Physical Proportions of the Typical Man," these pieces introduced readers to anthropometry and mechanized training, complete with physical charts, pictures of the measuring machines, and examples of ideal physiques.[81]

Sargent's equipment was also featured as part of the Narragansett Machine Company exhibit at the 1893 World's Fair in Chicago. The display's location, inside the building Anthropology: Man and His Works, highlighted the machine-body connection (fig. 8). As visitors passed by numerous ethnological exhibits listing the cranium and skeletal measurements for ethnic groups, they were encouraged to consider how their own bodies measured up. Sargent's equipment allowed them to find out: they could step into an alcove and be anthropometrically charted. Results in hand, visitors could then try out the machines, possibly remeasuring themselves after a brief workout.[82]

Though perhaps unaware of it, the majority of East Coast, middle- and upper-class Americans had had some contact with Sargent's systems by the early 1900s. Many already knew of the machines by the time they visited the fair; according to one historian, Sargent's apparatuses were widely sold in the United States after the Narragansett Machine Company marketed them in the 1890s.[83] According to Sargent's own estimate, by 1890 his machines were being used by 100,000-plus people in 350 institutions across the country.[84] The proliferation attests to the dramatic change that physical training and physical evaluations had undergone over the half century preceding 1920. By the early twentieth century it was commonplace for students to exercise on machines. Anthropometric studies, if increasingly designed for posture work or eugenic data, continued to rely upon mechanized equipment to evaluate the physical form. Sargent's work effectively made machines guides in the quest for physical health. No longer would individuals measure strength solely by means of boxing matches as had his Bowdoin students. Along with sawing, rowing, and other manual tasks, hand-to-hand combat had become antiquated for followers of Sargent's system.

Traditional athletics and daily labor may have made men appear strong, they may have even allowed men to do a great deal of work, but they did not build "scientific" strength. As Sargent told readers in his *Scribner's* article in a statement that would have pleased George Windship, it was not uncommon for exceedingly strong-looking men to fall into

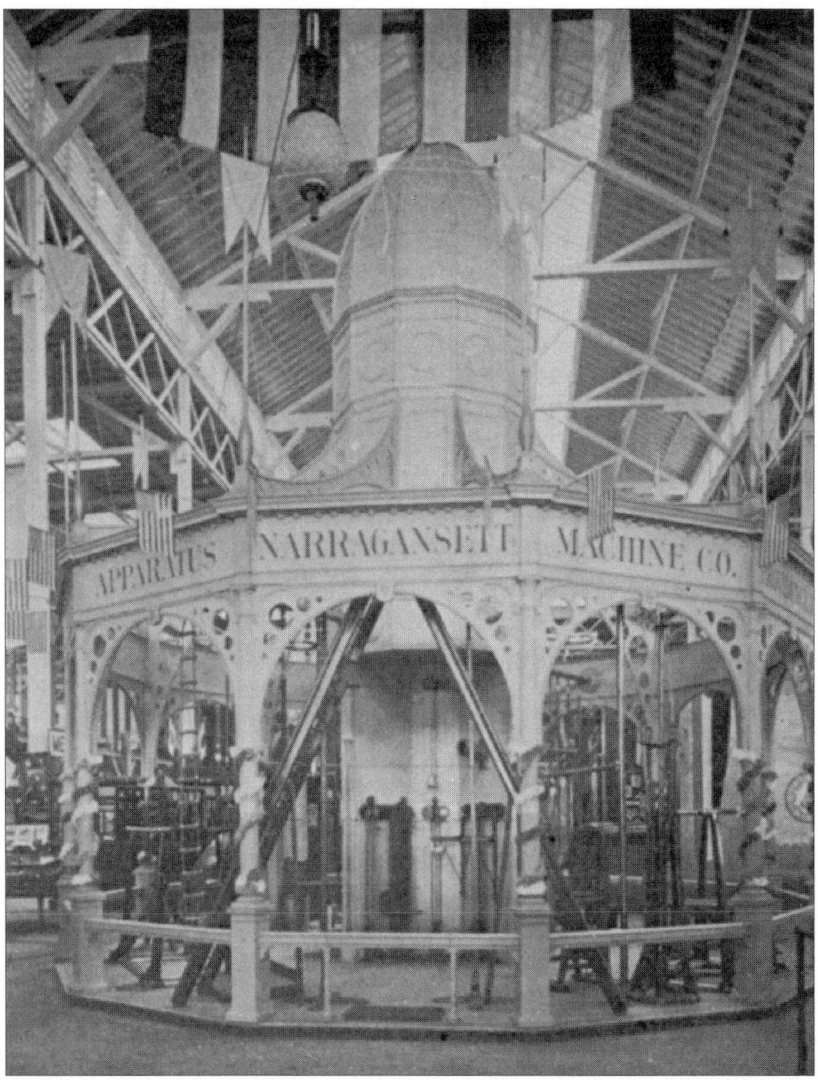

Fig. 8. Sargent's apparatuses as displayed by their manufacturer, the Narragansett Machine Company. Hubert Howe Bancroft, *The Book of the Fair; an Historical and Descriptive Presentation of the World's Science, Art, and Industry, as Viewed through the Columbian Exposition at Chicago in 1893,* vol. 6 (Chicago: Bancroft Company, 1893), 637.

the lowest 5 percent of strength when dynamometered. It was a weakness, he observed, that would not be readily detected without the use of machines.[85] This connection between machines, strength, and class would not end with Sargent; in the 1910s it was reinforced by Gustav Zander in American health spas.

Gustav Zander and Spas: Trotting Toward Modern Energy

Visitors to the 1876 Centennial Exhibition in Philadelphia had ample opportunity to observe mechanical progress. The Corliss Engine commanded the center of Machinery Hall, presiding over the spin and hum of the machinery while providing fairgoers with an imposing central power source for the surrounding commotion. Much has been written about the Corliss; it is often said to have elicited the same awe that would later inspire Henry Adams to write about the virgin and the dynamo.[86]

The Corliss and its mechanical entourage were not the only impressive machines at the fair. Several buildings away Sweden's exhibit displayed a miniaturized version of Stockholm's Zander's Therapeutical Institute. Twelve of the institute's fifty machines sat arranged around a central motor, offering a Machinery Hall in miniature for visitors to test. Their appearance was probably striking; ominous dark hues and imposing gadgetry strangely contrasted with a nearby exhibit of a Laplander carting animal skins in a hand-made sled.[87] Those who stopped to talk with the institute's director, Dr. Gustav Zander, or to browse the brochures, learned that the machines were designed to improve upon previous gymnastics methods. As Zander's fair brochure explained, it was important to deliver to the body a precise amount of muscular resistance; "too much would cause a strain, too little would be useless." His machines, powered by electricity or steam, regulated each user motion, thereby eliminating variation. Such precision and regularity led to "a slow and gradual increase in the use of muscular power."[88] Visitors probably gave added weight to his theories because Zander was reported to have nine hundred patients under his care at several European institutes.[89] At the very least, the exhibition judges were impressed, awarding Zander a gold medal for his machines, a feat he repeated that same year in Brussels and two years later in Paris.

Americans first heard of Zander's work at the Centennial Exhibition, but he had been developing machines and theories of physical training over the previous decade. In many ways his life bears striking similarities to Sargent's. Like Sargent, Zander invented his first machines to train himself as a gymnast. And like Sargent, he had a medical degree, having enrolled in medical school only to better pursue his interest in health machines. Shortly after graduation, Zander opened his Stockholm institute, outfitted it with machines he had invented and offered a program of regimented physical exercise.[90] Zander enjoyed enormous popularity; by 1906, he had established institutes in 146 cities in Europe and South America.[91]

Designed primarily to rehabilitate the sick, Zander's machine-based system received a boost from Germany's Act for Insurance against Accidents. The 1884 statute made it state policy to rehabilitate and return injured workers to their jobs as quickly as possible. This affected the lives of fourteen million workers within the empire's one hundred trade associations. Patient records at Zander's institute in Utrecht reveal the statute's role in Zander's European success. The majority of care in 1897 was paid for by the state; patients arrived through doctor referrals, the local military hospital, the Dutch railway's Health and Support Fund, and the state insurance group.[92] State support for Zander treatments extended to children as well, with the Society for the Free Treatment of Children of Insolvent and Poor Families in Utrecht covering forty-five children's Zander treatment for an hour each week.[93]

Zander's legacy has not received the attention in the United States that it has in Europe. It is, in fact, easy to assume that he had little impact in this country. Sources as late as 1904 declared his machines of little interest.[94] Combined with reports from European historians that his institutes began to close in 1910 and were almost entirely obsolete by the 1930s, there appears to be little chance that they could have enjoyed American popularity.[95] Yet Zander's European demise actually marked his American ascension. The earliest record of Zander machines in this country dates to 1906, when Zander institutes were opened in Baltimore, Chicago, Boston, New York, San Francisco, St. Louis, and Wauwatosa, Wisconsin.[96] There are no records known to have survived from these institutes, but their proximity to major urban centers suggests that ample numbers of Americans were familiar with the machines by 1910. Health studios also purchased the machines; a floor plan of Dr. Savage's New York Health Studio shows devices in the "mechanical room," including developers similar to Sargent's and a Zander "horseback machine" (fig. 9).[97] Americans also saw Zanders outside the studio: reports indicate that

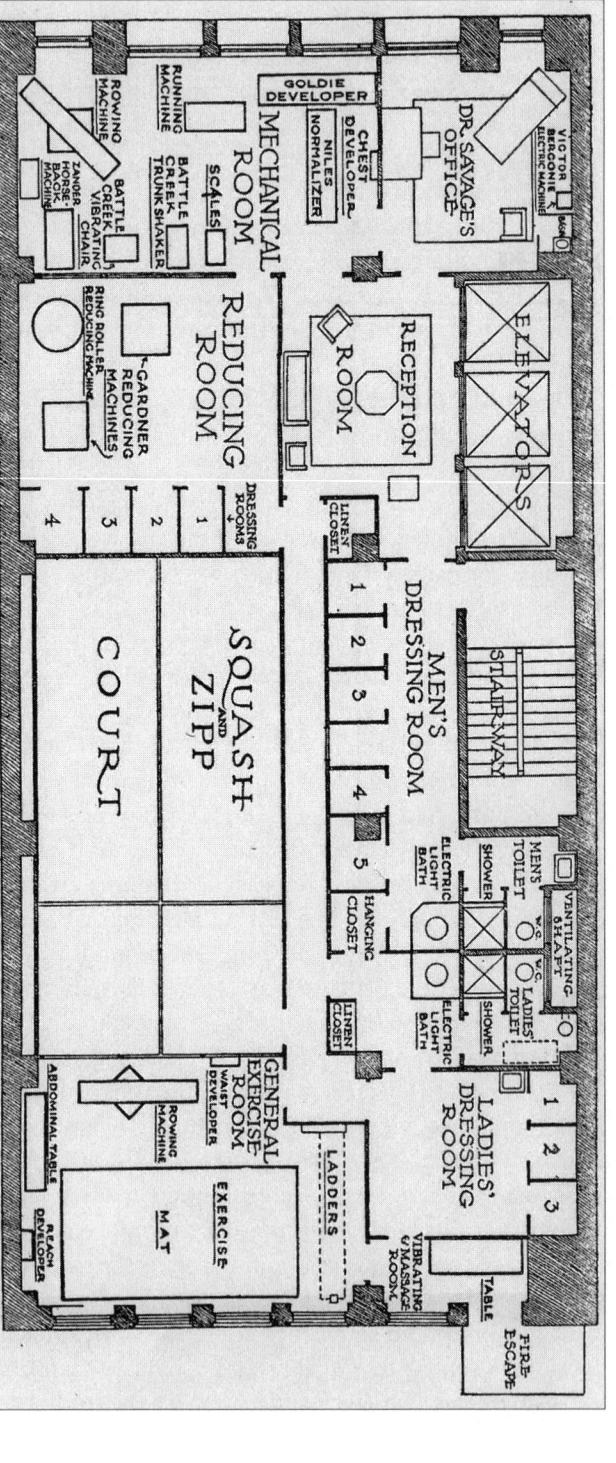

Fig. 9. Dr. Savage's health studio featured a Zander "horse-back machine" in the mechanical room next to two machines from John Harvey Kellogg and what was probably a Sargent rower (see lower-left corner of floor plan). "The Dr. Savage Health Studio," undated brochure, Warshaw Collection of Business Americana, Physical Culture Files. Courtesy of the National Museum of American History, Smithsonian Institution.

74

individuals in New York and Philadelphia purchased machines for their private use from the European distributor Rossel, Schwartz & Company in Wiesbaden.

Zander's home machines would have been expensive, far beyond a working-class budget. Yet working people, specifically those of the white-collar class, made up the majority of Zander machine users, thanks to the numerous spas in the early twentieth century that installed Zander machines. The Greenbriar Hotel in West Virginia, the Homestead Resort in Virginia, and the Fordyce Bathhouse in Arkansas each installed full Zander rooms between 1913 and 1915. As to their reasons for purchasing Zander machines, we can only speculate, but the 1914 agreement allowing the Kny-Scheerer Company of New York to produce and market Zander machines in the United States probably played a role.[98] According to attendance and therapy records, American health spas exposed more than 80,000 visitors to Zander machines each year between 1913 and 1925.[99] When compared with the 185 individuals who used the Rotterdam Zander Institute each year in the late nineteenth century, it is clear that Zander machines had at least as much of an impact on Americans as they did on Europeans.[100]

The Homestead resort in Hot Springs, Virginia, provides clues as to why spa owners acquired Zander machines and how customers used them. First established in 1766, the Homestead was one of many late-nineteenth-century spas to attract visitors looking for restorative vacations. Although its mineral baths had been praised for their medicinal properties in the early 1800s, by the 1890s the Homestead's offerings were more social than medicinal.[101] It was a place where members of the middle and upper classes could come for mineral baths, healthy meals, and, above all, the opportunity to meet influential members of the eastern business class. At the Homestead, Americans who could not afford to attend elite institutions such as Harvard or Bowdoin could still be exposed to mechanical training similar to Sargent's.

In 1902, the Homestead's owners rebuilt much of the hotel, seeking to keep pace with resorts in other parts of the country.[102] It is unclear how the Homestead learned of Zander's machines, but in 1911 Dr. Kurt Linnert traveled to the resort from Vienna, Austria, to install thirty-six Zander devices and train attendants in their use. The Homestead's Zander room represented a tremendous investment: at $50,000, the machines cost nearly half of what other spa owners had spent rebuilding their entire facilities.[103]

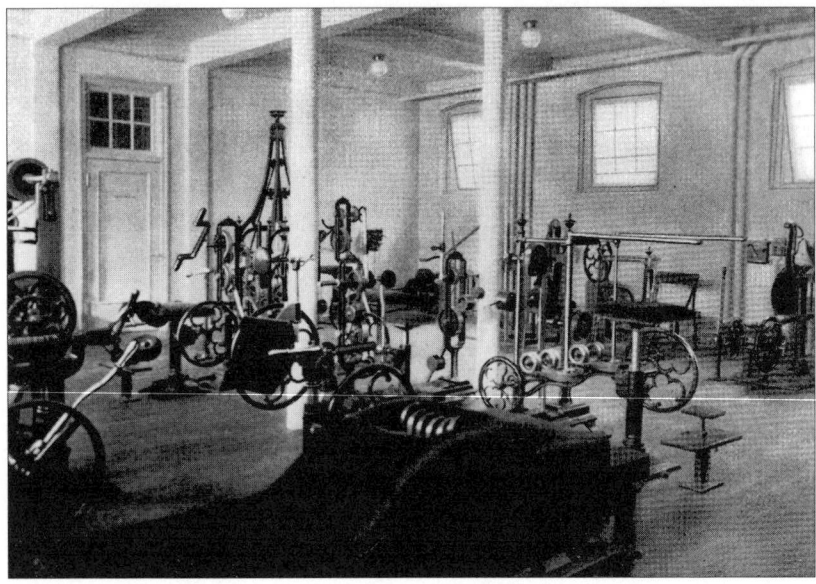

Fig. 10. The Zander Room at the Greenbrier Resort. George D. Kahlo, "A European Cure in America, White Sulphur Springs: Climate' Waters' Baths' and Other Curative Resources" (March 1915, reprint May 1916), 22.

The Homestead hoped that these machines would attract people and create revenue. To this end, between 1913 and 1920, its promotional booklet printed a feature on the benefits of Zander therapy.[104] Conceivably, many of the estimated 62,000 resortgoers each year used the Zanders; usage was free of charge to any who paid for the basic spa treatment. The location of the machines, on the top floor, may have reminded visitors of their presence; they were visible from the verandah, one of the resort's prime sightseeing spots. In any event, the Zanders would have been memorable and probably worth seeking out, so startling were they in design and presentation. All frames were of cast iron, and each pulley, pivot, and lever was steel or brass. Although the image shown here (fig. 10) is of the Greenbrier's Zander room, that room was similar in size and arrangement to the Homestead's. Packed into a space smaller than the 3,000 square feet that Zander deemed the minimum for an institute, the machines appear to be a jungle gym of metal and motors.[105] Trained attendants worked the room, preventing injury and providing a guide to machine use.

At the Homestead, as at most spas where they were offered, the Zander machines included active and passive devices. Among its active machines was the hip-knee flexion (fig. 11), which exercised the pelvis, spinal column, hip, and upper thigh. A precursor to the StairMaster, the machine provided resistance to the familiar motion of climbing a staircase.[106] The lever on the far side of the machine could be adjusted to increase or decrease resistance. Zander considered the lever principle central to the machine's curative abilities because it provided the benefit of

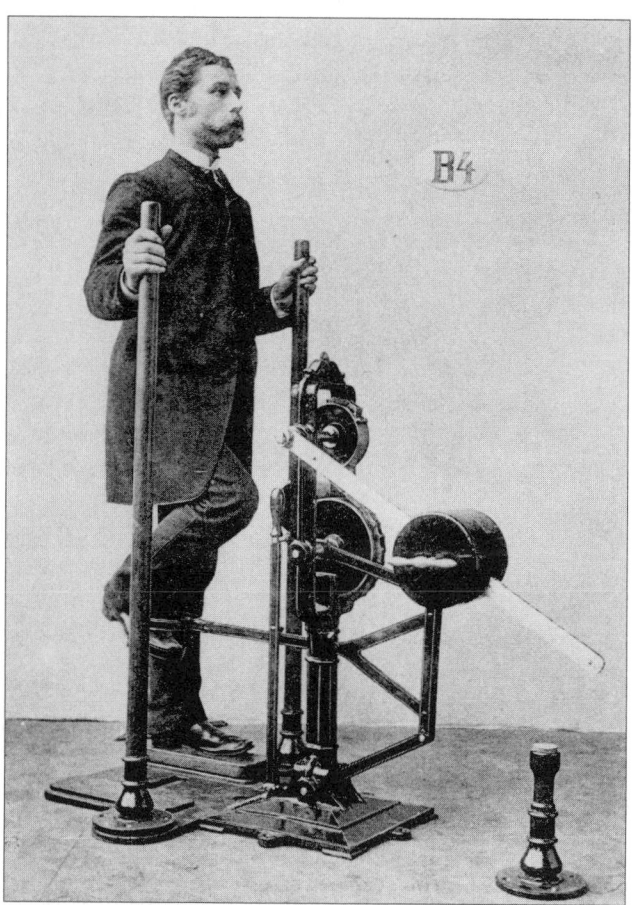

Fig. 11. Zander's knee-flexing machine. A. Levertin, *Dr. G. Zander's Medico-Mechanische Gymnastik* (Stockholm: P. A. Norstedt, 1892).

circular force. Muscles encountered the least resistance when they began the motion. As they pushed down, the lever reached a more horizontal position and more strength was required. This varying exertion rate, Zander argued, allowed muscles to develop evenly without undue exertion at the start of an exercise.[107]

The Zander machines for vibration and percussion were the resort's most mechanized offerings. Each machine required a connection to an outside power source such as a steam engine, a gas engine, or a four-horse-power electric motor.[108] The user would hear the machines humming and often, as with the device for leg percussion, see the belt running from the machine to an electric engine located at the center of the room. The machines asked little from the user, who could sit or stand and enjoy the purported health benefits of vibratory motion. The chest expansion machine, for example, had a comfortable chair from which the user could raise and lower its metal arm holders, pushing the chest up and down to the machine's cadence. Together, the active and passive Zanders formed a central part of physical treatments in resorts like the Homestead; thanks to attendants' training in Zander methods, each user learned that receiving the full benefit required using Zander machines two or three times a day.[109]

Zander Case Studies: Mechanizing the Business Body

Massage had been a treatment at American resorts since their inception in the mid-nineteenth century. John Harvey Kellogg, director of the Battle Creek Sanitarium, asserted that he had treated "thousands of cases" with hand massage by 1906.[110] For Kellogg, massage was the key to maintaining good health. He prescribed it in particular for patients suffering from exhaustion, arguing that massage could actually infuse the body with increased energy. "Mental fatigue is relieved through massage, through its effect upon the circulation and the eliminative organs," he stated. In an explanation that conjured up mesmerist practices, Kellogg declared that massaging the body with one's hands or with a percussive machine actually carried "toxic substances produced by mental activity" out of the body and sped up the flow of blood, leaving "wearied nerve tissues" repaired and cleansed.[111] He connected his massage theories to the more-well-known rhetoric of muscle building. Massage, administered correctly, provided the body with more energy than did exercise. In Kellogg's mind, by exercising muscle without exhausting it, as weight training was prone to do, "massage produces an actual increase in the size of the muscular structures."[112]

In spite of manual massage's popularity at Battle Creek, Kellogg replaced it with Zander-like machines in the early 1900s.[113] His analysis of these machines hints at how users would have experienced Zander vibratory machines at health spas. Machines, Kellogg reasoned, were more efficient than hands at producing energy. They could move at a more rapid pace for a longer period than could even the strongest human masseur. At fifteen oscillations a second, Zanders outpaced even a resort's John Henry, the nineteenth-century legend who died trying to defeat his machine competitor. Kellogg and other spa owners promoted this theory of superior mechanized massage in their literature. If users did not grasp the concept by reading, they had another opportunity when they encountered the machines. For example, a user stood directly against the machine called "vibration of the heart," embracing a round metal pad, and looking forward as it applied rhythmic punches to the chest. Another person could use the machine simultaneously by resting his feet against the machine's leather bench. The apparatus, advertised in one promotional brochure as "working accurately, never wearying and never deficient," continued unfatigued in its motions, reportedly pushing out toxins and increasing mental capacity.[114]

Supplanting the nineteenth-century mesmerist practice of improving one's energy through a laying-on of hands, Zanders transferred users' allegiances from human bodies to machines.[115] Numerous reports of patients' experiences emphasized their increased relaxation at the hands of the machine. "Patients after one trial have no fear that the machine may go beyond the fixed limit in making the movement, and feel in consequence an assurance that they do not have in the hands of a masseur," commented a popular writer on health and disease.[116] Patients enjoyed a better treatment, sources explained, because they could stop anticipating the "well-meant but sudden and painful increase in the range of movement" experienced in many manual massages.[117]

By installing Zander machines, resorts like Kellogg's taught patients that machine power was both superior in its prophylactic effects and gentler than human touch; just as Butler Health Lift users had rejected Dio Lewis's partner exercises, patients progressively moved toward machines and away from human contact. A striking example of this comes from Kellogg's own description of his mechanotherapy room. Machines filled the room in the basement, each of which offered a different percussive effect: kneading, shaking, vibrating, or rubbing. As users stood beside their machines, they could see the centrally placed electric motor that powered all appliances. The "therapist sat elevated in a chair watching the proceedings from a far corner," now more machinist than masseur.[118]

Nature's Energy under Man's Control: Zanders in the Spa Context

Zander users may have observed machines replacing men, but they did not see them replacing nature. On the contrary, the environment surrounding Zander machines stressed the interconnectivity of nature, machine, and physical energy. The interior décor at most resorts, such as that of the Fordyce in Hot Springs, Arkansas, was saturated with natural symbols. Fountains, mosaics, statues, and exhibits featuring Native American bathers provided a natural context. Further, the remote location of most spas strengthened the connection between the treatments within and natural world outside.[119] In an apparent contradiction, machines themselves reinforced this connection to the natural world. Similar to their "improvements" in human touch, by replicating natural motions, Zander reminded users that machine technology did nature's work, only better.

Zander's "trotting motion" machine was one of his most popular (fig. 12). Offered at the Greenbrier, the Fordyce, the Homestead, and several New York City health clubs, the "horse," as it was usually called, appears intimidating at first glance. It stood as tall as most users and was accompanied by a driving motor almost as large as the machine itself. Users had to step on a box to reach the stirrups and lift themselves over the machine's metal body to mount. From a user's perspective, however, the horse was less mechanistic than one might assume. The machine displayed detailed craftsmanship; the soft leather saddle was etched in gold, with intricate patterns running from the base of the seat to the top handle. According to one source, it revealed "the spirit of the age" in its embossed scroll, rosette, and urn patterns.[120] Made of expensive materials, it was packed with layers of straw to ensure a soft seat.[121] Even the board on which the machine was mounted was oil finished to give it a shiny veneer. The costly embellishments suggest that the trotter was designed as more than an efficient machine; it was meant to evoke associations with quality tack and fine furnishings.

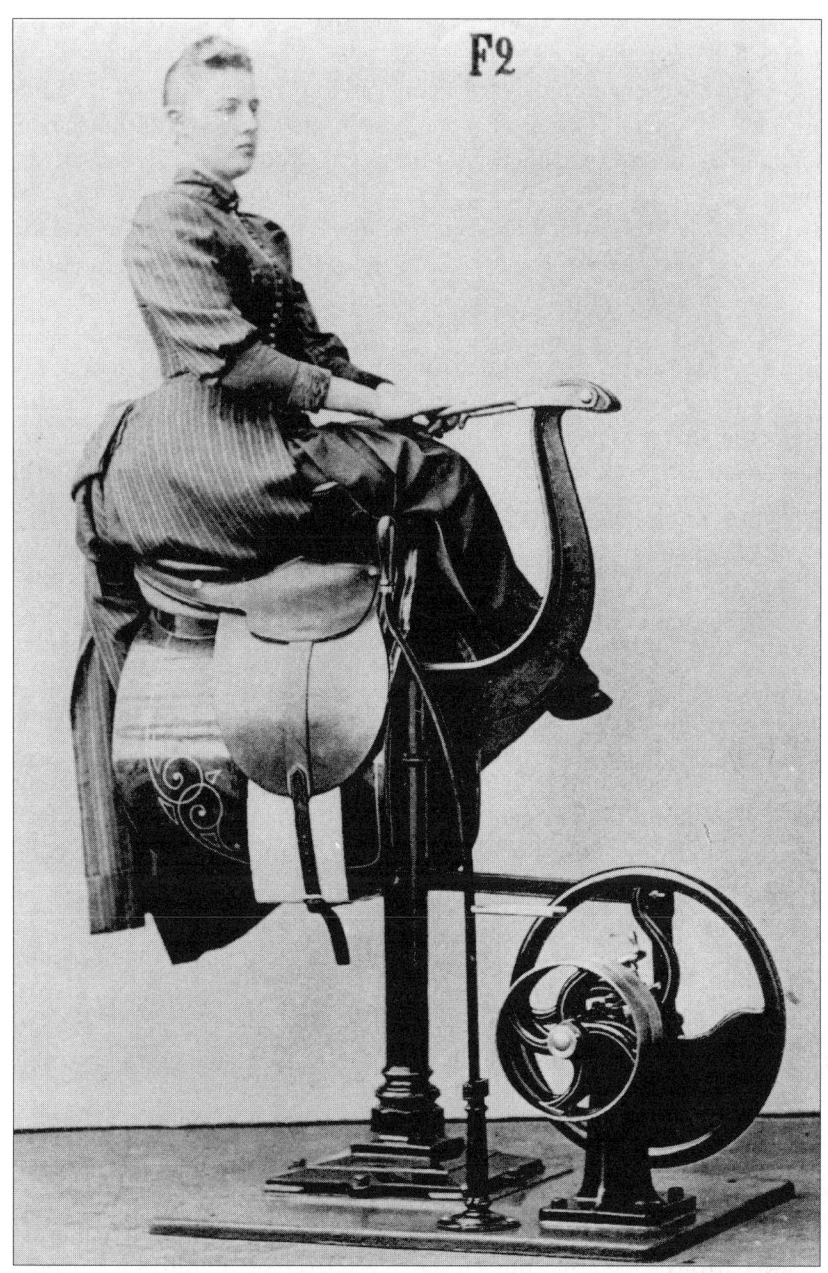

Fig. 12. Zander's mechanical horse. A. Levertin, *Dr. G. Zander's Medico-Mechanische Gymnastik* (Stockholm: P. A. Norstedt, 1892).

Users experienced a fusion of mechanized process and natural sensation when using the trotter. The "horse" was unmistakably a machine. Its large drive wheel and pulley belts connected to an exterior power source evoking industrial imagery. Especially to users familiar with horsemanship, mounting the machine would have evoked contradictory sensations: one rode a horseless saddle and traveled without getting anywhere. Yet the trotter actively attempted to mimic a real horse in sensation and appearance. Designed to stimulate "the vegative nervous system, in particular the intestinal function," it subjected the user to the up-and-down motions of a trot in the country during a two- or three-minute treatment.[122] Like a horse, the trotter could be prodded into faster action simply by using a rod, here by adjusting a lever at the machine's base rather than applying the crop to its hind quarters. One observer called the Zander machine a "mechanical horse" with the ability to "rock, trot, pace or canter."[123] The leather reins of the machine connected to a curving iron stern that resembled an animal's neck and head. The curve was not a functional requirement of the machine; the reins could have been attached in a more straightforward fashion. Although the Zander appears more ostrich than horse, the anthropomorphizing may have reminded users of riding in the outdoors. Though few would have recognized it as such, the machine achieved Butler's model of a perfect body-machine relationship: to be as "horse and rider."

Zander designed his trotter and many other active machines to mimic natural motions. Like Sargent, he believed that many daily activities produced muscle, but unless undertaken together, they did not create complete physical health. Zander's machines took the best of each world, replicating the natural motion and doing so with machine efficiency. The trotter did not grow tired; it did not spook on the trail; it did not require food. One account, which seemed to overlook the trotter's external power supply, said that using the machine was like entering a magical world: "All you need to do is sit down on this saddle and the invisible steed gallops away with you."[124]

It is significant that trotters were most popular in rural resort settings. Spa brochures instructed visitors on the importance of taking long walks in nature to augment their massage and bathing routines. In spite of what must have been ample opportunity for outdoor activity and actual horse rides, patrons sought out these mechanized trotters. If visitors were looking for psychological along with physical relaxation, the combination makes sense. By taking the machine treatment and the "natural" water and outdoor treatments together, resort visitors could affirm that machines need not replace natural exercise; they could improve upon it.[125] Machines were not to be feared when placed alongside Mother Nature, in a clear continuum of care. Like a Trojan horse delivering modernity to the unsuspecting, the Zander lay tethered in the Fordyce, fully domesticated for human use.[126]

The Mental Benefits of Zander Therapy

Zander machines affected more than users' bodies. Their intricate weights, gears, and belts engaged minds. Arguably, putting one's body in the midst of an unmistakably mechanized process offered mental benefits to a class of individuals whose sense of physical well-being had diminished in the age of the machine. Few records exist from Zander users. Those that do, however, suggest that these machines produced an attendant "mental effect." Men who put their bodies in contact with Zanders placed "dangerous" and "foreign" machines in a productive, familiar context. This intimate experience may have provided physical proof that a world of machines could simultaneously produce healthy economies and healthy men.

By 1915, men made up the majority of clients in America's resort spas. Whereas early water therapies, stemming from Vincenz Priessnitz's cold water cure, had attracted reform-minded women, modern bathhouses attracted men seeking rest and relaxation away from the working world. An article written in 1913 to debunk the curative effects of twentieth-century bathing recognized the new male clientele, suggesting that primarily "tired business men" sought spa cures to make up for "over-dissipating" throughout the year.[127] This change in patronage manifested itself in the design of facilities. The Fordyce maintained twenty-one tubs in the men's facility, seven in the women's; men bathed in a grand hall with an ornate centerpiece, women in a hall small and simply decorated.[128] Women still frequented the resorts, but the target patrons had become men from the growing white-collar class.[129]

By 1915, the Homestead, like most spas, had become a gathering place for the aspiring office worker as well as the distinguished businessman. With hotel rates as low as six dollars a week and rooming houses in which, one physician reported, "one can live as cheaply as any city in America," even the average office clerk could take the occasional Homestead vacation.[130] At the same time, John D. Rockefeller, Andrew Mellon, and Henry Ford were reportedly frequent guests. By 1920, so much business was transacted at the Homestead that a broker's office was opened, its chairs filled to capacity early each morning. One proprietor reported that in April and October, so many of the brokers and their wives had taken up Homestead residence it seemed as if the New York Stock Exchange would have to close.[131]

That Zander machines arrived just as businessmen were becoming these resorts' primary patrons was not a coincidence. Promotional materials suggest that the machines were actively marketed in the United States to relieve the stresses of business life. One promoter declared that Zander machines returned the body to its natural physical development by struggling "successfully against overexcitement of the nerves," which accompanied "a present school-education with its great demands."[132] Others made their intended users more explicit. Zander himself asserted that his machines should be used in the United States to augment office life. Speaking specifically to the new business class, Zander referred to his machines as "a preventative against the evils engendered by a sedentary life and the seclusion of the office."[133] Fifteen years later, he made the connection even stronger: although men might prefer the convenience of pills to treat ill health, "the increased well being and capacity for work" from his machines offered "rich compensation for the time bestowed on them. For a man of business, that health is money may be as great a truth as that time is money."[134]

Using the Zander machines may have afforded businessmen more than money; it also may have offered a chance to defuse fears of industrialization through their own bodies. Like Sargent's students, men who used Zander machines were taught that the graduated movement of machines offered the best means to increase muscular energy. Yet whereas Sargent's system had relied on simple pulleys and weights, Zander's placed the user in the heart of a machine's intense power. The abdominal massage machine, standard equipment in both the Fordyce bathhouse and at the Homestead, placed users directly in the path of the engine's pummeling force (fig. 13). To operate, the user stood between two vertical iron pipes. One supported an engine-driven wheel, and the other, a back support. When adjusted, the support pushed the user's stomach up against a pair of fist-sized rollers. A lever extended from the wheel at groin level. When

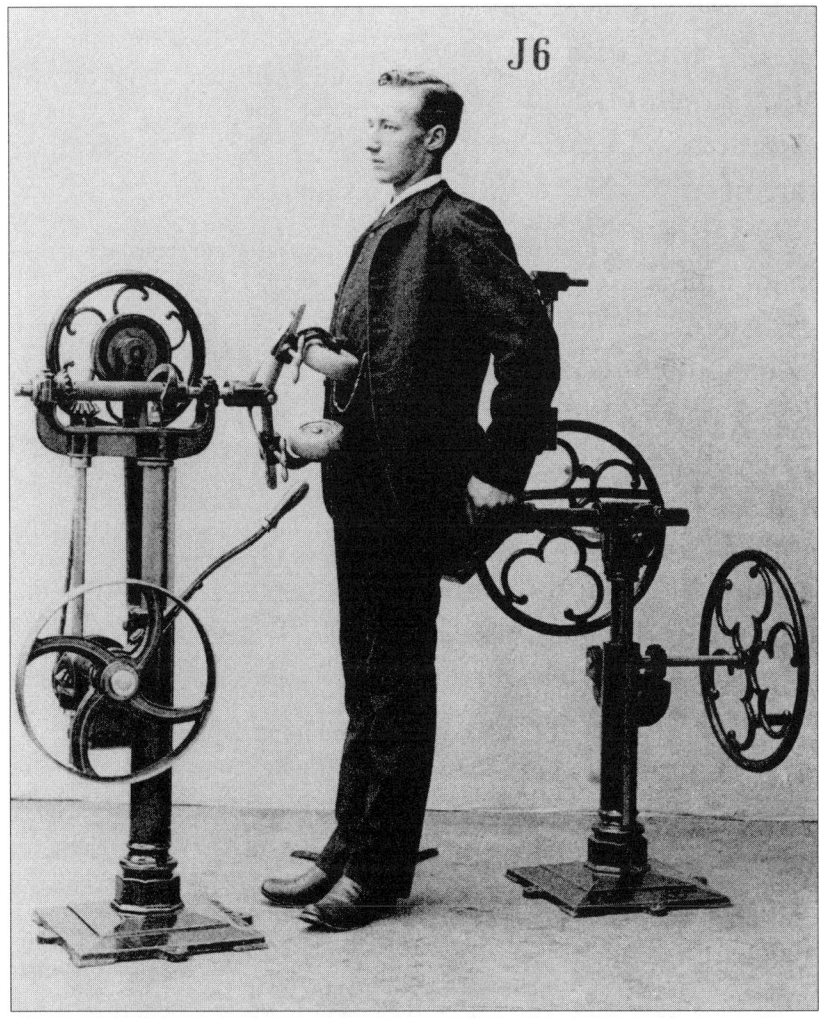

Fig. 13. Zander's machine for passive abdominal conditioning. A. Levertin, *Dr. G. Zander's Medico-Mechanische Gymnastik* (Stockholm: P. A. Norstedt, 1892).

engaged, it unleashed two fists in a rotating and thrusting motion, turning the patient into a human punching bag. Brochures explained by striking the stomach in a repetitive fashion, "sunken vital energy is raised by strengthening the abdominal muscles."[135]

Testimonies from patients at Zander's European institutes provide a sense of what this experience was like for American patients. Many patients could vividly recall years afterward the intense sensations they felt during treatments and the way the sensation connected them to a mechanized system. One remembered sitting at a machine that bent and straightened his injured knee:

> I was intrigued to trace back the origins of the pain in muscles and joints via an almost infinite sequence of counter-weights, truss beams, gear wheels and transmission belts to the mighty, lonely axis, which slowly revolved in the shadowy heights. That was the law of laws, the ever resting, well-oiled pivot of all, the origin of all grunting and groaning.[136]

The Zander therapy described here affected the user's body at a physical and an emotional level. The engine assumes an almost primal significance, a force whose agents exacted its unyielding power upon its captive users. Another man's account of a childhood Zander treatment echoes this interpretation of the machine as an outside force acting upon the body: "In synchronicity with the movements of my shoulders, my back was fiercely pushed forwards by a wheel, which rolled up and down. . . . [I]t was impossible to invent a comparison for this complicated and dual action."[137] At first glance, this account diminishes the power of users by making them, literally, "cogs in the wheel." To be a cog, however, is to be part of the machine itself. In fact, both of these accounts suggest that the user is not a victim, but rather a product, or beneficiary, of the machine.

In a time characterized as an "era of gears and girders," the opportunity to merge with mechanical energy so as to emerge with increased physical energy may have been important mental therapy.[138] For many spa and resort patrons, the pace of mechanized life was unsettling. White-collar workers sought refuge from the business world where they themselves increasingly functioned like well-oiled machines.[139] Although they could have been treated just as effectively with manual therapy, such as slow massage or stationary weight lifting, these individuals increasingly sought Zander therapy instead. Absent a physical explanation of why the machines were conducive to well-being in these situations, promoters began to advertise the special mental benefits of the Zander approach. One brochure suggested that patients who were treatable with more traditional methods should use Zander machines to augment regular therapy because of "the mental effect produced by the huge and complicated machines," which it termed "a valuable adjunct."[140]

The "mental effect," it could be argued, was a side effect of repositioning the body with respect to the machine. If one imagined oneself to be a mere cog in the wheel, be it a literal wheel of a factory or a figurative wheel of a machine-like office environment, then one spent days expending energy on external products. Zander therapy reversed this process, placing the body itself on the assembly line as product. The switch rendered machines the agents to welcome rather than fear; the more powerful and complex the mechanism, the better the "effect."

As a user sat in a machine, he listened to the whir of gears and belts; he watched the central engine drive the motion of a room full of machines; and he felt the energy act upon his body. The tables were turned on technology: the result was not physical diminishment but physical expansion. For men of the rising middle class, Zander treatments offered a chance to turn the precision of modern systems, feared as the cause of ill health since George Beard, into a source of vitality. After undergoing a day of rejuvenating manipulations, many may have believed that instead of draining their energy to produce products, the modern age might instead harness energy to produce men.[141]

Historian John Kasson provides evidence that suggests that the resorts' Zander machines would not have been the first to produce this valuable "mental effect." His study of Coney Island shows that entertainment places have frequently served the twofold task of physically releasing individuals from workplace stress while redefining that source of stress as a means for pleasure. While Kasson is looking at the working class, it is possible to connect the cultural function of Coney Island to that of health spas. In rides that mimicked taking an elevated train or tumbling down coal mines, amusement parks turned Americans' real-life fears into anxiety-decreasing entertainment.[142] In like fashion, Zander users could escape the pressures of an increasingly efficient and physically taxing working world by engaging in an explicitly mechanized world of relaxation. Examined in this light, the Zanders' ability to "renew" their business-class patrons extends beyond their energy-enhancing properties. They rejuvenated both body and mind by uniting physical efficiency and mechanized order.

When considered together, the machines systematized by Dudley Allen Sargent and Gustav Zander helped acclimate members of the middle and upper classes to the new pace of modern life. By pitching their products to men and making efficient muscle the offspring of machine training, these inventors encouraged those of the rising business class to look to machines for the energy modern life demanded. Further, by arguing that their machines offered the benefits of nature intelligently applied, they inserted mechanized processes into the natural order. Their most far-reaching effect, however, may be in a subtle redefinition of masculinity. In an age when the majority of American men neither attended college nor traveled to distant resorts, defining the energized body as one specifically trained by machines made "real manhood" the prerogative of the middle and upper classes. As historian Carroll Pursell has pointed out, the scientific elite have often used technological knowledge to protect their privileged status; in this case it was machine designers whose systems allowed only those with access to be deemed sufficiently "energetic."[143]

Both Sargent and Zander argued that full physical development required machinery based upon scientific principles. Each would have heard his own philosophy echoed in an advertisement for Eugen Sandow's developer: "Every man who has not gone through such a course, no matter how healthy or strong he may be by nature, is still an undeveloped man."[144] Men who walked away after Zander's trots and Sargent's pulls could rest assured that though they might not ever outbox, outlift, or even outride the average working man, their bodies alone possessed machine power for the modern age.

3

Exploring Electric Limits

In 1887, the *Electric Review* reported to an emerging professional class of American electricians that something new was powering the bodies of the nation's congressmen. Those who found themselves lethargic after "receptions and suppers all night" or who had "exhausted their brain power by speechmaking," were retiring to the basement to be "filled quietly with electricity." Someone had rigged a primitive electrical device in the capitol's engine room that allowed lawmakers a direct, invigorating connection to the power behind the building's lights, heat, and machines. A serial electric jolt was transferred to any who held the wire that emerged from below the engine wheel belt. By merely grasping a "small brass chain attached to the railing around the engine's wheel," one completed the electric circuit. The sensation, which would last as long as one held the wire and grasped the chain, would have felt like a rapid succession of tiny pinpricks through the hand and up the arm.[1]

This congressional invigoration reflected the late-nineteenth-century vogue of electric-energy devices. Unlike health machines in design and function, these devices were typically simple, more portable, and less expensive. As such, they were more accessible to the general population. One needed little more than a wire, a source of electric current, and a physical leap of faith to take part in a technological treatment. Even manufactured devices were inexpensive enough to be purchased by working-class consumers.

Electric devices differed as well in their reported impact on the body. Whereas health machines had claimed to harness "force" to unblock internal energy and free it for productive use, the devices promised to transfer energy directly from device to body, actually increasing the total energy within the body itself. With the help of electric technology, lawmakers and laborers alike could avoid strenuous, time-consuming exercises with machines. A trip to the basement, a grab of a wire, or a quick cinching of a belt made it possible to take in electricity faster than one could eat a meal. Electricity's seeming ability to infuse the body with additional power quickly and efficiently delivered, or so many believed, an actual deposit of physical strength.

Building the Body Electric

Long before the nineteenth century, electric experimentors sought ways to convert static force to physical power. The novelty of the devices and the actual physical effects they imparted certainly influenced the methodology of these early investigators. But the ultimate direction of experimentation was at least equally affected by many researchers' predispositions to connect electrical power to human force.

The Leyden jar, for example, illustrated a basic, though newly conceived, principle of static electricity. Developed in the 1740s, it was one of the first devices to capture and redirect electricity.[2] By transforming a familiar physical sensation into a regulated process, researchers were able to scientifically investigate the relationship between electricity and the human body. They, and hobbyists alike, almost immediately sought ways to apply this newfound technology to improve human health. In one application, a patient sat next to the Leyden jar while conducting instruments transferred a spark to a particular part of his body. Used to treat ailments such as muscle weakness, neuralgia, ulcers, and skin adhesions, the current would have been clearly felt by the user. Strong currents applied directly to the arms, legs, or torso emitted a spark and gave a palpable jolt. The fact that such contact could cause a great deal of pain if administered incorrectly attests to the powerful sensation imparted by treatments.[3]

As the technology was disseminated, researchers with their own agendas transformed and reapplied it. One was the Italian Luigi Galvani, known today as one of the fathers of electrical theory. In the 1870s, he was a physician and a professor of anatomy. Although the accounts differ, legend has it that Galvani stumbled across a correlation between nerve force and electricity while preparing a frog's leg for dissection. A metal scalpel, it seems, conducted an electric current to the frog, making its leg muscle twitch. Convinced that he had found the source of animal vitality, Galvani began a series of experiments with muscles, nerves, and metals. Using Leyden jars and other electrostatic machines, he sought to prove that the vital force behind all animal power was electricity. This "Animal Electricity," he postulated, was a fluid that was transferred between the brain and the muscles via a network of nerves. The electricity produced by mechanical means was interpreted to be an artificial form similar to the naturally found "animal electricity," which explained why muscles contracted with electrostatic contact.[4]

Galvani's theories, though partially incorrect, provided the foundation for future research on electricity. The greatest academic challenge to them came from a contemporary physicist, Alessandro Volta, who correctly identified the source of muscle contraction in Galvani's experiments as an electrical reaction that occurs when two dissimilar metals come into contact. Galvani's frog challenged Volta to develop his theory further because the two metals never actually touched. Volta hypothesized that the muscle itself, or rather the liquid within the muscle, acted as a conductor between the two metals. As such, he continued, the muscle could actually store electricity. Galvani's frog leg, then, was the first electrical battery.[5]

Volta would develop this idea into an actual battery, called a Voltaic pile, which alternated copper and zinc in a saline solution. The invention, capable of delivering a constant electrical current, would be used by the next generation of electrical researchers and tinkerers in their physical-electric experiments. Dr. A. Paige, an electrotherapist practicing in Boston in the 1840s with both Leyden jar and galvanic batteries, described his work in terms Galvani would have well appreciated. He used electrotherapy primarily to open what he called the body's "avenue to electricity."[6] Paige's prescription for brain fever, a form of dementia first diagnosed by Hippocrates, suggests his conviction that electricity drove the body's functions: "The exercise of the mind induces electrical action in the brain," causing the brain to become "congested with blood, and heated by electrical action." A patient could be cured by a physician who regulated "the electrical forces of the body" by applying a positive current to the head and a negative current to another part; electric currents would thereby be carried away from the affected area, restoring the brain's electric balance. Using a slightly altered version of Galvani's theory, Paige concluded that only electricity gave patients "renewed power, more of the element of life."[7]

Paige was neither an amateur nor a charlatan. His degree in medicine, even in the pre-Flexner era, vouched for his familiarity with the workings of the nervous and cardiovascular systems.[8] Yet Paige, like many physicians in that time, used electricity and physiology, both nascent sciences, to explain each other. Few contemporary physicians understood the complexities of the human system; it was not until 1860, for example, that the role of the blood in fighting disease became known.[9] During this scientific infancy, the body electric emerged as a viable entity.

E. J. Fraser, a successful homeopathic physician and graduate of a Chicago medical school, pronounced in an 1863 text aimed at a lay audience that the human system could be "best understood if looked upon as a voltaic pile . . . the brain is the great central organ, and the positive pole of the organic battery. From it springs the whole nervous system. The nerves, after leaving the spinal column, are disseminated through the entire body. These termini constitute the negative pole of the battery."[10] Given Fraser's analogy, it is not surprising that he believed electricity was the only agent capable of regulating the body's internal force. A medical practitioner, he argued, knew that there were "electro-vital forces" in the body that could be "augmented or diminished at pleasure, by the application of artificial electricity."[11]

In their attempts to understand the human body, the nature of disease, and the properties of electric force, mid-nineteenth-century American physicians left much room for readers to conflate physical energy with electric power. Even as early as the pre–Civil War era, Americans had begun to extend electrotherapy's potential toward the supernatural. Fraser himself knew that among his readers, many were eager to believe that electric currents could fundamentally alter the human body. So accepted was this concept that Fraser issued a warning to those who asserted that they had been "charged with the battery." "[I]t must be remembered," he said, "that nothing is imparted to the system by a current of electricity. All that it can possibly do is to regulate the already existing forces and assist them to assume a healthy action."[12]

Mesmerism, Popular Culture, and the Electric Hand

It is probable that late-nineteenth-century Americans believed that electricity could augment the body before they knew of these medical debates. The claims were similar to those made by mesmerists a generation earlier. Introduced in Europe by Franz Mesmer in 1778 and brought to the United States by Charles Poyen in the 1830s, mesmerism, sometimes called magnetism, posited that disease was the result of internally obstructed "universal fluid," an infinitely fine material comparable to electricity.[13] Mesmer's cure for disease involved moving his hands in a circular pattern over patients' bodies or directly touching them to move internal electrical force. In the United States, where mesmerism's popularity was greater than in Europe, his method was often referred to as animal magnetism.[14] Practitioners used a grassroots approach to demonstrate its effectiveness: in town meetings throughout New England, mesmerists gave well-publicized demonstrations of healing practices.[15]

Mesmerism's popularity provided the underpinnings for how electrotherapy would be marketed and accepted in the mid-nineteenth century. Magnetism established, for believers, that the body was composed primarily of electrical fluid. In his 1845 text *Bagg on Magnetism*, J. H. Bagg described the body as "a galvanic battery, an electrizing machine, a great magnet."[16] Most practitioners, like Bagg, used electric and magnetic theories interchangeably, arguing that the body was made up of "magnetic fluids," which often manifested themselves through electric charges.[17] Brochures sensationalized such claims, often featuring large magnetic hands shooting out lightning bolts of electric fluids (fig. 14). Performances yielded more than memorable stories; audiences saw bodies transformed electrically before their eyes. One of Bagg's stories often told during performances concerned a "respectable" lady who became charged during a display of the northern lights in 1839; for months after, she was able to shoot sparks from her fingers, sending shocks from her body to those around her.[18]

In a similar way, magnetists claimed, their own hands could act as an electrical source to cure others. A patient's body, viewed as a container for electrical fluid, could be adjusted for optimum performance. The magnetizer's skill was judged by how well he or she could redirect a patient's energy. Bagg proudly tells of how he cured a young girl of "scaratina," a nervous weakness. Taking her wrists in his hands, he created a circuit with his own magnetic body, continuing to do so for two days as she fell into a "magnetic sleep" and eventually awoke restored. By using the "medium of the will," Bagg argued, he allowed his body's magnetic force to communicate with another's, leading to an improvement in a patient's mental and physical abilities.[19]

Mesmerism gained popularity across the country in the nineteenth century even though it was dismissed by regular physicians who considered it a useless elixir of performance and mysticism.[20] For individuals like Phineas Parkhurst Quimby, mesmerism was among the questionable

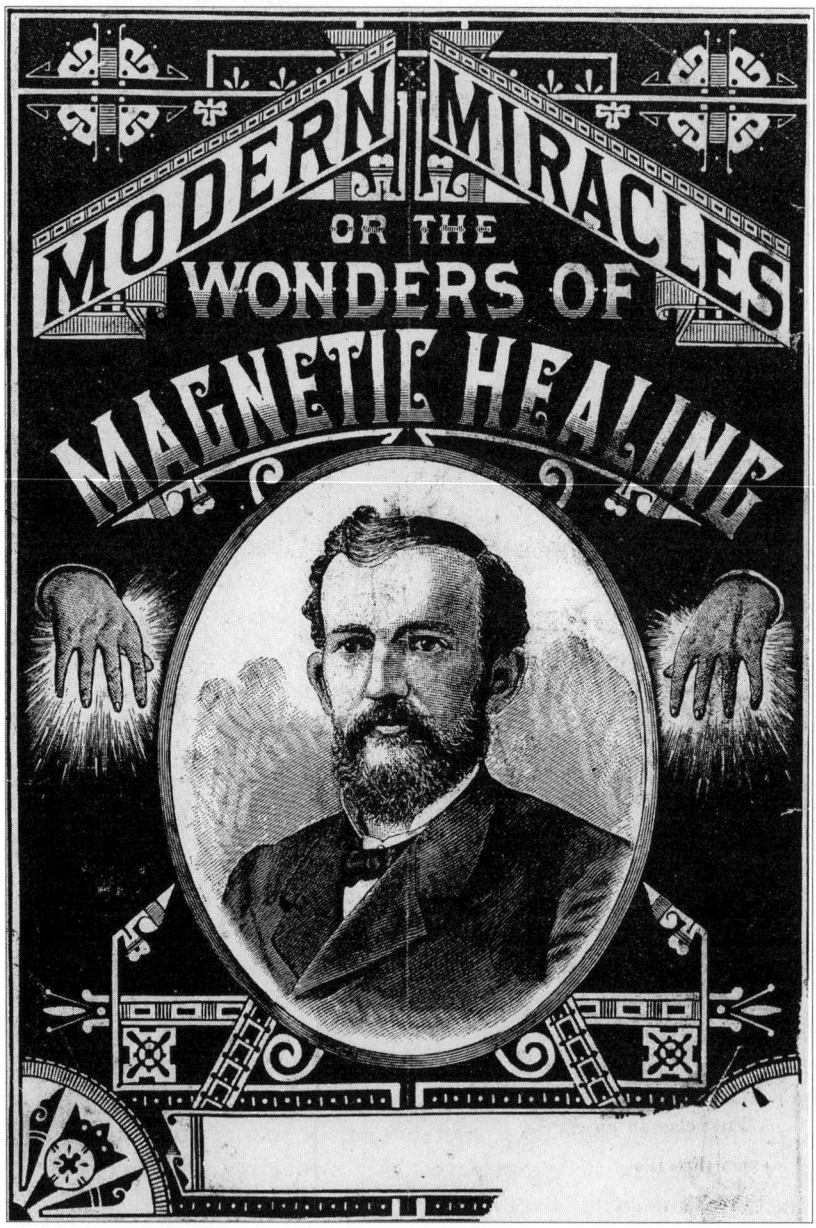

Fig. 14. "Modern Miracles or the Wonders of Magnetic Healing," miscella-
neous pamphlet cover, no author or date, Electricity, box 1, loose pamphlets,
Warshaw Collection of Business Americana, Archives Center. Courtesy of the
National Museum of American History, Smithsonian Institution.

practices that convinced him that a patient's belief in the efficacy of treatment was, in itself, an effective treatment. Quimby became one of the first proponents of the "mind cure" that Mary Baker Eddy would make famous. For individuals interested more in mesmerism's effect on the body than on the mind, the urge to increase energy found a home in electrotherapeutics, as the practice divided along the lines of legitimate and illegitimate electric treatments after the Civil War.[21]

By the 1870s, regular electric treatments had largely been standardized. Physicians used galvanic currents, which required only a galvanic power source, and faradic treatments, which utilized an "alternating" induction coil. In the 1880s, companies like Jerome Kidder manufactured battery systems specifically for physicians. Their price, roughly twenty-five dollars for a combined galvanic/faradic battery and from ten to eighteen dollars for a galvanic or faradic model, made the devices affordable to most physicians, and their compact design made them especially attractive to those who made house calls.[22] Static or Franklinic electricity, though used on occasion to stimulate a particular muscle with a visible shock, had mostly been abandoned. Physicians used easily controlled direct, or galvanic, currents to create localized muscle contractions, to stimulate digestion and evacuation, and to remove or reduce moles, ulcers, and tumors. The currents could be stimulants or sedatives, depending on whether one used the positive or negative electrode in contact with the affected part. Faradic currents issued a more powerful jolt to the body and were therefore given primarily as a nerve tonic or general stimulant. Electrotherapists used galvanism as their primary tool; one basic machine with attachments for internal treatments and a special battery for galvano-cautery used in internal surgery could constitute a physician's electric toolbox for less than one hundred dollars.[23]

Whether something fell into the category of "regular" or "irregular" electrotherapy had more to do with the credentials of the person administering the treatment than with the treatment's effectiveness. Electrical therapy did work in many instances, particularly in relieving pain, treating partial paralysis, and as an aid for cauterization in surgery. These, however, were only a few of the ailments that physicians "cured" with electrotherapy. By the 1880s, electrotherapy manuals held that physicians could cure everything from poor eyesight to sexual dysfunction with a small battery-powered device. We know now that electric currents were ineffective cures for the majority of these conditions. Pain might have been temporarily relieved or sensation restored for the duration of the treatment, but electricity could neither rebuild nerve endings nor restore damaged tissue.[24] Electrical professionals, however, were not constrained by the limits of their method's efficacy; by the turn of the century, it was common to find a plethora of urban and rural physicians offering electric treatments that went well beyond relieving pain and stopping blood flow.

The claims of licensed physicians were not markedly different from those made by "irregular" therapists.[25] For physicians struggling to make a name for themselves, particularly in crowded urban centers, proclaiming fantastic electrotherapy cures was good for business. This was especially true in an age when there was little to distinguish licensed and unlicensed practitioners, either in skill level or social prestige. Arguably, in order for licensed physicians to compete with self-identified "physicians," they had to offer what patients called for. Regrettably for them, once they opened the floodgates of electrotherapy enthusiasm, there was little they could do to ensure that the money would flow in their direction.

Regular physicians' attempts to compete with irregular electrotherapists were actually counterproductive. By offering the technique in their own practices, they legitimized portable electric health machines that could easily be purchased by unlicensed practitioners or by individuals for home use. Thanks to catalogue sales, anyone with mail service could purchase batteries similar, if not identical, to those used by regular practitioners. All that was required was a familiarity with electric principles and a desire to tinker.[26] In 1888, Professor W. R. Wells offered his battery for home use, complete with instructions on how to connect the wires, add sulphate of copper solution, and increase the machine's power if needed by changing from primary to secondary current production. Not only was the battery almost identical to those marketed to physicians by McIntosh and Jerome Kidder, one could even purchase a case of specialized instruments to use in treating the eye, throat, ear, rectum, and vagina.[27] The fact that few individuals understood electricity and therefore relied upon battery manufacturers for supplies and information left the field wide open. This was only furthered by the lax standards for medical licensing which allowed medical degrees to be bestowed by diploma mills after a six-month "correspondence course."[28] For those interested in electrical treatments, there was little reason to pay a physician's price.

Companies that sold batteries to the general public placed few limits on their products, either in packaging or promises. Consumers eagerly purchased the most "limitless" products. D. C. Moorhead's Graduated Magnetic Machine, first manufactured and sold in 1847 in New York

City, combined galvanic technology with mesmerist principles. Moorhead himself professed neither medical credentials nor extensive electrical knowledge; primarily a tinkerer, he borrowed from popular electric lore and emergent electric science. He associated his invention with those used by regular physicians, asserting that it was being used by American and European scientists and would "ultimately effect a complete revolution in the practice of medicine and surgery."[29] Who the physicians were and how the revolution would take place, he left to the reader's imagination.

By claiming the endorsement of unnamed physicians, Moorhead used a technique common to medical charlatans since early-nineteenth-century snake-oil vending. Yet Moorhead's product differed from previous elixirs. Unlike products composed primarily of water or stimulants like cocaine, the Magnetic Machine was essentially the same as the machines physicians purchased from medical supply catalogues. This would have been apparent to patients who tried both. The Magnetic Machine sent constant currents to the body; turning it on and gripping two metallic handles released a sensation that could be adjusted from weak to strong. The charge would have been similar to using a portable galvanic-faradic machine, though perhaps more localized to the hands. Moorhead included neither illustrations nor technical details of his machine's operation, perhaps preferring to rely upon readers' familiarity with medical batteries rather than promoting his machine as a departure. The Graduated Magnetic Machine profited from regular medical devices, thanks to the wide dispersal of electrical "knowledge" in American popular culture.

Moorhead sold his invention through the mail for twenty years, enjoying success even as electrotherapy professionalized and was more easily accessed. Given the choice, many Americans purchased the Graduated Magnetic Machine instead of medical batteries, owing, arguably, to the machine's "magnetic" component. Moorhead was not interested in exploring the science of his machine; he admitted outright that he would leave understanding how electricity worked to "future investigation." All that the buyer needed to know was that "it had been generally admitted by scientific persons that galvanism or magnetism is identical with vitality."[30]

Reflecting the teachings of mesmerists a decade before, Moorhead declared that disease was the result of imperfect vital force. As users placed their hands on the machine and felt the current become stronger, many were probably reminded of the mesmerist promise: internal electric force recharged for better health. The tingle they felt running from the metal handles into their fingers, wrists, and forearms perhaps conjured up the stock electric hands used in mesmerist advertisements. After a ten-minute session with the Magnetic Machine, users might feel themselves filled with the energy of regular and irregular science; here was a place where the physician's electricity and the mesmerist's magnetism could coexist.[31]

Moorhead's promise, aimed at a popular audience, reflected Americans' desires to see electricity as a cure-all, and their propensity to reward manufacturers who gave them products purported to do just that. By the late nineteenth century, those who willingly embraced the electrical fantastic were not necessarily acting outside the medical model of electrotherapy. The stream begun a generation earlier with theories of electric vital force emptied into a hearty river, as physicians increasingly described the body in electro-mechanical terms.

By 1871, Albert Steele, a doctor with an established New York practice, declared that his extensive research with electricity on the body led him "irresistibly to conclude that man is but an electrical Machine, and that disease is simply a disturbance or diminution of the electrical forces in the system."[32] Many of the best medical theorists of the day offered some version of "man the electrical machine." As they debated whether latent electricity in the body was released by contact with electrical current or whether the nerves were enhanced by electrical charge, many late-nineteenth-century regular and irregular practitioners agreed that the body's future lay in applied electrical power.[33]

Fantastic Spaces, Neurasthenic Bodies, and the Rise of Electric Theology

The period between 1880 and 1920 has been called the "Golden Age of Electrotherapy."[34] Earlier reservations about electricity's therapeutic efficacy fell by the wayside; physicians increasingly purchased and applied galvanic and faradic currents in their offices and in patients' homes. Manuals contained lengthy lists of ailments to be treated and methods for electric application, and many physicians shared their knowledge gained mainly from experimenting with electrical current as amateur electricians. For fifty years, they had tapped spines with static sparks to cure paralysis, applied galvanic currents to the temples to relieve headaches and improve eyesight, and used general faradic currents to cure constipation and chronic fatigue. A cultural shift around 1880, however, changed what had been a profitable, if limited, side business into a therapy upon which one could build an entire practice, with or without a medical license.

Not surprisingly, the "Golden Age of Electrotherapy" coincided with the "Golden Age of Electrification" in the United States. By the 1890s, electricity was transforming the pace and nature of urban life. City centers that had been dark after sunset became lighted spaces for strolls and window shopping, thanks to illuminated displays. Amusement parks, Coney Island among them, attracted evening patrons who marveled at hundreds of thousands of lights. As early as the 1890s, many urban dwellers had heard about home electrification, though it was still a luxury of the upper class. The gray pallor of gas lamps was giving way to the advance of bright-white electricity. Americans of all classes were eager for even more electric ingenuity.[35]

One did not need to live in the city to see the old world slowly being eclipsed by electrical power. Magazines brimmed with articles contemplating an electric future; popular novels wove electric fantasies; and cheap goods illuminated like treasures in the neighborhood five-and-dime whispered the grandeur of electric consumption.

The parallel ascent of electricity and electrotherapy in the popular imagination was no coincidence. Electrotherapy, by promising that the body could improve as a physical entity with the application of electricity, quieted fears about an encroaching electric modernity. If the body's full capacity for health and strength could be reached only by connecting it physically with electric currents, how could one not feel an odd kinship with the telephone, telegraph, and streetcar? Experts on the period have long discussed the electric dynamo's ability to awe a late-nineteenth-century audience. The reasons behind that awe are perhaps more complex than mere appreciation of the human ability to exert power upon the material world. Once added to the mix, electrotherapy may have added to that awe. Many Americans eagerly sought a material world that, once transformed electrically, could make human power superior to the most modern machines.

In the late nineteenth century, few Americans had access to electricity in the home. Most middle-class homes received electric power in the decade after World War I; many farm families went without electricity until the rural electrification projects of the 1930s.[36] Not until the 1920s did Americans read by electric light and eat bread from an electric toaster.[37] From 1880 to 1910, electrification was, according to David Nye, "almost exclusively a public, urban experience."[38] As a result, electricity appeared first as a visual or emotional force and only second as a utilitarian tool. For more than twenty years Americans saw electricity at work from a distance, in city lights, animated signs, amusement parks, and theaters. This distance played an important role in the popular reception of electrotherapeutics; it was easy to invest a new technology with unlimited, fantastic powers if one had never had contact with it in its mundane form. Exploring electricity in its urban incarnation provides an important backdrop for concurrent theories concerning its effects on the body.

Cities struggled to outdo one another with turn-of-the-century electric displays. A "great white way," or street fully illuminated with electric lamps, was requisite for downtowns large and small.[39] Night lighting was, above all, a practical endeavor. Stores could stay open late with streetlights and interior lighting. Electricity brought people into urban centers for longer periods, providing more time to purchase than when sunset had meant closed doors. Functional explanations, however, do not fully explain electricity's appeal. Americans' use of electricity during this period far exceeded what was necessary to illuminate space. A city's association with electric illumination became a source of pride; the larger the display, the more status it conferred. Paris planners took this to the extreme in their unsuccessful plan to install thousands of arc lamps downtown, thereby creating an artificial sun that would turn night into day.[40]

If American cities did not manage to entirely banish the night, amusement parks did create fantasy worlds that rose from the darkness. At Coney Island, Luna Park's technicians installed a quarter million electric lights in 1903 to attract visitors to evening offerings. A year later, Dreamland opened, not merely matching Luna's electric display but topping it; a million-plus bulbs covered the buildings, shrubbery, and fencing on the park property. Visitors could probably feel the heat from the 100,000 bulbs crammed onto its 375-foot central tower.[41] Such dramatic lighting would have appealed to the senses in two ways. First, the illuminated outlines of buildings, and in particular the central towers, would have dramatized the pure lines of their classical Greek forms. Under parapets and amid colorful cacophony, columns and arches emerged as pure in form as those in the Columbian Exposition's central court. A powerful physical sensation was also manifest. Alfred Paine, describing the park in *Century* magazine, captured the moment when dusk gave way to illumination:

"Tall towers that had grown dim suddenly broke forth in electrical outlines . . . as the living spark of light traveled hither and thither, until the place was transformed into an enchanted garden."[42] Luna lights did not merely turn on; they broke free from their motor and brick moorings, like untamed energy. Paine's words evoke the physical properties of electricity that visitors sought in parks like Luna and at World's Fairs in Chicago, Buffalo, and St. Louis.[43] Watching the lights go on at night was like watching the world grow modern. Standing in the middle of the electrical shower, one might for a moment absorb a spark before it escaped into the night sky.[44]

Not all Americans would have correlated this pageant of light with their own bodies. It is probable that many visited expositions and amusement parks and enjoyed electrical displays for what they could do: the light they could create and the machines they could power. Yet it would be incorrect to assume that Americans were interested in disembodied electricity.[45] Even a stalwart intellectual such as Lewis Mumford found himself, on occasion, blurring the lines between electrical grandeur and physical power. He remembered that as a young man he had crossed the Brooklyn Bridge and viewed New York's skyscrapers lit up in the distance: "Here was my city, immense, overpowering, flooded with energy and light. In that sudden revelation of power and beauty all the confusion of adolescence dropped from me, and I trod the narrow, resilient boards of the footway with a new confidence."[46] The mesmerizing properties of electricity provided a bridge between material phenomenon and physical sensation. In urban environments saturated with electricity, it was sensible for dwellers to seek their own betterment by merging with the source.

George Beard: Disproving the Electric Evil

Mumford was not the first to sense a connection between urban electricity and the physical body. In his 1855 *Leaves of Grass*, Walt Whitman celebrated technology's physical possibilities by referring to "The Body Electric."[47] Physicians sought to make the link more than rhetorical. One of the most active in the endeavor was George Beard.

Since the 1960s, scholars have credited Beard for coining the term "neurasthenia" to refer to a variety of nervous, or fatiguing, disorders appearing in urbanized post–Civil War America.[48] More attention, however, has been paid to how he diagnosed the disease than to what he saw as its cause and cure.[49] Modern life, with its educational, navigational, and production demands, had overtaxed the body's limited energy reserves, resulting in ill health. "Nervous diseases scarcely exist among savages or barbarians," Beard explained in a talk before the Baltimore Medical and Surgical Society in 1879, citing their premodern lifestyle as cause.[50] He physiologically distinguished between "brain workers" who did white-collar work in urban environments and "muscle workers" who labored primarily with their bodies in rural settings. Beard read contemporary physical decline through the lens of thermodynamics, the principle that matter is constantly in a state of increasing entropy. Only the laboring class, whose lives Beard believed were unchanged from the century previous, avoided critical entropy and continued to enjoy good health.[51]

Beard's 1880 *American Nervousness* blamed Thomas Edison for much of the problem, citing his electric light as one of the "new functions . . . interposed in the circuit" of the body that overtaxed and led to decline.[52] Modern civilization's inventions, which had eased the lives of many, posed a dire threat to the body. In invited appearances across the country, Beard told perplexed physicians to look at the less benevolent side of the marvelous electric light to understand their growing neurasthenic clientele. Similarly at fault were the telegraph, railways, and periodicals. "The introduction and popularization of the railway and the telegraph and the development of the periodical press, belong, it will be observed, to the nineteenth century; and they have intensified in ten thousand ways cerebral activity and worry."[53] The common link among these elements was electricity: the telegraph used electrical power to increase communication, as did the modern printing press. Railways, which ran at first on steam, expanded exponentially with the advent of electric systems. By the 1880s, Beard had become convinced that Edison's electric light was dealing a fatal physical blow, an allegation he substantiated by citing a parallel rise in electric wattage and neurasthenic Americans.[54]

Such statements suggest that Beard campaigned against electricity. Yet he remained hopeful throughout his career that bodies could transform electric energy from an agent of degradation into a means of salvation. In fact, he saw more similarities than differences between himself and Edison, with whom he developed a friendship in the 1870s.[55] Both were entrepreneurs, both had suffered a hearing loss, and both were fascinated by electricity's ability to generate power in the body. For Edison, the fascination meant using his body as a testing ground for new theories.[56] Edison's interest in the physiological workings of electricity extended well beyond laboratory experiments to his inventions such as the "inductorium," an induction-coil device that administered electric shocks and offered, as Edison stated, a "specific cure for rheumatism."[57] Edison originally agreed to meet Beard only after Beard offered, through a mutual friend, to meet and "exchange views" specifically on more general medical uses of electricity.[58]

Beard held that electricity alternatively condemned and redeemed American bodies. Along with his partner, Alphonso Rockwell, he ran the foremost electrotherapy practice of his day and published the main text in the field, *A Practical Treatise on the Medical and Surgical Uses of Electricity*.[59] For twenty years Beard had experimented with electricity and the body, using static, galvanic, and faradic currents to treat nervous ailments that he believed stemmed primarily from excessive electrical force in the body.[60] In his general faradization treatment, Beard attached one copper electrode to a patient's feet and put the other in his hand, allowing the current to run for ten to twenty minutes to induce muscular contractions (fig. 15).[61] The procedure's purpose was to restore healthy circulation by replenishing it if diminished and redistributing it if excessive.[62] Whether the electric current did combat the effects of overelectrification in the late nineteenth century is difficult to ascertain. Patients like Enoch Seals of New York, however, believed. Having suffered for sixteen years from neuralgia of the head, a common neurasthenic illness, he underwent faradization by Rockwell. After four treatments over eight days, the headaches disappeared and Seals considered himself cured.[63] Whether Seals correlated the electric current run through his body, the electrifying city he lived in, and Beard's theories of overcharged American bodies is unknown.

There is evidence that even those most familiar with electricity were likely to perceive the body as electric. J. Emmett O'Brien, author of the 1903 text *The Identity of Nerve Force and Electricity*, echoed Beard in his comparison of the body to an electrical system.[64]

[When] I picture the nervous system and its mechanisms in living action before my mind I see beside it the central telegraph system of New York or London, with its radii of lines and cables, telephonic and telegraphic; its multiple switches, arteries, relays, transformers, condensers, resistances, shunts, duplex and automatic circuits . . . and in a hundred ways doing what is done in the nervous system, and always by means of the same force, the only form of force capable of such vast and varied service.[65]

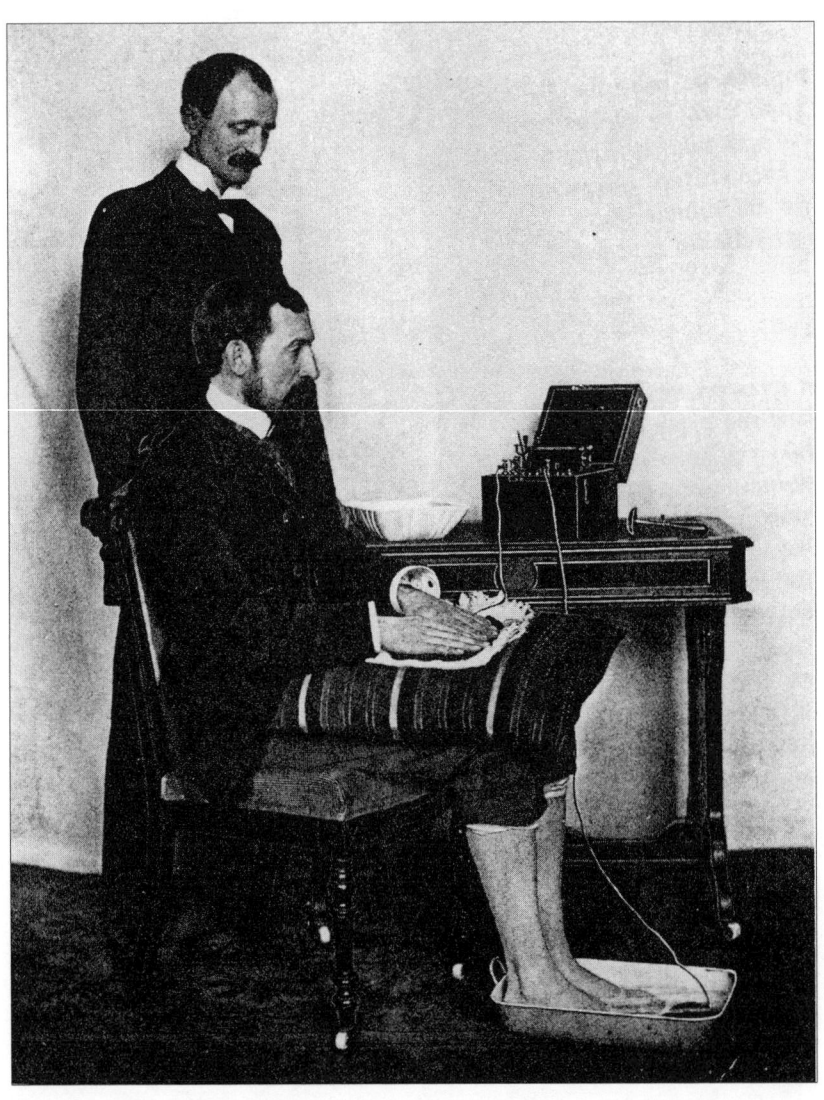

Fig. 15. An example of the general faradization treatment commonly used by George Beard. *General Faradism, A System of Electrotherapeutics as Taught by the International Correspondence Schools*, vol. 4 (Scranton: International Textbook Company, 1902).

His metaphor is no accident: before he became a physician, he worked for the army's telegraph service. O'Brien did in writing what other Americans likely did in their heads: translated his experience with electricity into a modern understanding of the body. Certainly this task became easier for anyone who underwent Beard's treatments.

By the time Beard reached the height of his popularity in the 1880s, physicians and laymen alike had been influenced by the idea that electricity rebalanced bodies made ill by urban life.[66] By 1881, his patients and followers had been exposed frequently to his definition of the body electric. Speaking to readers of his best-selling *American Nervousness,* Beard explained the necessity for electrical treatment, allowing the body and electric light to merge into a single technological entity: "Sooner or later . . . when the amount of force is insufficient to *keep all the lamps actively burning,* those that are weakest go out entirely, or, as more frequently happens, burn faint and feebly, they do not expire, but give an insufficient and unstable light."[67]

Beard's evocation of health and light did more than recall a popular analogy. It alluded to scientists' efforts to connect electricity, light, and the body, efforts that would be rewarded when Niels Ryberg Finsen won the Nobel Prize for physiology of medicine in 1903. Medicinal electricity, when considered as the aggregate of devices marketed and consumed in the United States, was a phenomenon more popular than scientific. Yet this should not obscure the real advances made during this period in treating the body with electric currents. Beard's findings introduced a generation of physicians to electricity's ability to alleviate pain and treat paralysis. Finsen's work revealed that exposing the skin to electrically generated light, or phototherapy, could cure dermatological ailments. Scientific advances in electrotherapy gave a popular audience reason to believe in electricity's remarkable curative potential. The devices that actually reached the hands of the multitudes would not have been regarded as "cures" had they not basked in the glow of these scientific successes.[68]

From Prizes to Products: The Popular World of Electric Cures

By 1900, the American public was familiar with fantastic electric cityscapes and electric neurasthenia cures. These provided a foundation for the rise of what one historian has called a modern "electric theology," the belief that electricity was a spiritual triumph of mysterious power with unlimited potential.[69] Yet the true ramifications of this spiritual phenomenon cannot be understood without understanding its resonance in the popular culture. For Americans of the 1890s, electricity's relationship to the body went beyond metaphorical descriptions. Popular literature, entertainment, and even food products revealed a concerted effort by Americans to imbibe electrical power directly.

The displayed body, the expanded body, and the powered body emerged as three distinct physical-electrical tropes in late-nineteenth-century life. The first became a common feature in public entertainment and private novelty. Dancers like Loie Fuller attracted audiences by adorning their bodies with electric lights and styling new dances out of darkened stages.[70] The practice became popular with society hostesses and working girls alike. Women from New York socialite Mrs. Cornelius Vanderbilt to the wife of South Dakota industrialist E. E. Gaylord donned dresses and robes fitted with electric lights and held electric torches in tableau portraits of the dazzling technology embodied.[71] One could even rent "electric girls" for special occasions from the Electric Girl Lighting Company begun in 1884. All one needed, presumably, to ensure that any party would be memorable was to rent a serving girl whose dress was illuminated with "fifty candle power each in quantities to suit householders."[72]

Most of the bodies on electric display were female, a fact that can be attributed to standards of dress allowing women greater adornment and the importance of electric domestication. Certainly the image of a bedecked Mrs. Vanderbilt, wife of the leading railroad magnate, holding on high a massive electric torch evoked the extravagance of the nation's expanding industrial power. At the same time, by having a woman's body display electric power as a decoration instead of a man showing electricity's utilitarian function, the technology's inventors positioned electricity as a force compatible with safe domestic consumption.

Men also sought ways to display their bodies electrically, if less dramatically. The electric tie light, a phenomenon of the 1890s, allowed men to cloak a love for the illuminated aesthetic in practicality. Advertised for their "efficient beauty," the ties fit close to the neck, presumably illuminating the body and the space just in front of it. The four-inch battery hidden in a coat pocket enabled concealment of the power source, making the body seem self-illuminated. Advertisements suggesting that engineers should purchase the lights for their "emblematical" value reveal that men saw electric technology imprinted on their bodies as marks of status.[73]

Theories also abounded that electricity would expand the physical body internally and externally. Electricians asserted that electricity would soon maintain life, just as the sun maintained plants; it was merely a matter of time until it would be absorbed directly into the body to provide all necessary nourishment. In an interview in *Western Electrician,* Amos Dolbear, a Tufts professor of physics and astronomy, saw a future without food, when humans would simply "absorb energy from space" in unlimited supply.[74] In Europe, researchers studied the effects of electrical stimulation on children's growth. One study, in which a schoolroom was fitted with a high-frequency electric current for six months, found that children grew an average of 20 mm more than those unexposed to electricity. These "electrically charged children" were probably also smarter after exposure, assuming that they shared in the benefits of their teachers, who reported their own faculties "quickened" by the experience.[75] Such studies, covered in magazines like *Scientific American,* reflected the plots of popular juvenile literature. For example, in L. Frank Baum's *The Master Key: An Electrical Fairy Tale,* a boy unleashes his own personal genie, the Demon of Electricity, from an electrical set. In John Trowbridge's *The Electrical Boy,* a young orphan manages to climb electric wires to reach his mother in heaven. Both stories' heroes increase their physical power by commanding electric technology. The lesson for young and old was the same: a bit of electrical know-how allowed one to transcend physical limitation.[76]

According to historian Carolyn Marvin, the desire to see technological changes in the physical world reflected in people's bodies drove much of the fascination with electrical technology.[77] Dressing in electric lights and pondering electric growth were ways to physically connect to electricity, to see a new physical reality accompany advances in industrial power. This impulse appears strongest in accounts of superpowered bodies, those endowed with supernatural ability courtesy of electric currents. Turn-of-the-century circuses featured "Electric Boys" who shocked those willing to spend a few cents to touch them. Accompanied by stories of their original "electrification," these human attractions were proof that the body could store and generate electric power absorbed from external phenomena. Probably those who paid money to experience the sensation saw what they wanted to see; typically an Electric Boy's electricity came from nothing more fantastic than the metal plate upon which he stood.[78] Professional journals perpetuated these anecdotal accounts even as they sought to condemn them. One 1886 story in *Electrical Review* related in order to dismiss the rural legend of Willie Brough, an "extremely nervous boy" from Turlock, California, who purportedly could set things on fire with his eyes.[79] Yet many readers, especially those who were merely skimming the pages, were as likely to walk away believing the story as they were to dismiss it.

By the 1890s, researchers were seeking ways to grow food electrically by applying currents and artificial heat to greenhouse plants. If successful, they reasoned, modern foods would no longer face restrictions of climate and season.[80] Yet it was not merely harvesting flexibility that these experimenters were after. Electrically grown food would contain actual electrical energy that would be taken up by the body during digestion thereby making eating a way to generate physical power. Just as plants transform the sun's energy into chlorophyll, the body would transform the plants' energy into usable electric currents.[81] In 1887, a variation on this theme, the Electric Cocktail, grew fashionable at parties. There one could bypass the hassle of actually growing electrical food and eating it: an electrolier, or an electrically heated rod, could do the trick, reportedly transforming a mixture of alcohol and sugar into an energizing beverage.[82]

Turn-of-the century popular culture teemed with electric facts, fads, follies, and, above all, fantasy. Tangible and intangible factors embedded the electric body within the very idea of modern progress. Physical limitations, endemic as they seemed to twentieth-century life, seemed ready to be overcome by healing currents; long-traded tales of electrified bodies could now be realized at home with a copper handle, wire cord, and home-made galvanic battery. Folk beliefs, unsettled medical knowledge, and an ill-defined technology combined to create a space for unbridled electrical enthusiasm that, with phrases such as "recharging my batteries" and "short circuiting," crept into colloquial speech.[83] This was the landscape that "quack" physicians and manufacturers entered, providing an eager public with the products it had been implicitly promised. To the horror of regular physicians, the cult of the electric body had emerged.

Electric Belts, Ozone, and the Cultural Cure

One can gauge the impact of nonlicensed or irregular physicians by the volume of protests against them. Once confident that time would distinguish electricity's healers from its frauds, American physicians had relied upon furthering their own science and complaining about charlatans amongst themselves in professional journals. Yet by the late nineteenth century, physicians found that instead of sealing their grip upon electrotherapy practice, they had begun to lose it entirely. The idea of electricity as a vital power and curative agent, a notion they had long promoted, took on a life of its own in the hands of "quack" marketers. M. Allen Starr, a professor of diseases of the mind and nervous system at the New York College of Physicians and Surgeons, admonished the sensible readers of *Scribner's Magazine* to sift the good from the bad in electrical treatments. Starr was probably unfamiliar with the habits of his congressmen when he cited, in 1890, the problem as ignorance. Why else, he asked, would people fall victim to street promoters proclaiming that "electricity is life" and inviting them to enjoy a quick pick-me-up courtesy of current-generating metal handles?[84] Physician S. E. Morrill agreed. Current machines, electric hairbrushes, and galvanic belts appealed to people who were easily led. Speaking of the traveling shock machine popular on urban street corners, Morrill blamed its success on its "all-powerful influence on the invalid," suggesting that those who believed in its efficacy must be of feeble constitution.[85]

Given the relatively equal influence of regular and irregular physicians, Americans found it easy to ignore the advice of experts and to pursue alternative electrical therapies. Between 1890 and 1930, as physicians waged war upon the makers of these unapproved electrical devices, an eager public decided to cast its lot with the unlicensed, lining up to purchase their wares, the more outlandish the better. Electric belts, ozone generators, violet rays, vibration devices, and current collars made their manufacturers wealthy, despite the American Medical Association's best efforts to discredit such individuals through a combination of press releases and prosecution for postal fraud.[86] By promising an attentive audience that they could "revitalize nerves" and "reinvigorate tired muscles" with inexpensive, easy-to-use products in the privacy of their own homes, the quack promoters had tapped a market ready to see electric theology realized. Unlike physicians, quacks realized that many Americans sought electrical cures more cultural than medicinal, cures that could place the body at the center of a dizzying, modernizing electrical age.

Between 1880 and 1930, irregular electrotherapists offered three types of cultural cures for the travails of modern life. In the late nineteenth century, these were gendered according to male and female prescribed roles; only in the 1920s would an electric device apppear that considered men and women equally in need of energy transfers. Electric belts and batteries, aimed primarily at men, allowed individuals to hook into electrical sources directly, placing their physical bodies in the metaphorical center of modern life. Ozone generators and violet-ray machines, for which women were the primary consumers, washed away Victorian germs, disease, and decay, suggesting that electric technology brought physical life back to an original purity. Low-level electric harnesses, such as the I-ON-A-CO, offered men and women an exposure to imperceptible vibrations designed to bring the body into harmony with the modern era.

It is obvious in hindsight that few of the above products actually cured bodies. Physicians were right to argue, in print and in court, that such items possessed little medicinal value beyond slight stimulation and mild air purification. One ought not confuse, however, medical facts with physical realities. As recent research on the placebo effect has suggested, physical cures can be as much psychological as physiological.[87] Americans had myriad reasons to want electrical devices to relieve physical weakness, disease, and depression. For those who believed Beard's thesis or knew of the second law of thermodynamics, electricity would have been a logical place to look for relief. Even those unaware of Beard or thermodynamics had reasons to be curious about electricity's curative abilities, given its proven strength as an industrial and domestic energy source. Sales records, advertising materials, and biographical data can recreate the role these products played in acclimating bodies to the modern landscape.

Electric Belts and Industrial Supremacy

Wearable electric devices were available for purchase as early as the 1870s. Some of these were novelty items, such as the electric tie light; most were medicinal. The most ubiquitous and most long-lived of these was the electric belt, which, in 1875, was first successfully marketed in the United States by the British electrician J. L. Pulvermacher.[88] The belt's charge emanated from what Pulvermacher called the 120 "elements," spools of copper wire wrapped around rods three inches in length. In order for it to conduct, the entire belt had to be soaked in vinegar before each use. Later versions of the belt contained small galvanic batteries, but their intended benefit was the same. In advertisements, Pulvermacher enouraged people to buy and wear the belts by describing electricity as "the prime motive power for promoting circulation, assimilation, secretion, and excretion."[89]

By the turn of the century, many companies joined Pulvermacher in the belt business, including German Electric, Dr. Crystal's, Dr. Horn's, Addison's, Edson's, and Edison's (started by Thomas Edison's renegade son Tom), Owen, and Heidelberg.[90] There were slight differences among the belts, but most looked and worked similarly. A typical belt was made of cloth with interior metal wires that connected to galvanically charged disks. As in the Owen belt, consumers usually could choose between basic and deluxe models, which gave off a greater charge. Wearing a belt created a light buzzing, or tingling, sensation under the skin where it came in contact with the current-conducting wires. As objects, the belts were unlike other clothing of the era in that they were fairly unisex in design, although they were marketed more frequently to men.

Unlike regular physicians, whose professional status kept them from advertising electric machines, electric-belt makers were heavy promoters locally and nationally. Manufacturers cast their nets widely by advertising in popular magazines like *Harper's Weekly* and *The Illustrated News*, and specialized publications like *The Graphic*.[91] By the turn of the century, even rural Americans with little use for urban magazines saw the belts in general supply catalogues like those of Sears, Roebuck and Co. Still, one need not to have read periodicals to know about the belts. The manufacturers also employed direct-mail campaigns, peppering communities with letters that hawked belts and their healing properties.[92] These were augmented by door-to-door sales, where customers could see the belts and examine the gadgetry while hearing the pitch.[93]

Given that electric appliances were not available in most homes until after World War I, the chance to own an electric product must have attracted many buyers. It is difficult to locate company records to prove precisely how many belts were purchased, but the sheer number of belt manufacturers permits speculation that there was money to be made. Companies like A. P. Owens of New York not only maintained businesses well into the 1920s but also expanded from their East Coast origins. Before being shut down in 1922 for postal fraud, Owens had selling and distribution centers in Chicago, Buffalo, Miami, Indianapolis, San Antonio, and Woodcliff Lake, New Jersey.[94] As late as 1926, the Iona Company, manufacturers of the I-ON-A-CO electric belt, earned $36,000 in net profit from the 2,445 belts sold in the first five months of the year.[95]

Electric belts succeeded, in part, because of salesman tenacity. Working on commission, and frequently purchasing belts at cost before earning anything from sales, salesmen reaped no reward from making the rounds of a neighborhood and ending up empty-handed. A successful salesman could earn extraordinary commissions. Addison's Electric Belt salesmen, for instance, sold a basic belt for as little as $1.10, but the cost of the belt to the salesman was $2.50 a dozen.[96] It must have been tempting to exaggerate the benefits of the belt to prospective customers. The belts were often packed in boxes printed with outlandish claims. Addison's, for instance, declared that its belt, after having been soaked in "good cider vinegar" for ten minutes, would exhibit "the life principle, the nerve force, the crystallized energy, or the health element of our being."[97]

Even the best salesman cannot make a consistent profit from a product that fails to meet popular demand. Belt manufacturers built their promotions on physicians' enthusiasms voiced in previous decades, often embellishing them. Most makers went well beyond what physicians were willing to promise, capitalizing on people's fears of disease and fantasies of electricity.

To readers of electric belt advertisements, electricity seemed a simple, painless key to health. It "puts life and force into anything it touches," was how Addison's put it.[98] German Electric explained that by running a current through the body, one was "removing the cause of disease and strengthening and invigorating the nerves that control their action."[99] Although belts were constructed of prosaic materials—copper, wire, galvanic batteries, leather, and cloth—what was actually being sold was a vision of physical electric abundance. The body was not merely a vessel containing a set amount of energy that, in Beardian fashion, could be depleted at any moment. Nor was it a collection of nervous forces that had to be redirected at the electrotherapist's office. It was, in the words of Dr. Bell's Appliance Company, which sold belts for more than twenty years, a collection of sponges waiting to be saturated by electric energy. As one promotional letter declared, "Electricity, the basis of human vitality," washed over the body during electric treatments, "like water running down hill."[100]

Electricity had not only fascinated turn-of-the-century city dwellers with light displays and transportation marvels, it also had made them fear for their physical health. Electrical accidents became commonplace in cities and towns with the arrival of electric wires and speeding electric trains. In one of many court cases involving electrical accidents, the Kentucky Court of Appeals ruled in 1899 that electricity was "the most powerful and dangerous element known to science."[101]

Doomsday predictions were made by those fearful of electricity's deviation from their perceived natural order. Clergymen were particularly prone to this view; as community leaders, they helped influence countless others to feel the same. According to Bishop Turner of the African Methodist Church of Georgia, Kentucky, and Tennessee, there was much to be feared from "the invention of the white man in controlling electricity." As reported in *Electric World*, Turner predicted an imminent "unbalancing of the air currents," which might cause "whole cities to be blown away at a time, and floods unlike any save Noah's."[102] His prediction was outdone by the Reverend A. C. Johnson's proclamation two years later: a modern Armageddon was coming when "the electricity stored in the earth will come in contact with the heated matter inside and blow the whole world up."[103]

Electricity's position between physical fears and physical fantasies is nowhere more evident than in its controversial use for capital punishment in the 1890s. Proponents of electric execution argued that the method was quick, relatively painless, and spared the victim slow strangulation and horrific decapitation at the hands of incompetent hangmen. Yet counter to the assurances of experts like Alphonso Rockwell that alternating current could kill quickly and humanely, Albert Kemmler, the first to receive the "electric chair," did not die after the first jolt: he required two separate electric charges. According to witnesses, the process appeared neither efficient nor painless, given the smell of his skin burning under the electrodes and the sight of blood flowing from his nose.[104]

After the Kemmler execution, few could doubt that electricity was as dangerous as rumored: it was a force that even the experts could not control. Thomas Edison's efforts through much of the late 1880s to publicize the lethal power of George Westinghouse's AC generator in order to ensure that it would be used in executions instead of his own DC generator only strengthened this perception. Still, the very mysteriousness of this "executional" force may have increased its demand as a curative agent. This is particularly likely in that Kemmler's execution and its expansive press coverage coincided with a surge in popular electrotherapeutics in the early 1890s.

Advertisements for electrical products often assuaged electric fears by portraying electricity as dominated by the physical body. On company letterheads and in advertisements, it was common to see electricity "captured" by human force. One advertisement for American Electrical Works relates an allegorical story to its audience of electricians and tinkerers: professionals harness violent electrical force without fear. Set against a mundane textual explanation of the company's products lies a captivating image of electrical force: a jacketed and cuffed fist reaches out as if desiring to soar beyond the wires and cables being sold, shooting into the air and gripping electricity's bolts. The image suggests that electrical experts positioned themselves on the front line of electric power; owing to their superior education ("the suited arm") and their physical prowess, they dominated electric force.

Electric belt advertisements used the same symbols to extend "physical expertise" to men and women of the general public. The lightning bolt was ubiquitous; it appeared more often in advertisements than the belts themselves. Pulvermacher Galvanic Company, for example, often used it to dramatize and exaggerate the power of its product. In an 1882 brochure, lightning is the sole light source in a dark universe, coming from the sky toward the earth (fig. 16). The cover's bold electricity would first attract the attention of the reader, who might assume lightning was for sale. The iconography established a close connection between the belts and electricity, suggesting even to the casual reader that the belts might control that most deadly of forces.

Most belt companies made sure that readers made the connection between lightning's power and their products. In illustrations, lightning frequently emerges in the form of sparks that leap from the belts. Lightning bolts showed up on company stationery and in advertisements, strikingly similar in appearance from one manufacturer to the next. In each case, the lightning emerges from the conducting disks attached to the belts. The more disks, the more lightning. Some models, such as Owens' Gent's Belt No. 4, had so many conductors that the entire belt became illuminated with electricity (fig. 17). Such illustrations had no basis in fact; electric belts did not emit sparks of any sort. Their galvanic batteries created low-level charges, perceptible only to the touch. The illustrations implied that belts used static electricity, or sparks, an antiquated technology inferior to galvanic currents in therapeutic applications.

Unlike regular physicians, belt manufacturers were not limited by accuracy. By portraying their products as powerful conductors of bursting electrical force, they appeared to be allowing consumers to absorb dangerous quantities of raw electricity. The intent is manifest in the illustrations that appeared in product instructions. In those for the Gent's Belt,

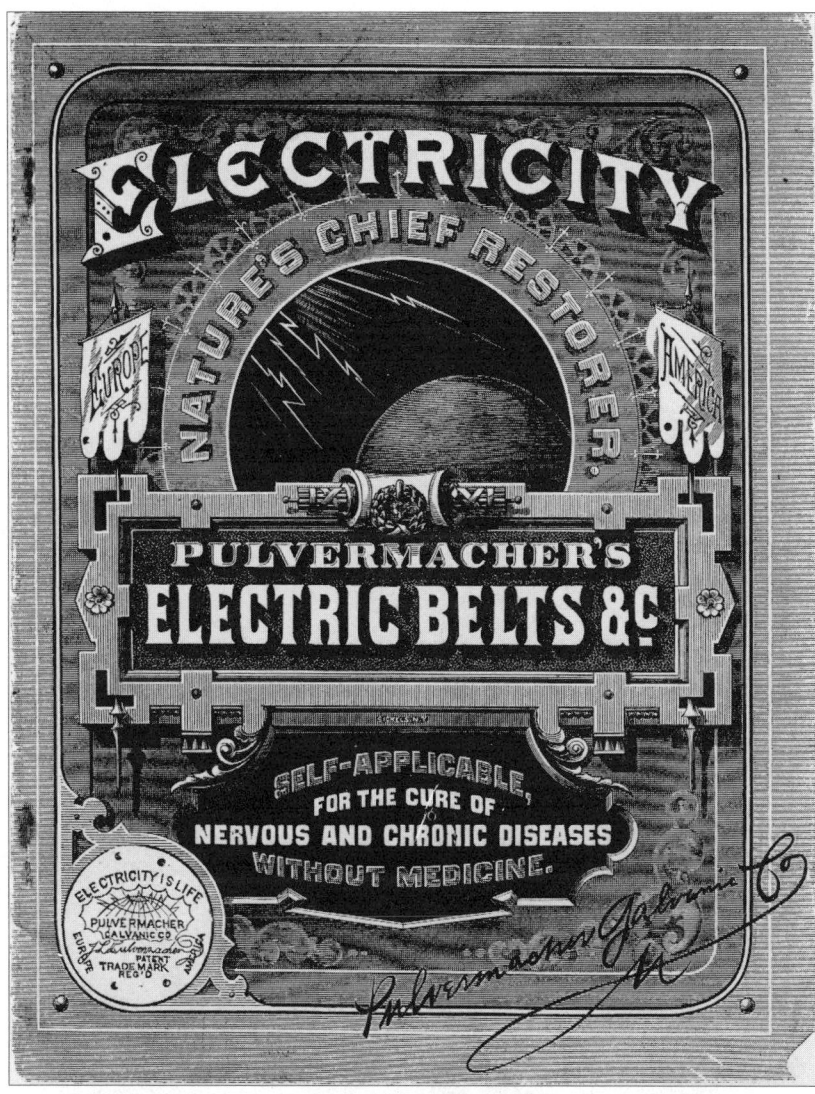

Fig. 16. "Electricity: Nature's Chief Restorer," cover of brochure for Pulvermacher's Electric Belts and Company (Pulvermacher, 1882), ephemera collection. Courtesy of the Bakken Library and Museum of Electricity in Life, Minneapolis.

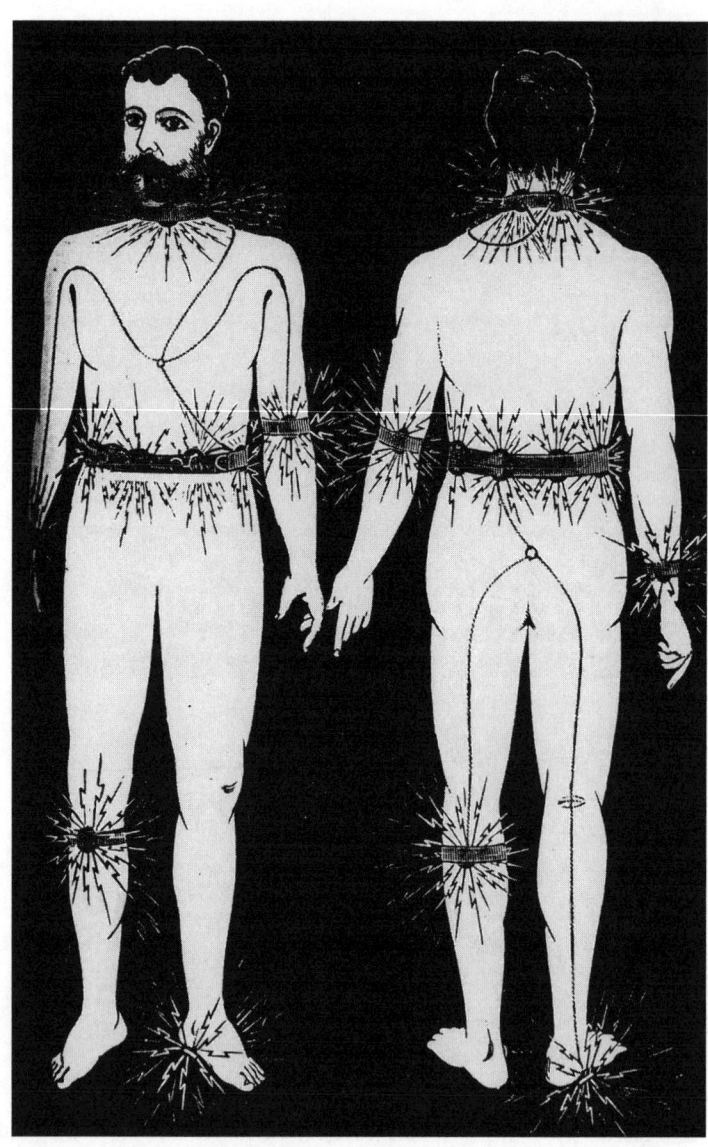

Fig. 17. Gent's Belt with Special Appliances, Dr. A. Owen, *Catalogue of the Owen Electric Belts and Appliances* (Chicago: Owen Electric Belt and Appliance Company, ca. 1890), ephemera collection. Courtesy of the Bakken Library and Museum of Electricity in Life, Minneapolis.

an individual is surrounded by a circuit of visible electric shocks. To the uninitiated, such a scene might resemble one of the electrical accidents referred to by the Kentucky court or perhaps an electric execution in progress. Carried from the belt by small wires draped over his body, electricity is emitted by the subject's neck collar, his arms, knees, and even below his feet. Given that the illustration is supposed to be instructive, belt purchasers may have believed that it would yield such dramatic results at home.[105]

Owning an electric belt placed a consumer at the top of an electrical hierarchy. Advertisements frequently compared the power of the products to commercial electrical applications. The London Electric Fabric Company of New York advertised its "Edson Electric Garter," which promised to develop the ankle into "perfect form," in *Frank Leslie's Illustrated*. Encouraging readers to misread the item as the "Edison" electric garter, the ad stressed that it was "as Wonderful as the Telephone and Electric Light."[106]

The German Electric Belt Company also connected its belts to Edison's marvels. "We have now arrived at what may properly be termed the *Electric Era*," it informed readers in its 1890 belt brochure "German Electric Era." "Everything is done now by Electricity; our streets are lighted by it, our engines run by it, it carries our messages in the twinkling of an eye under the broad Atlantic and conveys our voice from city to city by telephone." Yet these, it declared, were not the greatest applications of electric force.

> While the Electric Light, the Electric Telegraph and Telephone were all great discoveries in their way, it remained for a famous German Electrician to invent a simple method to apply Electricity to the human body in the shape of a Belt for the removal of disease, and we question if this discovery will not be of more real benefit to the human race than all the others mentioned, put together.[107]

The appeal of the belts' technological aesthetic probably explains why manufacturers did not differentiate between men's and women's models in their design. Androgyny had other benefits, of course, namely, lowest cost; perhaps uniform belts were simply the cheapest option. The ornamental nature of the belts, however, suggests that cost was not the most important consideration. Manufacturers knew that their belts sold first to the eye and then to the body; the decorated electrodes and engraved metal batteries also meant added cost, but most companies applied ornamentation even to their base model. More likely, belts were gender neutral because a technological aesthetic was more desirable than a gendered one. Later, appliance manufacturers would realize that they could sell to women by means of decorative colors and soft, streamlined edges, but such modified products would appear only after electricity had already been introduced into the home and domesticated. The age of dangerous lightning and electrical deaths called for a belt that confronted the risks while delivering on the promise of ultimate electrical potential.

Balancing this sense of newness and danger were the titles belt companies gave themselves to connote history and prestige. The German Electric Company, it must be noted, was based in New York City, not Europe; likewise Pulvermacher's of London was based in Cincinnati. Manufacturers used Continental language to describe products made in the United States even though the belts were far more popular in this country than abroad.[108] Companies consistently evoked a European heritage, often more contrived than real. Certainly their inclination could be viewed as simply part of the cultural moment: Americans tended to regard European artists and scientists as superior well into the twentieth century. Yet it is probable that some manufacturers used European heritage as a weapon against Americans who would label them "quacks": belts from Heidelberg may have been harder to label fraudulent than were those from Cincinnati.

Belts appealed across classes. Expensive models such as the I-ON-A-CO were aimed primarily at the middle class. Sales prices suggest that it was the primary market for most belts; with prices ranging from ten to thirty dollars, most were out of range for working-class incomes. Yet evidence suggests that working-class men bought belts as well. One physician employed in a charity dispensary at the turn of the century recorded his frustration that patients with little money for food often came in wearing electric belts. Some, made of chamois, had cost them as much as twenty-four dollars.[109] Advertised high prices went out the window when, typically, belt manufacturers cut deals with customers based on ability to pay. German Electric, for one, sent out general letters advertising its wares. If a recipient did not reply, successive letters with dramatic discounts in price followed until the recipient capitulated or moved.[110] Belts could easily be purchased from the Sears, Roebuck and Co. catalogue and delivered to one's home for as little as four dollars.[111] In fact, belts could sometimes be had for free. Promotional programs, like a 1903 program of the St. Paul office of Heidelberg Electric Belts, occasionally offered belts without charge.[112]

For many working-class Americans, electric belts may have been cheaper alternatives to often expensive and sometimes fraudulent medical treatments. Certainly manufacturers believed they had a viable consumer base among the working class and immigrants. The most profitable belt manufacturer of the era printed a detailed brochure in Chinese for his Los Angeles and San Francisco salesmen that carried an illustration of a Chinese woman in traditional dress promoting the product.[113] The chamois belt suggests that the devices may have functioned as middle-class status symbols for working-class buyers. One would not invest in a high-quality belt if it were not something of which one could feel proud. Wearing an electric belt may have had a twofold appeal to working-class and immigrant Americans: they could simultaneously harness a potentially dangerous energy within the body and effectively "Americanize" themselves. Like the expert engineers, they too could join the elite class of those who understood and commanded electrical power.[114]

By associating their invention with the marvels of modern electric life, belt manufacturers appealed to white- and blue-collar workers who were captivated by technology's mystique. It is no coincidence that belts sold best to people whose lives inside and outside the workplace were being rapidly altered by new technologies. Belt promoters actively sought to contextualize belts as a means for restoring balance between the body and the environment. In text and iconography, their messages told consumers that the true purpose of electric technology, from its directed form in the telephone to its chaotic essence in the lightning bolt, was to make bodies powerful.

Were one to believe the claims of German Electric, all applications of industrial and domestic electricity paled in comparison to the power of the belt one could wear. This was obvious in advertisements, such as the image on the back cover of one brochure that was meant to attract prospective salespeople (fig. 18). Here a man, wearing the company's electric belt, literally on the top of the earth, exposes his body to what should be deadly electric currents from surrounding electric lines lightning bolts. He stands at risk from neither the bolts emanating from the earth, nor those coming from the sky, nor the modern inventions around him. Holding another belt above his head like the Holy Grail, its bolts simply ricochet off his frame, having been confronted by the superior

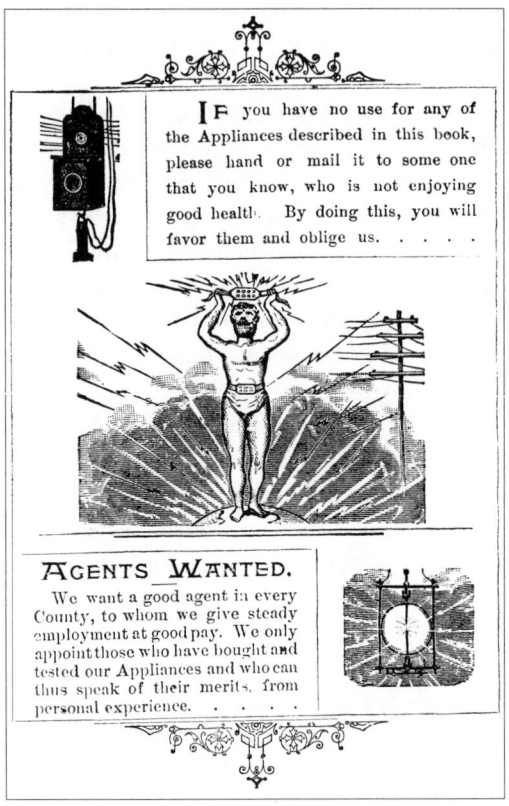

Fig. 18. "Agents Wanted," "The Electric Era" (German Electric Belt Agency, 1890), ephemera collection. Courtesy of the Bakken Library and Museum of Electricity in Life, Minneapolis.

electrical force he now possesses. In what German Electric termed "the Electric Era," belts were the next step in technological progress, a step that allowed the body to rightfully claim the industrial energy it deserved.

In the world of electric belt promoters, the body was not eclipsed.[115] Advertisements suggested that doomsday prophesies had not come true. Instead of succumbing to the technological taxations of modernity, the body would use technology's energy to become a superior being. Pulvermacher's description of its electric current, in fact, could be read as an inversion of Beard's "neurasthenic" electrical paradigm. If one was exposed to regular, intermittent electric currents, the blood globules would slow and the body would weaken. But, it declared, if the current was continuous, it would increase "the normal speed of the movement of the blood-globules, in other words, the circulation will be accelerated." Thus the device allowed a user to take deteriorating electrical forces in urban life and make them invigorating. The telephone, telegraph, and electric light, in this context, were all harbingers of the body of tomorrow.

An electric belt, by fastening directly to the body and requiring through an intricate buckling system that the wearer be conscious of its presence, brought users into even closer contact with potentially frightening technologies. This confrontation with fear, controlled as it was by the electric belt, inoculated users against electricity's potential for harm. Until the belts' popularity diminished in the late 1920s, wearers could cinch their bodies into the awesome power of dynamos, electric lights, and lightning bolts.[116]

The Electropoise, Violet Rays, and the Beautiful Death of Decay

By wearing electricity, individuals staved off fears of corporeal obsolescence, fortifying their bodies with an extended armor of energizing materials. There were also active efforts to bring electricity beyond the body's surface and into its interior. As befitting a culture that dictated "separate spheres" for men and women, medicinal electric gadgets were marketed differently to each gender based upon cultural ideals of health and power. If men were the targets of electric belts to face the outside world, then women were the targets of devices that were tailored to their domestic needs.

Between 1880 and 1930, electric-remedy manufacturers advertised two products primarily to women to combat the effects of fatigue and aging. The Electropoise, a device manufactured in New York and promoted by the aptly named Hercules Sanche, declared that it did so by "inducing oxygen directly into the entire circulation" through a "treating plate" that could be fastened around the "naked ankle."[117] The Violet Ray, manufactured by a variety of companies in the early twentieth century, pronounced that it applied a "huge voltage" of violet-colored electricity to the body, which, through rapid vibration, restored youthful skin and cured rheumatism by stimulating circulation and eliminating cell waste.[118]

Little has been written about these products, in spite of their popularity.[119] As artifacts, the Electropoise and the Violet Ray offer insight into how electrical products were marketed differently to men and women. They also suggest that electric energy interacted with bodies even more intimately than was possible through belts; the Electropoise and the Violet Ray went deeper than the skin's surface, the electric energy purportedly seeped into cells and sped their renewal.

In 1912, the American Medical Association's guide to fraudulent medical practices listed fourteen oxygen-related products. Machines like the Oxypathor, the Oxygenor and the Oxybon promised to improve health by increasing the body's oxygen, a process, according to one advertisement, that would "burn up wastes and poisons in the blood, thus leaving it rich and pure."[120] It would be easy to dismiss such products as "hokum," in the language of contemporary critics. Oxygen infusers had no curative properties. Each was a simple metal cylinder called a "polarizer," which was empty or filled with sand or carbon, from which emerged a cord called a "conductor," that fastened around wrist or ankle. To release healthful oxygen into the body, the user placed the cylinder in water, attached the band to her body and waited. Immediately thereafter she would feel the "profound, restful slumber" that accompanied the body's internal restoration.[121] In spite of infusers' questionable medical value, between 1909 and 1914 alone more than 45,000 Oxypathors were sold.[122]

Hercules Sanche, who first marketed his oxygen inhaler in 1892, long resisted the AMA's best efforts to expose him as a fraud. His device, a frequently copied cylinder and cord attachment, worked by increasing what Sanche called an "electric force in the system." Not only would the equipment he described be able to improve physical force, it was desperately needed by a body in a constant state of degeneration. "The gases from decaying food are positive in their electrical quality and cause disease. With the Electropoise we cause the negative elements so abundant in the atmosphere to be attracted into the body in sufficient quantity to consume the accumulation of combustible matter stored up by the imperfect action of the vital organs."[123] In two sentences, Sanche turned negative and positive energies into potentially life-threatening elements requiring the technological intervention of the Electropoise. Like a magnet drawing in negative charges, the device restored the body to a state of balance.[124]

Sanche's explanation resonated with an age when oxygen absorption was deemed essential for preventing consumption, or tuberculosis, a prevalent, little-understood, and often deadly disease. Physicians commonly saw air as the cause, and cure seekers went on extended trips to mountain or coastal areas whose air was considered more healthful. Given that the Electropoise did not have an attachment for breathing the "electrified" agent it contained, it may seem unlikely that the device was marketed to consumption sufferers, yet its promoters did, however, attribute to it increased lung capacity: "The Electropoise applies the needed amount of electrical force to the system, and by its thermal action places the body in condition to absorb oxygen through the lungs and its pores."[125] Here was a product that required neither the discomfort nor the vulnerability of traditional treatments, and that did not rely upon unhealthy lungs alone to infuse the body with healing oxygen. Suggestively, it was also one that allowed women to follow culturally prescribed behaviors and undergo their treatment at home rather than heading west, away from domestic responsibilities.

Hercules Sanche never said that the Electropoise cured tuberculosis.[126] His imitators, who were less skilled in walking the fine line between advertising freedom and postal fraud, did. E. L. Moses of New York, inventor of the Oxypathor, spent eighteen months in prison for false claims made in 1915, among them, that the device enabled the body to cure diphtheria and tuberculosis. Sanche, on the other hand, trusted users of his device to make the connection for themselves.

According to historian Katherine Ott, by the 1880s, there were more than thirty vaporizers and atomizers on the market aimed at increasing the lung capacity and oxygen absorption of consumptive patients.[127] Patients could, however, choose to undergo "electric gas" treatments in physicians' offices, typically by inhaling carbolic acid or creosote.[128] Given the "regular" options, it is easy to see why people may have preferred treatments like Sanche's water and blissful rest.

Advertisements for the Electropoise often included images that evoked lounging "Gibson Girls." Women were shown in finely decorated parlors, wearing the devices around their ankles (fig. 19). Their pale complexions, thin bodies, and theatrically fatigued facial expressions exemplified the "consumptive look" characteristically praised for its delicate feminine beauty.[129] Americans who came upon Electropoise advertisements in popular magazines like *McClure's* and *Cosmopolitan* would have recognized the suggestion that the product was ostensibly an "oxygen" cure for consumption.[130] At a time when, as Ott has described, "everyone was a little bit consumptive," it was an effective pitch.[131]

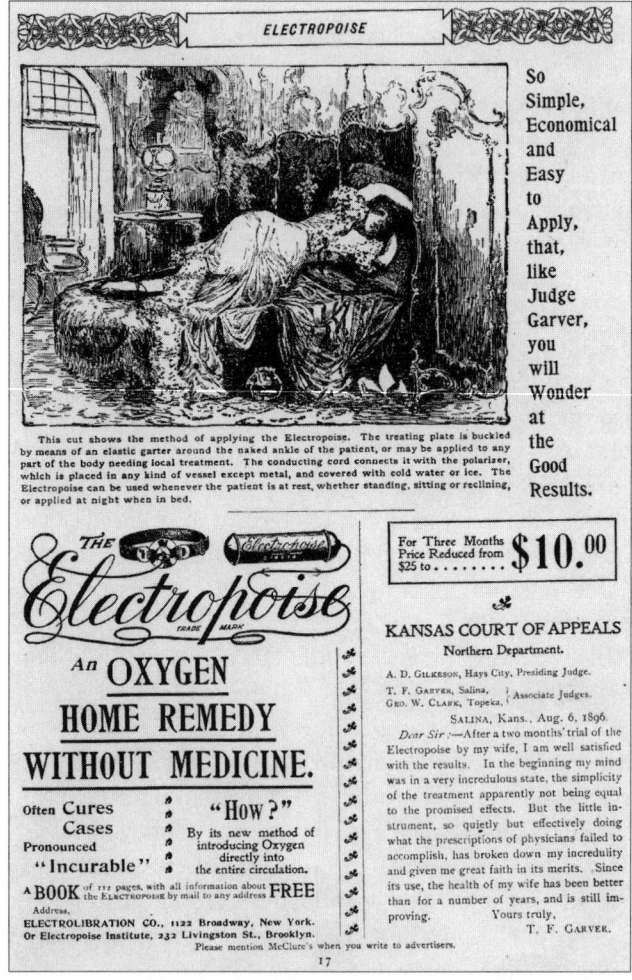

Fig. 19. Electropoise, *McClure's Magazine,* undated, ephemera collection. Courtesy of the Bakken Library and Museum of Electricity in Life, Minneapolis.

Such devices did not challenge the cultural ideal of a delicate femininity. Belt advertisements typically featured muscular men taking visible electric shocks to the body; Electropoise and Violet Ray, hand-held devices that produced streams of purple light and purported to enhance one's appearance, showed women of average build using invisible electric power. Although some manufacturers stressed the "huge force" Violet Rays could impart, advertisements rarely illustrated electric power emanating from the products, nor did they make a connection between the dangerous, impressive electrical forces of industry and the products' ability to power bodies. Electricity, as introduced in these products, warded off death and decay, elements that destroyed youth and beauty. The Violet Ray was sold to consumers specifically to treat insomnia, headaches, nervousness, sallow complexion, weak lungs, hoarse voices, dandruff, gray hair, and premature baldness. Many of these "diseases" were cosmetic, a fact attested by the "attachments," including steaming combs and facial massagers. The emphasis on physical beauty is reflected in typical advertising images. Women are frequently seductively posed, looking out at prospective consumers as if sexually enhanced by electric devices. In some cases, such as the advertisement for Roger's Violet Rays in 1915, a male hand holds the device on a woman's body, perhaps suggesting to the male consumer that he could participate in this intimate exchange (fig. 20).

The sexual imagery does not distinguish Electropoise and Violet Ray advertisements from those for men's belts. Where they differ, however, is in the way that sexual power should be used. Turn-of-the-century promotions of electric products for men showed the body visibly charged by external forces. It was an energetic potential that radiated outward, from the devices' emanating "lightning" to their users' expanding muscles. Women's "electrified" bodies were rendered relaxed, soft, beautiful, and often prone. Fully powered, they radiated not an external change but an internal glow. As contextualized by imagery and rhetoric, electric products for women defined a healthy body as one that resisted age and decay and maintained its appeal to the male gaze.[132] This gender distinction would endure until challenged by products like the I-ON-A-CO, which combined the power of internal, youthful vibrations with the charge of a vigorous, visible belt.

Henry Gaylord Wilshire's I-ON-A-CO: "Plugging in" to the Modern Era

In 1926, roughly twenty San Franciscans gathered in an office on the city's Powell Street. In a photograph, they appear to be a middle-class cross section: ranging in age from thirty to sixty, white, and properly

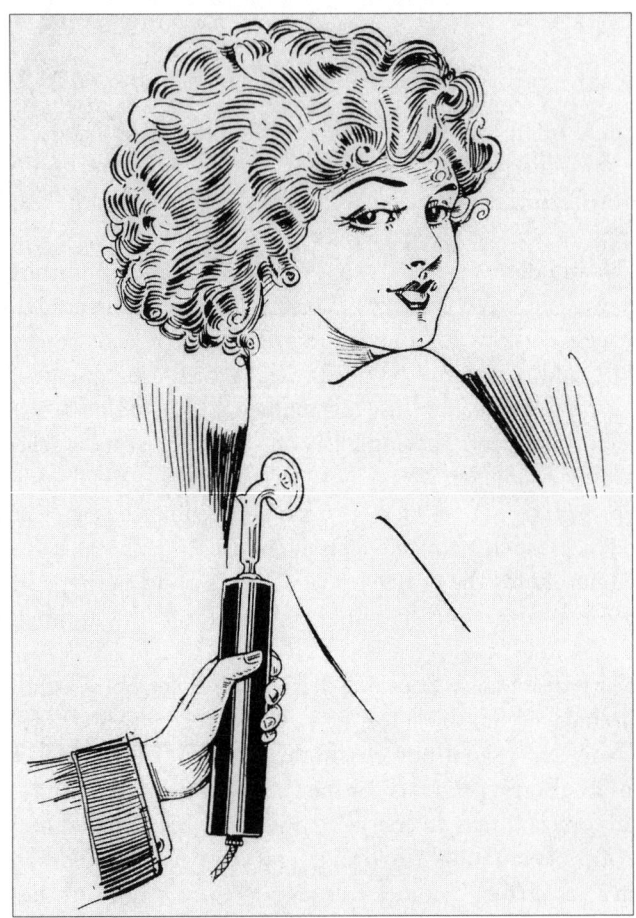

Fig. 20. Demonstrating the Violet Ray to prospective buyers. "Rogers' Violet Ray" (Rogers Electric Labs, ca. 1910), ephemera collection. Courtesy of the Bakken Library and Museum of Electricity in Life, Minneapolis.

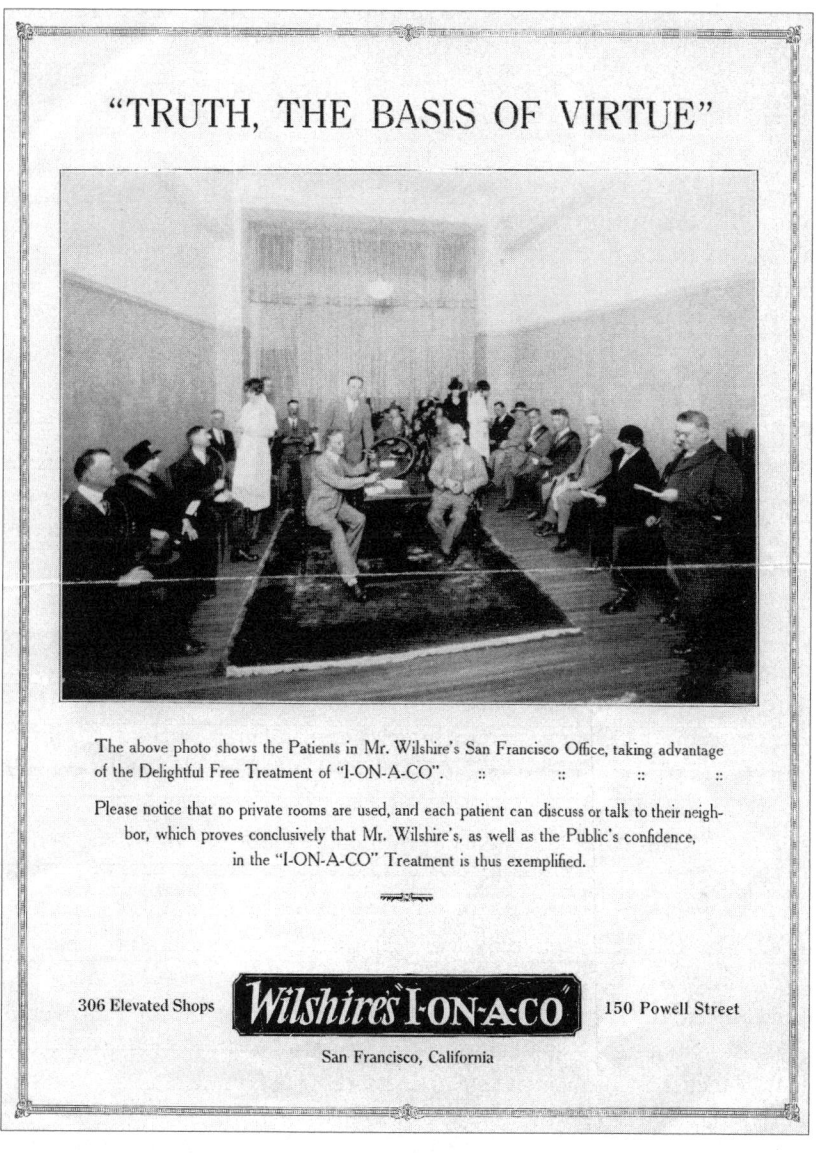

Fig. 21. "Truth, the Basis of Virtue," advertisement for Wilshire's I-ON-A-CO, San Francisco. Wilshire I-ON-A-CO correspondence, p. 2, The Iona Company, folder 0403-13. Courtesy of the American Medical Association Archives.

dressed (fig. 21).[133] Were it not for the women, one might incorrectly suppose a meeting of Rotarians had come there to be treated with the new I-ON-A-CO, a device that reportedly cured disease by electrically magnetizing the body's iron. It was a scene repeated from Los Angeles to Rochester between 1925 and 1930. Bringing with them diseases confirmed and suspected, men and women assembled in the hope that Gaylord Wilshire, explorer, entrepreneur, and failed statesman could extend his Midas touch to the body with three hundred feet of tightly wound magnetic coil.

The I-ON-A-CO consisted of about three and a half dollars' worth of insulated wire in a coil eighteen inches in diameter covered with hard leather. It looked like a cross between a steering wheel and a harness; its nickname, "horse collar," derived from the latter, suggesting the appeal of nostalgia in a rapidly modernizing age. Simple to use, the I-ON-A-CO required no electrical knowledge beyond the ability to plug its cord into an outlet. One could easily confirm that it worked. A secondary coil connected to a miniature light bulb that lit up when the device was in use. Adding nothing to the device's operation, the bulb "showed" the person being treated an otherwise unobservable force.[134] Once the bulb lit up, signaling that the device was ready, users placed the collar over their shoulders for the recommended daily ten-minute treatment.

The I-ON-A-CO presents an interesting challenge to the traditional trajectories of American popular electrotherapeutics. The vast majority of products that could be purchased from nonlicensed physicians, including electric belts and "oxy" products, had been dismissed by the 1920s as "fakes." One would assume from the American Medical Association's extensive records of its efforts to shut down irregular manufacturers that it had succeeded by 1920. By then, the AMA had been paying a professional prosecutor for decades to investigate numerous irregular electrotherapists. From his Chicago office, Arthur Cramp had answered citizens' letters to the associations' experts, always with a negative reply as to the curative powers of electric devices. He had also assembled extensive data documenting the false promises made by irregular practitioners, using them in lawsuits charging postal fraud. Cramp had largely been successful; by 1920 few unlicensed electrotherapists could use the mail to sell their wares, and consumers were increasingly mistrustful of unsubstantiated claims. Even so, the public's will to believe was not dead.

Henry Gaylord Wilshire entered the market in 1925, without medical training, promoting a product with few scientific merits. With the help of newspaper advertising and at least sixty agents who went door to door in California, Nebraska, Ohio, Oregon, West Virginia, Kentucky, Florida, and Washington, Wilshire sold in excess of three thousand I-ON-A-COs in the first year.[135] By 1927, he had expanded his operation from its Los Angeles base to twenty-three regional offices.[136] Just before Wilshire died late that year, he was running popular free clinics, placing full-page newspaper advertisements, and hosting coast-to-coast radio health shows.[137] Through the 1930s and 1940s, the I-ON-A-CO continued to draw users. And long after the AMA called Wilshire's death a victory for fraud fighters, imitation products like the Thernoid, Electronet, Magnecoil, Iona-tone, and Restoro continued to be profitable.[138]

Much about the I-ON-A-CO is curious. The device had less medicinal value than electric belts. The latter, by running on galvanic batteries, at least produced a perceptible electrical current. The I-ON-A-CO's low electrical charge generated neither vibration nor heat after its initial two-minute warm-up. It purportedly worked primarily not by changing the body but by infusing it with electromagnetic current which sped circulation and cured disease. Further, Wilshire's device lacked the theoretical possibilities of Sanche's Electropoise, which seemed similar to ozone, a substance that actually did exist. Yet even with a sixty-dollar price tag, the I-ON-A-CO was more popular than the Electropoise and outsold many competing electric belts.[139]

No single factor can explain the I-ON-A-CO's improbable success. The following factors, however, all contributed to it. Audiences were primed with forty years of electrotherapy promotion. Wilshire's advertising was extensive and sophisticated. Theories of magnetism had been circulating for a century. In addition, Wilshire himself represented a modern source of creative energy, the entrepreneur who was rapidly changing the face of urban life. But beyond all these, however, lies one explanation: the user's interaction with the machine itself. The first thing a user did with the I-ON-A-CO was to plug it in. The electric current flowed into two coils. One lit up a light bulb, the other powered the person. The effect of this physical electrical connection should not be underestimated.[140]

Wilshire seems an unlikely person to have devoted his last years to promoting an electric cure-all. Born in Cincinnati in 1861, he grew up surrounded by successful industrial entrepreneurs. His father had enjoyed high standing as a bank president and had grown wealthy as one of the original investors in Standard Oil. Wilshire's cousins experienced similar successes: one became president of Fleischman's Yeast; another, president of a large coal company.[141] Wilshire applied his business savvy to an unusual series of careers. After briefly studying economics at Harvard, and without a diploma, he set out for Los Angeles, where he pursued his theory that capitalism and socialism could coexist. Arguably, his success in the promotion of an electric cure-all was the perfect marriage of the opposing philosophies: he dreamt of wealth by bringing health to the masses.

When Wilshire arrived in Los Angeles in the late 1880s, it was a capitalist's frontier. He was able to buy immense tracts of land for relatively little money following the first southern California boom and bust. Most of the land lay between Los Angeles and the Pacific; other scattered holdings would later become Orange County. For several years he occupied himself with real estate. Long before Ford's Model T would make automotive travel the norm, Wilshire bought billboards and arranged to have them placed alongside the region's first highways. He also engaged in city planning by founding the town of Fullerton, turning hundreds of acres of unpopulated orange groves into a center for industry and commerce. Wilshire would become best known for commercial developments, including the downtown Los Angeles shopping district that would be known as Wilshire Boulevard. Its pricey shops, multilane thoroughfares, and first parking lots attracted tourists from all over the world.

Had Wilshire's only goal been to get rich in real estate, his life would have been a success story. Yet, his utopian schemes, some more successful than others, made it difficult to lionize him as a capitalist "founding father." He ran, unsuccessfully, for Congress on the Socialist ticket numerous times over a twenty-year period, financing his own campaigns. He kept company with radicals and progressives, among them William Morris, Havelock Ellis, H. G. Wells, George Bernard Shaw, George Sterling, and Upton Sinclair.[142] In the late 1890s, when his real estate profits grew substantial, he founded *Wilshire's Magazine*, a forum for his socialist opinions and those of his friends. At the age of sixty-four in 1925, he put the remainder of his fortune at the service of the I-ON-A-CO.

Wilshire apparently based the I-ON-A-CO on the work of a German biologist who had discovered that the body's iron helps tissue absorb oxygen and regenerate. Drawing a connection between this new information and theories of magnetism, Wilshire arrived at his theory: in a fashion similar to nineteenth-century magnetic treatments, electricity could create a ring of magnetic force around the body.[143] Within the ring, the body's iron would be compelled to greater action, thereby speeding up the cat-alyzation process and increasing the body's absorption of healthy oxygen. Absent the increased magnetic effect, which only the I-ON-A-CO could produce, the body suffered from what he called "auto toxemia," a disease caused by poisons trapped in the tissues.[144]

There is some evidence to suggest that Wilshire had more faith in his belt's ability to generate a profit than to effect a cure, but he seems to have made his claims largely in earnest.[145] Not only did he ask some of his clos-est friends, including George Sterling and Upton Sinclair, to risk their rep-utations by endorsing his product, he himself did so in extensive radio broadcasts and speaking tours.[146]

The close association of developer and product undoubtedly ac-counted for much of the I-ON-A-CO's improbable success. Unlike other electrotherapy promoters, Wilshire remained the front man for his oper-ation throughout the three years he promoted it. He appeared on radio shows and in demonstrations in most towns where he ran newspaper ad-vertisements, augmenting the printed word with his own reputation.[147] If advertising material is any indication, his radio shows reminded listeners that this was no ordinary product: it was the healing discovery of Gay-lord Wilshire, described by one advertisement as "originator of the Fa-mous Wilshire Boulevard of Los Angeles" who now "Revolutionizes Treatment of Disease."[148]

Wilshire was a master at attracting a crowd. He typically drew up-wards of 150 people to his frequent lectures at Los Angeles hotels like the Fairmont and the Biltmore.[149] Further, even those who had not antici-pated attending a Wilshire demonstration often found themselves in the thick of one. During a 1925 food exposition at the Ambassador Hotel, for example, Wilshire was reported as having convinced "thousands" to try his device by touting it as a five-minute-rejuvenation session. He did not mention later how many actually purchased his device at the exposi-tion, but stated that the vast majority had left "completely restored to their original vitality."[150]

If Wilshire's reputation gave his product its legitimacy, his treatment centers gave it exposure. Other belt manufacturers had relied exclusively on local advertising and salespeople; Wilshire added street-front therapy centers to the mix. These spaces in Pasadena, Seattle, and Portland of-fered prospective I-ON-A-CO buyers a place to try a treatment in a vari-ety of ways.[151] The tentative prospect could test the device with the help of a trained salesperson. There was no obligation to purchase, but there were payment options. More important, patients could come for weekly or daily I-ON-A-CO treatments without having to purchase their own device.

The centers make it possible to argue that the I-ON-A-CO affected far more people than sales records might suggest. It enjoyed healthy sales between 1925 and 1927, often more than 8,000 a month. This figure, however, pales in comparison to the number of people treated.[152] The Pasadena office, for example, reported selling 26 belts in March 1926 and administering 539 treatments.[153] Using this ratio of sales to treatments as an average, and assuming that as many as half of the 539 treatments were given to repeat customers, we can estimate that for the 8,000-plus belts purchased nationally each month, 80,000 individuals received I-ON-A-CO treatments. In other words, nearly one million people came into direct contact with Wilshire's device during that one year, a figure of far more consequence than the 96,000 belts purchased.[154]

What is significant about the figure is not merely that millions of Americans wrapped themselves inside an I-ON-A-CO coil and "plugged in." The centers provided not only the means for electrical treatments but, more important, a context in which the treatments could be understood. Home users were free to interact with the I-ON-A-CO as they chose; people treated in centers had carefully controlled experiences. Simply by entering a center, they situated the imminent physical experience within the context of the surrounding urban world. Once they sat down to undergo the treatment, a salesperson familiarized them with Wilshire's theories, making sure that they understood that any physical benefit they received would be due to the surrounding electrical current. Further, during their five or ten minutes with the device draped over their shoulders, there were few distractions and ample opportunity to watch fellow citizens "plugged in." Many probably took note of the cord running from their bodies to the nearest electrical outlet. Whether they believed themselves cured after such treatments or not, the connection between electrical energy and physical energy had been intimately reinforced. And when one factors in the centers' urban locations, it is easy to imagine the treatments as subtly reinforcive of the compatibility of urban development, electrical energy, and the vigorous body.

Whether the centers influenced their reactions, I-ON-A-CO consumers, male and female, praised the device to a greater degree than users had praised previous electrotherapy devices. The accolades varied in intensity, from that of a Mrs. Wolford who in 1926 told a son the I-ON-A-CO was "doing wonders for people" in California to that of E. K. Cassab, fruit grower and melon namesake, who declared himself unwilling to part with his I-ON-A-CO for ten thousand dollars.[155] Individuals wrote to the American Medical Association in response to articles in the *Journal of the American Medical Association* and *Hygeia* warning against Wilshire's fraudulent devices. Many claimed to have been cured of physical and psychological ailments, including hemorrhoids, stiff necks, goiter, earaches, vision problems, and nervousness.[156] There is every reason to believe that the I-ON-A-CO cured people. Not only were people buying contrary to the advice of medical experts, they were defending their actions to those very experts. Margorie Speed, a teacher and university graduate, found *Hygeia*'s warning inaccurate and insulting, complaining to its editors that the article "smells to high heaven with the stench of hidebound smuggosity and narrow-mindedness." After months of visits to doctors to cure a sore throat, Speed's mother had been cured in three short I-ON-A-CO treatments. In the opinion of this user, doctors who condemned the device were simply afraid to admit that their competition did have medicinal value.[157]

Speed was probably correct. Physicians had every reason to fear this fast-selling placebo that would not die. Thirty years after the first campaigns against electric belt manufacturers, the American Medical Association was still fighting a battle to prove that low-level and no-level electrical treatments were ineffective. Physician Anna G. Lyle of California, for one, roundly dismissed Wilshire's device without firsthand knowledge of it or its patients. After a year of hearing about its cures, in 1926, Lyle wrote the Association's fraud division that the device was pure "hokum": without medical value and administered by storefront technician. "Who could foresee that 'I-on-a-co' would so fire the imagination of the medieval-minded multitudes that they would cease celebrating, slip their necks into a noose, turn on an ordinary light-switch, and claim to be cured of every known ailment from cancer to catarrh?"[158]

Lyle's rhetoric reflects the dichotomy physicians saw between electric science and electric superstition. Her use of the word "noose" suggests that she believed I-ON-A-CO buyers were dangerously duped. While they thought they were being made well, they were actually facilitating their own demise, literally from the ailment left untreated and financially from the money paid. To Lyle, the whole I-ON-A-CO success story merely affirmed that ignorant producers and "medieval-minded" consumers were well matched. Neither seemed able to distinguish between therapeutic electricity and an "ordinary light switch."

Lyle thoroughly dismissed the I-ON-A-CO without disproving its effectiveness. There was no room in the minds of professional physicians to even speculate that the I-ON-A-CO might somehow cure. Scholars also have deemed Wilshire and other electric product purveyors conscious of their deception, and eager to prey upon an ignorant and gullible public.[159] This is to believe, as well, that people like Speed and Dr. A. G. Emerson of the Las Vegas tuberculosis facility who asked, in 1926, to become a salesman for the "great" device, were either lying or mistaken.[160] The AMA's collection of folder upon folder of letters from people who had heard of the device's effectiveness suggest that many had witnessed their own reasons to believe.

Although electromagnetic currents are not sufficient to cure major diseases, the I-ON-A-CO's light electric massage, if applied directly to accupoints, could have remedied minor ailments like fatigue, hemorrhoids, goiter, earaches, stiff necks, and sore throats. Electric massagers continue to be marketed to ease tired feet and increase circulation. Electrodes, applied directly to affected muscles and tendons, are used by physicians to alleviate chronic pain and tendonitis. TENS, or transcutaneous electrical nerve stimulation, machines are available in the United States and Europe to ease the contraction pain of women in labor. With its low-level electromagnetic current, the I-ON-A-CO lacked the force of current medicinal devices. As a result, it did not have the ability to relieve intense pain or permanently cure a condition; it may, however, have been sufficient in some cases to temporarily relieve a patient's suffering.[161]

What Lyle was reacting to was probably not the idea that the I-ON-A-CO or any other electric product could help ease minor ailments but its portrayal as a miraculous cure-all in the press and in popular culture. Her refusal to recognize the possibility that it might have some health benefit is illustrative of the immense threat licensed physicians perceived. In 1926, when American physicians had been regularly licensed for little over a decade, Lyle might have been recalling when mail-order "degrees" were available to anyone with ten dollars and postage. There was no room for a medical professional to concede that an unlicensed, former real estate mogul turned health expert could offer a product that did some bodies some good some of the time.

In so quickly dismissing the claims of Wilshire's followers, physicians also overlooked the possibility that belief can cure.[162] The I-ON-A-CO has never been proven to cure any ailment, let alone "every known ailment," but for some users simply connecting their bodies to an electric outlet—the 1920s technological equivalent of hooking oneself to mechanized Zander systems—may have been enough to inspire them into recovery.

For many other users, the Wilshire device may have worked, at least in small increments, because Wilshire said it did. Promotional material actively countered doubts by reminding readers that this product was only one in a long line of technological marvels. "Naturally all of this seems beyond belief," a brochure told readers, "but the radio, sending winged words around the world, the airplane, carrying Byrd to the North Pole, would have been beyond belief a few years ago."[163] In a world changing so quickly, who was to say what was possible or probable where the body was concerned? It was a time of amazing inventions from heroic men like Volta, Edison, Ford, and the Wright brothers. Wilshire, it seemed, was just another link in the chain, a man who built a metropolis out of the desert and envisioned the highway before Ford. It was wholly plausible, then, that he could invigorate the body through a power outlet. It is also plausible that Wilshire counted on this "mental effect" as an important component in an I-ON-A-CO cure. His wife, Mary McReynolds Wilshire, was an eminent psychoanalyst during the years of the device's popularity. The correlation suggests that Wilshire would have been well informed on the relationship between psychological and physical health.[164]

By 1930, it was possible for middle-class men and women to frame their bodies in the center of a powerful electric future. Generations of regular and irregular electric medicine had promised the body a position of primacy over efficient machines. Electric medicine contextualized the body and the world it would inhabit in the modern era. For some, the experience took place in physicians' offices; for some, it occurred via inherited magnetic machines or during street-corner electric demonstrations; for others it was felt through electric belts, oxygenators, or I-ON-A-COs.

When electric lights began to turn night into day, electric machines promised to cure disease. When electric machines began to increase industrial and domestic production, electric belts and electric oxygenators promised to help the body keep up the pace. Even the modern cityscape, with its electric streetcars and electric consumer palaces, symbolized the body's potential, a lesson one might have reinforced after an afternoon on Wilshire's miracle mile followed by a rejuvenating session with his I-ON-A-CO. The body was not left behind in the rush toward electric modernization. To the contrary, it was now the recipient of an "energy transfer," an actual infusion of energy produced outside the body and ingested for productive gain. There was reason to believe in the limitless energetic future of modern men and their machines.

4

Powering the Intimate Body

For many American men early in the twentieth century, their most intimate moment with technology came while wearing an electric belt. This is not to say that electric belts were the only products to necessitate close contact between technological materials and human bodies; I-ON-A-CO collars embraced their users; Oxygenators slid under women's clothing, clamped around skin, and pressed metal to flesh. The experience of contact, however, was not the same. Whereas collars and oxygenators "held" body parts one might share publicly, belts, as well as electric prostate massagers, treated private body parts. By surrounding the penis and scrotum with low-level electric currents, and massaging the prostate with electric power, these devices inserted technology into the intimate body, uniting modern man, sexual vigor, and electrical power.

Rachael Maines has argued that American women used electric technology for sexual satisfaction during the early twentieth century. Her work reveals that women purchased and used vibrators to masturbate, effectively rebelling against inadequate male partners and a social imperative to put men's sexual satisfaction above their own. Although numerous women undoubtedly did realize that "medical vibrators" could be used to reach orgasm, medical literature, product promotional material, and archival materials tell us that women were not the primary benefactors of technological sexual enhancements.[1] Invigorating sexual performance with electric currents was largely a male domain.

There was something particularly American about the marketing of electric belts. In Britain, belts sought a market composed equally of men and women; in the United States, the vast majority of advertisements were aimed at men. Belts for women, as with Violet Rays and the Electropoise, were usually placed within the context of accepted gender roles. As a result, nineteenth-century women could find electric belts that looked much like men's, but most belts appeared closer to corsets. Such products claimed to increase energy, but did so within a restrictive, energy-depleting costume. One scholar has supposed that the difference is due to America's "less matriarchal society"; a careful consideration of gender dynamics and consumer materials reveals a different reason.[2]

Between the late nineteenth century and the Great Depression, products that promised to improve men's sex drive and performance flooded the American marketplace. Many, such as pneumatic penis enlargers, functioned without outside power sources.[3] Yet the most enduring products, some of which sold in the hundreds of thousands over a thirty-year period, were those that used electric technology. One might dismiss artifacts such as galvanic suspensory belts and prostate massagers as novelty items, examples of sexually stimulating or perhaps humorous applications of technology. That view, however, is decidedly anachronistic. Men turned to electrical products because they promised a modern solution to a modern sexual problem. Electricity's perceived ability to "transfer" energetic power into the body solved three crises in contemporary male sexual performance: masturbatory depletion, perceived sexual inadequacy, and glandular limits. In an age that demanded increased virility in the boardroom and bedroom, many men found themselves physically unfit for the task. By infusing their bodies with electric technology, men could redefine normal sexual performance while concurrently "normalizing" electric power.

The Seed of Modernity: Why the Penis Must Be Powered

In the late nineteenth century, the Pulvermacher Galvanic Company sold belts of varying sizes and shapes to men and women. Its brochures stressed the benefits of attaching around one's waist a set of coils connected to a galvanic battery to achieve increased physical energy, relief from a series of illnesses, and clearer mental states. To say that Pulvermacher was an equal-opportunity manufacturer, however, would not be true. For each advertisement that specifically marketed belts to women there were roughly four aimed at men. When read as a compilation of images and text, the advertisements consciously promoted Pulvermacher's product as capable of creating a new man by electrically powering his genitals. The key to this interpretation is the suspensory sack, an optional accessory to the belt. The appliance was a light-metal woven pouch that, when connected by clips to the lower part of the belt, surrounded the

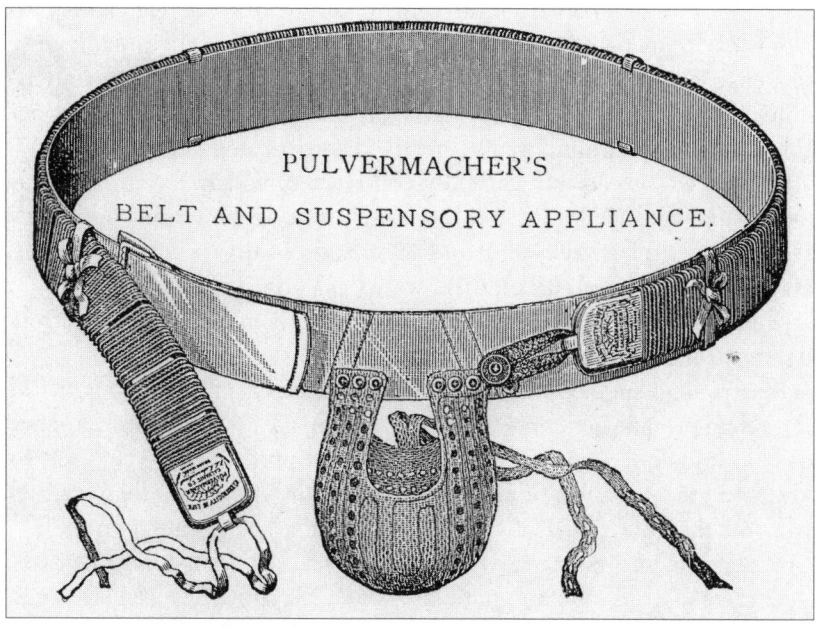

Fig. 22. The early Pulvermacher belt. "Pulvermacher's Belt and Suspensory Appliance," 26, ephemera collection. Courtesy of the Bakken Library and Museum of Electricity in Life, Minneapolis.

penis and testicles with galvanic current (fig. 22). As an artifact, the appliance lends itself to multiple interpretations. It could have been used as a reinforcement weapon to fight the same general debility that the belt did; with more of the body's surface exposed to the wires, perhaps, there was a greater opportunity for it to absorb healing currents. However, the appliance's location suggests a more complex rationale. Pulvermacher could have sold upper-thigh attachments just as easily, perhaps following the lines of Sanche's ankle cuffs. They would have provided even more of a surface area "infusion," had this been what Pulvermacher was after.

A further clue to the connection between the electrified penis and the healthy male body lies in textual description. In a late-nineteenth-century advertisement, Pulvermacher told prospective purchasers that the suspensory attachment's efficacy lay in its ability to cure "nervous and general debility, lost vigor, decline, and the whole train of gloomy attendants."[4] The description leaves a modern reader confused; how are these symptoms any different from the general fatigue that the belt claimed to cure for both men and women? The answer lies in the intentionally gray area ensconced in terms like "lost vigor," "decline," and "gloomy attendants." Americans of the time rarely directly discussed sexual dysfunction. Descriptions of impotence, erectile disorders, and lack of sexual desire appeared instead in a carefully constructed, widely recognized, and coded language. We know that the terms "vim, vigor, virility, and vitality," when used between 1850 and 1930, almost always referred to sexual power.[5] The attachments, then, were explicitly aimed at men who desired to reach beyond general electric transfer to enhance sexual performance through technology.

Illustrations suggest that using the suspensory appliance would do more than provide better erections; it would make the entire body a more visibly masculine terrain. It is significant that illustrations were used to advertise the appliance; typically they cost more to include than written text. Yet the advertising of each of the leading belt manufacturers featured sizeable images of male bodies wearing electric belts. In some cases these were clinical, diagrammatic half torsos to show proper belt placement. More often, they were full figures of male bodies being powered by belts and attachments (fig. 23). What is striking, however, is how little the advertisements focus on the galvanic product itself. The majority highlight instead a naked, visibly muscular body and allow the reader to make the connection between this "product" and the one ostensibly being sold. One first notices, for example, the strong arms and muscular thighs and buttocks of Pulvermacher's belt model before noticing the belt around his waist and genitals. Most belt advertisements feature a variation of this or a more overtly "virile" illustration, such as Dr. Sanden's, where the model, shown from the back, flexes his shoulder and arm muscles, clutching what appears to be a spear for some undisclosed purpose, all while receiving visible electric current from the waist and neck (fig. 24).

These images differ dramatically from accepted nineteenth-century presentations of the male body. As discussed in chapter 1, illustrated men were typically clothed and, mirroring their actual appearance, small in stature. These belt images, then, evoked ideals of the male body, not as most men who might purchase products were but as they hoped to be. Yet rather than suggesting that men lift weights or perform a localized muscular exercise that might create idealized bodies, the makers suggested instead that men electrify their genitals. That advertisements made electricity instead of muscular exercise the source of physique building was not

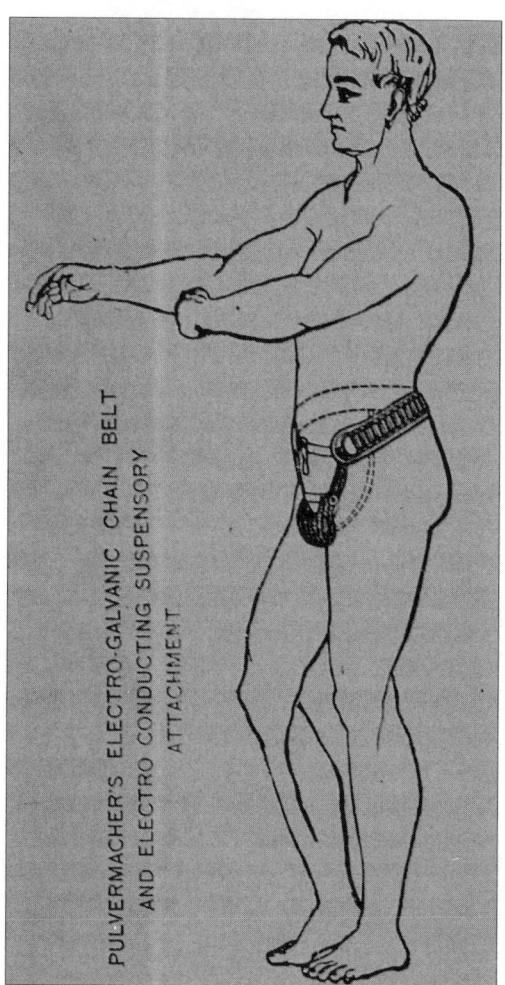

PULVERMACHER'S ELECTRO-GALVANIC CHAIN BELT
AND ELECTRO CONDUCTING SUSPENSORY
ATTACHMENT

Fig. 23. Demonstrating how to wear the Pulvermacher belt. "The Only Rational Means for Self-Cure," Pulvermacher Electro-Galvanic Belts, 27, ephemera collection. Courtesy of the Bakken Library and Museum of Electricity in Life, Minneapolis.

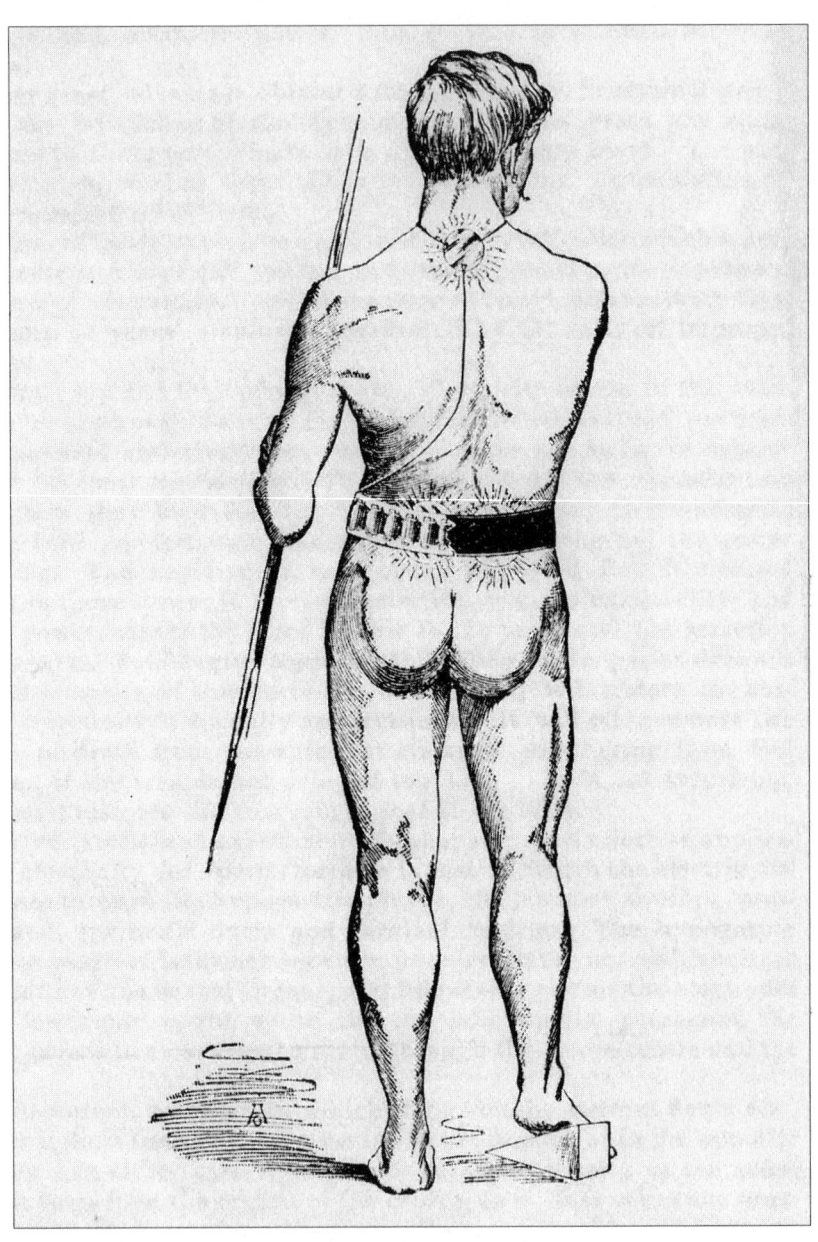

Fig. 24. Advertising the electric belt to prospective consumers. Brochure, Dr. A. T. Sanden (ca. 1910), 68, ephemera collection. Courtesy of the Bakken Library and Museum of Electricity in Life, Minneapolis.

surprising: by 1900, most people were cognizant of the fact that building a powerful body with weights or machines took hard work, dedication, and more than a bit of discomfort.[6] Given the other option, building muscle painlessly and almost effortlessly with electricity must have seemed attractive. This insight, however, does not explain why the genitals in particular were the recipients of electrically induced strength. We can only assume that there was a connection that readers would have understood, or been willing to learn, between powerful genital function and overall physical power or presence.

A careful reading of the historical evidence reveals that electric belts, precisely because they promised to improve erectile performance by infusing the penis with electrical power, promised to make men more powerful figures in the modern world. The muscular figures in advertisements were merely external symbols of the internal power that the belt wearer would possess. As the illustration from Dr. Sanden suggests, the electrified penis became a catalyst for the modernization of masculinity, one that could throw off nineteenth-century inefficiencies and meet twentieth-century demands.

Holding Back the Vital Force: Nineteenth-Century Impotence and Masturbation

As late as the nineteenth century, American physicians believed that women's bodies and minds were held captive by their reproductive functions. Hysteria, defined as a physiological disorder, was believed to be caused by the detachment of a woman's womb. Unmoored from its usual location, it traveled through the body wreaking havoc, causing normal women to behave in an extraordinary manner.[7] Women, though, were not the only ones believed to suffer psychological consequences from genital malfunction. For men, the malaise was impotence, an ill-defined diagnosis based on a collection of symptoms ranging from weakness and mental confusion to unsatisfying sexual performance.

Impotence has probably existed as long as there have been men. When one considers the physiological and psychological complexity of maintaining an erection, combined with a sufferer's reluctance to discuss his perceived "inadequacies," it is clear that impotence has long created a fraternity of silent sufferers. In the late nineteenth century those ranks swelled, challenging the silence and leading medical experts to declare an epidemic in their midst.

According to one American physician, impotence had become so common by the 1880s that "the ideal condition of virility [was] somewhat rare . . . and in any given case it will generally last for but a short time."[8] Among the men who sought help, physicians found two types. The first were those who suffered because of physical causes such as illness or venereal disease; its numbers were not on the rise. It was the second type that physicians singled out for the increase in reported cases. These individuals suffered from "psychic impotence," or what British physician James Paget called "sexual hypochondriasis." One physician, when comparing such men to the men affected with physical impotence, declared that "the former constitute a large portion of those applying for relief."[9] Paget told colleagues in the late 1870s that there was actually a pyramid of impotence sufferers: at its top were the most rare cases, men who suffered impotence caused by physical problems. Next down and more common, were men who suffered from impotence caused by nervous disorders and mental defects. At the bottom, in the most populous category, were men who suffered from impotence "complained of or dreaded" without cause.[10]

The definitive study of male sexual dysfunction has yet to be published. Nonetheless, we can use contemporary medical and advice literature to speculate that fears about masturbation's effects played a large part in convincing men that they possessed inadequate sexual power. If we consider impotence in the way it was defined by many of its sufferers, as a general loss of physical power, it makes sense to look to masturbation as a primary perceived cause. Experts throughout the nineteenth century warned young men of the dangers inherent in the vice and found ready audiences for their baleful predictions. In 1835, the Reverend John Todd published his *Student's Manual,* which went through seven editions in the next two years; by 1854, it had reached the twenty-fourth. Its chapter on "onanism," or masturbation, which stressed that the practice would lead to intellectual and physical ills, influenced many young men's attitudes toward their bodies. One physician, Dr. Gardner, considered himself among the "thousands [who] now live to thank this conscientious teacher" for lessons on avoiding a habit worse than tobacco and alcohol, substances not "so potent to rob man of all the high prerogatives of manhood, as this, humiliating, self-abasing vice."[11]

The connective thread between masturbation and physical decline thickened in the 1850s, when, like Dr. Gardner, physicians emerged ready to add the sanctity of science to earlier admonitions from ministers. This new group of decline harbingers transformed what had previously been a humiliating and self-abasing practice into a certain ticket to debility and death. One can partly attribute the shift to a cultural theory of scarcity that emerged in the mid-nineteenth century, which, in its various manifestations, encouraged conservation of natural resources, financial reserves, and physical energy.[12]

By the 1850s, physicians had supplanted preachers as the leading antimasturbation crusaders as concerns over the state of one's internal reserves became a more pressing question than the state of one's soul. Why this was so is hinted at by reformers like Frederick Hollick, an expert on sexuality and physiology, who could confidently declare by 1850, "[N]ervous substance and seminal fluid are . . . essentially the same thing."[13] The theory, commonly called "seminal economy," encouraged by reformers from Sylvester Graham to Henry Beecher, elevated the importance of seminal fluid beyond its role in procreation.[14] Ejaculatory fluid became life force, a precious substance to be lost only for the societal imperative of reproduction.[15] As its protector, the penis thus became a physical symbol of vital masculine energy.

Arguably, the theory of seminal economy created two imperatives for the man who would call himself healthy by the turn of the century. First, he would have to abstain from all sexual activity other than procreation. Masturbation was the worst waste of one's vital force, but gratuitous sex was not much better. Second, he would have to cultivate as much sexual force as possible to guarantee a strong vital reserve of energy for daily activities. Such a mandate would be difficult enough if young men had merely to make it through puberty before finding a marriage partner and beginning a sanctioned sexual life. Yet as Anthony Rotundo points out, late-nineteenth-century middle-class men married on average at age thirty, typically ten to fifteen years after puberty.[16] The sequence almost inevitably entwined men in a cycle of guilt and fear. Because they believed masturbation drained vital fluid, causing illnesses ranging from neurasthenia to insanity, those who masturbated, even once, often believed themselves permanently susceptible to such ills. Consequently, men of all ages and classes had reason to gauge physical or sexual weakness by the state of their semen supply.

Electrifying the Penis: A Modern Cure for a Victorian Malaise

Early physicians who experimented with electricity in their practices did not use it to treat sexual dysfunction. Long after inventions such as the Leyden jar and galvanic currents had brought electric therapies to physicians' offices and to private homes, electricity remained a tool more for general than sexual health. In 1863, one of the primary electrical texts in the field, Alfred Garratt's *Electro-Physiology and Electro-Therapeutics*, listed twenty-three conditions appropriately treated with the current.[17] Sexual dysfunction was not among them.

The situation began to change in the 1870s, when the first electric treatments for impotence appeared in the form of galvanic baths. George Schweig, a New York physician, was known for his galvanic treatments, in which patients were placed in tubs of water with electrodes submerged below the surface. The treatments, which lasted for several minutes, were given up to six times a week. They generated the first testimonials to electricity's impotence-curing powers, if we are to believe Schweig's text. One thirty-two-year-old man declared that before his treatments he "was able to perform the marital act at rare intervals only, and when he did, felt exhausted the whole of the succeeding day." After his sixth galvanic bath, he found his sexual power restored.[18]

By the 1880s, numerous physicians had begun to treat impotence with locally applied electric currents. Two of the most prominent, both for their practice and their writings, were Alphonso Rockwell and George Beard. Rockwell was one of the first to do so. In 1874, he described his typical treatments for spermatorrhoea and seminal emissions, conditions associated with impotence: a mixture of local galvanization, involving direct contact between the penis, scrotum, and an electric current, and central galvanization, whereby an electric current was applied to the entire body.[19] It is significant that Rockwell used both local and central galvanization in his treatments. Assuming that he shared his partner Beard's philosophy about the relationship between electricity, physical energy, and sexual dysfunction, Rockwell probably believed that impotence was more often than not a symptom of general energy depletion rather than the nucleus of a unique disease.

In George Beard's professional opinion, a man suffering from neurasthenia was a man suffering from sexual dysfunction. Famous for his diagnoses of this "civilized" disease that left modern men and women without sufficient physical energy to make it through a typical day, Beard's placement of the penis at the center of male physical decline has been oddly overlooked. Clearly, his fellow physicians paid attention to the connection. In a paper read to them at the New York Academy of Medicine, Beard recalled a typical treatment session for a neurasthenic: "When he first consulted me, I inquired into the condition of the genito-urinary system, as I always do in all cases of neurasthenia, not that it is the sole cause, but a very frequent cause of these troubles, or at least a complication of them."[20]

Beard's theory that the sexual organs were nearly always the source of nervous exhaustion was widely accepted by his contemporaries.[21] Physician C. L. Dana treated all reported cases of men's nervous weakness as veiled references to impotence. He typically initiated neurasthenia treatments with a special zinc cylinder filled with weak alcohol. Designed to fit over the penis, the cylinder was connected to the negative end of an electrode and the positive end was placed on the spine. If a man followed the regimen three times a day, Dana asserted, the general weakness would soon disappear.[22]

M. J. Grier, a respected American electrotherapist, expanded on the underlying connection between neurasthenia and male sexual dysfunction in a paper read before the American Electro-Therapeutic Association in 1891. It was up to the physician, he remarked, to see through the façade of incomplete symptoms that male patients presented. Typically, they "seek relief from a neuralgia, pain in the back, muscular debility, or some other cause leading easily and naturally from the ostensible to the real object of the visit."[23] He found his clients to be a mixture of men suffering from what he called "an appreciable physical failure" and men certain that "such a failure will certainly occur." The true culprit was not the sexual organs, it was the way they had been mishandled through masturbation. In the veiled language commonly used to refer to self-abuse, Grier explained that most patients actually suffered "from excessive and long-continued stimulation of special nerve endings, with consequent exhaustion of the spinal and cerebral centers controlling the parts involved."[24]

By the late-nineteenth century, physicians and patients alike knew the high price that American men paid for sexual urges. The body, limited by finite energy and driven to waste that energy on lust, progressed continually down a path to its own listless demise. By making the genitals the source of male physical power, Victorian culture demanded of men a nearly impossible restraint. The addition of electrotherapies suggested that there might a way to stay healthy without abstinence. As Beard reported and others confirmed, men could be cured of general weakness by taking direct current to their genitals. This combination of physiological and psychological treatment reached the majority of American men outside the boundaries of regular medicine. By purchasing electric belts, men acquired a technology that overturned Victorian theories of restraint and limits.

Electric Belts and the End of Masturbatory Decline

Electrotherapists may have begun to treat impotence by the late-nineteenth century, but the majority of American men suffering from the condition were not knocking on their doors. The reluctance can be explained, in part, by the fact that electrotherapists were often seen as irregular practitioners with ill-gotten diplomas. Yet, this does not explain why impotence treatments were not at least as popular as galvanic treatments for headaches and paralysis. Each was a common condition in men and could be "treated" by electricity equally effectively, meaning that symptoms occasionally could be relieved temporarily by electrical stimulation of the nerves. Admitting that one suffered headaches or paralysis, however, did not carry the same stigma as did admitting a problem with impotence. As neutral diseases, brought on by no doing of the sufferer, headaches and paralysis were occasions for sympathy. Impotence was a public admission of wrongdoing as much as it was a disease. To declare oneself impotent was to disclose two facts, neither likely to build a man's public esteem: he had masturbated at some time in his past, and, as a result, he did not possess the vital power to complete sexual intercourse.

Mail-order impotence remedies allowed men to go incognito for the cure. Many companies successfully manipulated sufferers' reluctance to seek medical help as a marketing tool. Zardon, purveyor of a mysterious nerve-stimulant pill early in the twentieth century, confided to men of "weak or erratic" desires that its experts knew all about sufferers' hesitancy to seek help. Its brochure asked on its front page, "Do you care to have your family physician whisper around that you are not as good a man as you once were? Do you wish to have the druggist laugh at you when getting a prescription filled? Don't you suffer rather than go to them for advice."[25] Belt manufacturers echoed such insider empathy. The German Belt Company sold its suspensory attachment as a completely confidential method for curing impotence. Because of its compact size, the company assured potential purchasers, "[N]o one, not even a person sleeping in the same bed need know you have one on."[26]

At a time when the majority of American men lived in rural areas and small towns, discreet local medical treatment could be an oxymoron. Mail-order remedies, much as on-line prescriptions today, offered a way to circumvent the traditionally busy mouths of small towns. Advertisements reinforced the notion that impotence was seen as a "fault" disease: the family physician would know you had wasted your vital force and the druggist would make fun of your dirty little secret. Were your wife to know, she might wonder about undisclosed indiscretions. Before innovations in printing technology made inexpensive mail advertising possible, most men probably suffered from actual or believed impotence in silence.

In such a climate, electric belts probably seemed a better treatment option than most. Secrecy, however, was not the only reason men purchased electric belts. Had men desired only that, they would have made successes of less expensive pill products like Zardon's. Electric belts became the most popular impotence cure between 1890 and 1920 by offering a unique combination of discretion, diagnoses, and deliverance. In addition to promising to treat impotence so quietly that even one's wife would not know, belt manufacturers defined the illness as a temporary, curable disease. Masturbation need no longer be the cause of permanent debility and lingering guilt; with an occasional electric charge, masturbation could be reimagined as a benign activity that left a man with plenty of energy in reserve.

Defining the Problem and Prescribing the Cure: American Electric Belts

Like physicians, electric belt promoters did not tiptoe around the cause of men's turn-of-the-century weakness. Impotence, declared the Pulvermacher Galvanic Company in an 1876 advertisement, was the clear result of "ruinous and prevalent masturbation among boys."[27] The diagnoses grew more pointed over the next twenty years. In 1901, the German Electric Company explained in its promotional material that "nervous debility is often produced by youthful excesses, but it is unfortunately to the vice of self-pollution . . . that we must in general attribute the moral prostration and physical incapacity now so wide-spread among the men of the present generation."[28] By 1910, Professor Crystal felt sufficiently confident to declare in his own electric belt promotions, "[N]ine out of ten times in men nervous diseases can be attributed to self abuse."[29]

The makers' reasons for identifying masturbation as the cause of ill health were not dramatically different from those of physicians. Both supported the nineteenth-century theory of seminal economy that posited seminal fluid as limited in quantity and identical to nervous force in function. Masturbation, explained Pulvermacher, was a terrible "drain on the vital forces." In one of the more graphic descriptions of depleted seminal economy in action, Pulvermacher declared, "[T]he male excretion embodies forty times more vital force than an equal amount of red blood right from the heart."[30] A male need not have masturbated recently to experience a dramatic energy drain. Most belt manufacturers referred to "youthful indiscretions" when looking for the cause of men's current weakness. "The germ of life, the seed of vitality, has been wasted in the spring time of life," explained Professor Crystal, "when most required for the development of a perfect and unimpaired manhood."[31]

In the aggregate, belt advertisements seem to have intensified fears about masturbation and its attendant debilitating effects. Their descriptions of drained hearts and wasted vitality seeds offered a far more graphic image of the debilitation suffered by masturbators than one was likely to receive from the family doctor. Further, the repeated emphasis on the correlation between masturbating occasionally in one's youth and impotence as an adult probably left men feeling even more helpless. As Professor Crystal told them, there was no returning youthful energy once wasted. As a result of those indiscretions, "the whole constitution has been weakened, the nerve forces enfeebled, [and] the genital organs shrunken."[32] Electric belt promoters provided a physical and moral diagnosis that although somewhat more private than that of the local physician, was hardly more comforting.

There were two fundamental differences between physicians and belt manufacturers: a clear diagnosis and a purchasable cure. Whereas physicians like Rockwell and Beard typically referred to their patients' illnesses using imprecise diagnoses of "masturbatory weakness" or "impotence," belt manufacturers codified specific diseases. In order for prospective customers to diagnose themselves, belt manufacturers described and illustrated specific ailments of the genital area. It was typical for advertising pamphlets to include, along with fancy illustrations of the belts, complete sections on how men might identify the disease by which they suffered according to specific symptoms. A typical reader of the most prominent belt advertisements would come face to face with three main causes of "male fatigue": spermatorrhoea, variocele, and seminal weakness.

Together, the three conditions presented symptoms ranging from those visible to the naked eye to those perceptible by only the sufferer. Spermatorrhoea was the most public of ailments. Described as an excessive secretion and discharge of semen, it was almost always attributed to masturbation during one's youth.[33] Advertisements made little attempt to differentiate between masturbatory ejaculation and nocturnal emissions; any loss of semen for a purpose other than procreation brought a young man one step closer to spermatorrhoea. Belt manufacturers such as Pulvermacher and German Electric stressed that although a man might choose to ignore his weakened state, others could be well aware of it just by observation. Sufferers, explained German Electric, bespoke their solitary vice in pasty skin and dark circles under the eyes, a look described as the "neurasthenic" pallor.[34] Some manufacturers' promotional literature carried entire articles on spermatorrhoea, complete with examples of the detectible pasty look. Pulvermacher's included two images of weakened men along with an article warning that "the eyes and countenances of most men are their own accusers." There was no place to hide from the truth, it warned, when "those black and blue discolorations under and around the eyes" were telling their own story.[35]

Were readers not to see their own condition in those descriptions, they might find a resemblance in varicocele or seminal weakness. Varicocele manifested itself in shrunken testicles, poor genital blood flow, and correspondingly imperfect erections.[36] It was probable that readers saw similarities between their physical condition and advertisements describing lumpy or "wormy" testicles and uneven testicular development; the connection may have convinced many that they had located the source of any present or future sexual shortcomings.

The most prevalent disease described in promotional materials was seminal weakness. It encompassed all general symptoms not covered under the first two. Nervousness, frequent headaches, fatigue, and low spirits were just as indicative that the ailment was present as was impotence. The disease was at once amorphous and specific. Within its etiology, any falling off from a state of perfect, energetic health could be attributed to masturbation. Dr. Sanden's three-stage description, more specific than most, captures the essence of a seminal weakness diagnosis. During the first stage, after infrequent masturbation, a man might feel timid, faint of heart, and uneasy. If he did not stop the practice, the second stage would bring on chronic irritation, urethra relaxation, nervous irritation, and lack of self-confidence. Continued self-abuse would eventuate in a complete "loss of manhood" followed by mania, insanity, and, in extreme cases, "a hurried removal to the confinement of the asylum."[37]

One might assume, at first glance, that these diagnoses would have intensified Victorian antimasturbatory fears while offering little hope for recovery from masturbation's effects. It must have been cold comfort for men who had heard repeatedly during childhood that masturbation was sinful to find it now to be the root of all physical degeneration. A perusal of Pulvermacher's or Dr. Sanden's materials left little doubt that the headache, tiredness, or ill temper one suffered was direct evidence that the antimasturbatory pundits had been right all along: its temporary pleasures were followed by enduring penance. In this way, the materials intensified fears well established in Victorian culture. Further, the graphic details of genital decay in these diagnoses seem not to have left readers much room to believe in quick or complete cures. Most followed a trajectory similar to Sanden's seminal weakness: minor symptoms came first, perhaps not even perceived by the sufferer; more obvious problems followed, such as sexual and psychological dysfunction. The whole process of physical degeneration happened so rapidly, were one to put stock in the promotional material, that one might easily ignore a symptom for a week or two and find the damage beyond repair.

Had belt manufacturers actually promoted this bleak prognosis, they would not have sold very many devices. In reality, their excessive emphasis on serious physical symptoms was meant to clearly identify the problem in order to sell items that cured it. This was a second difference between their treatments and those of physicians. After concluding a long treatise on the evils of advanced varicocele, Pulvermacher told its readers that the disease "can not be cured by supports, trusses, or compresses alone . . . the suffering parts must be subjected to the curative influence of the mild, continuous and prolonged electric currents."[38] Even Sanden, for all his emphasis on the slippery slope of seminal decline, stressed that masturbation's adverse effects appeared as a direct result of not having purchased a Sanden belt. At the onset of ill temper and weakness, "a moderate power Dr. Sanden Electric Belt and Suspensory should be used, for if the evil is not remedied, it passes sooner or later into another form of a greater weakness."[39] It was not, then, masturbation itself that brought the male body into a spiral of decline. The problem stemmed instead from failing to treat the resulting weakness with electric technology. In the world of electric belts, masturbation caused temporary energy depletion, not permanent debilitation. By emphasizing the body's internal balance of energy rather than the inherently sinful nature of the practice itself, makers' advertisements left readers free to take two routes to avoid what many believed to be the automatic illnesses that ensued. They could choose not to masturbate. Or, if it was already too late, they could choose to masturbate and recharge with the electric belt. Although one will not find belts advertised as devices for continually replenishing the energy of a "chronic" masturbator, it can be inferred that only a small leap in logic from the printed material was necessary to arrive at such a conclusion. Pulvermacher's advertisements for its suspensory sack, an electrically charged pouch within which the genitals were placed, underscored that its unique combination of design and electric current made depleted parts whole again: "In our treatment the Suspensory gives the necessary support to the scrotum; at the same time the electric-curative currents, which may be said to envelop the suffering parts, gradually equalize the circulation of blood in the enlarged veins, and effect a permanent cure."[40] German Electric, which promised that its suspensory device "drives out the stagnated blood and completely overcomes the disease," echoed such claims for electricity's efficacy.[41] Sanden made the connection clearer, suggesting that electricity applied to the genitals pulsed through the body combating all of masturbation's ill effects.

> In advanced stages of seminal weakness and nervous and sexual debility, electrical treatment with a steady, strong current pouring into the great nerve-centres and streaming out of them through every nerve and fibre of the body, to the vital organs, the heart, liver, lungs, stomach and kidneys, and to the generative organs, the bladder, seminal vesicles, prostate gland and testicles, renders powerful assistance in restoring the organism to health and vigor.[42]

One could read these advertisements as suggesting that an electrically treated body that masturbated would be more powerful than a normal body that did not. According to Sanden, the belt generates "new life and energy, and tones up the relaxed, weakened and shaky nerves, and gives them vigorous energy. . . . It takes away all that sense of weakness and irritability . . . and arrests the waste of semen and stops the emissions." Users were left with "a new sense of life and vigor." This

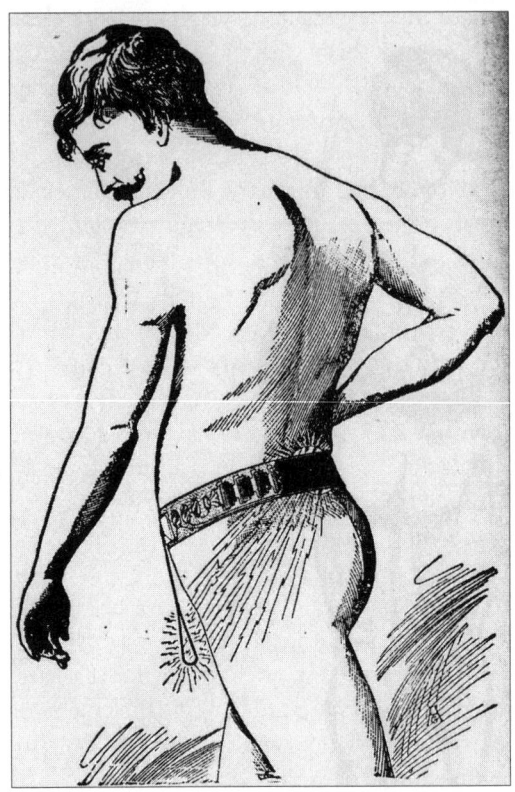

Fig. 25. Demonstrating the source of vigorous
energy. Dr. A.T. Sanden (ca. 1910), 36,
ephemera collection. Courtesy of the Bakken Library and Museum of Electricity in Life, Minneapolis.

rhetoric, combined with illustrations, suggested to readers that electric
treatments might leave one more masculine than even abstinence. The
message could be communicated literally, as in this common example of
the muscular, sexually posed belt wearer whose electrically powered genitals leave little doubt as to the source of his new sexual vigor (fig. 25).[43]
It could also be communicated by figurative images. The allegorical battle on the cover of Edison Jr.'s Magno-Electric Vitalizer shows the muscular, Anglo-appearing body slaying the "natural" body as represented
by the Native American (fig. 26).[44] The image would have been read as

one of many contemporary examples comparing Anglos and Native Americans, whether it was done to celebrate the Anglo ability to combine Native American strength and knowledge with "civilized" values in characters like Edgar Rice Burroughs's Tarzan or to celebrate the defeat of the threatening primitive as "progress" for a modernizing nation.[45] Here we can read the Native American body as symbolizing "nature," a nature that had demanded sexual restraint and energy conservation. With the help of the technology, the Anglo body is shielded from limits. It is noteworthy that this advertisement appeared at the same time that individuals like author and health advocate George Whorton James suggested that Anglos restore vitality by emulating the "primitive" lives of native people. The Vitalizer made it possible to eschew that suggestion; instead,

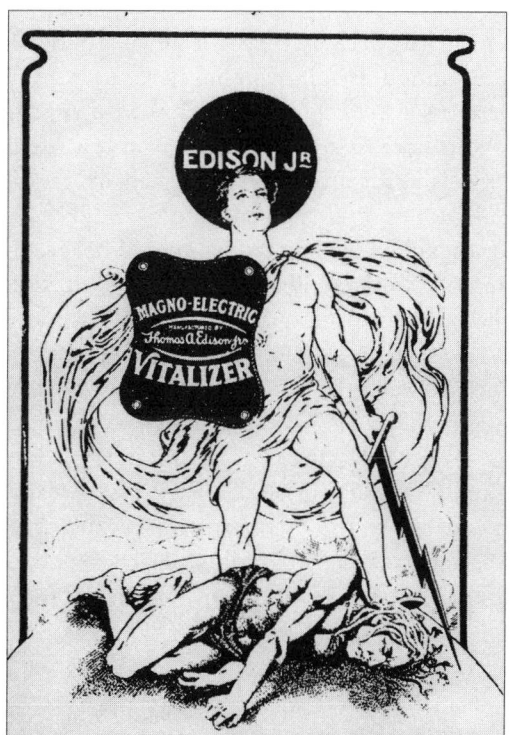

Fig. 26. Killing the Nineteenth Century with Edison's Magno-Electric Vitalizer, ephemera collection. Courtesy of the Bakken Library and Museum of Electricity in Life, Minneapolis.

those who embraced the future of plenty rather than the past of restraint would reign physically supreme.

Defining the illnesses caused by masturbation and allowing clients to treat themselves with electricity allowed belt manufacturers to do two things for users. First, they took masturbation out of its position as a sinful, degenerative practice that left permanent ill effects upon its practitioner. By defining masturbation's effects as specific diseases with clear symptoms, manufacturers allowed clients to identify whether they were sufferers and to take action. If perhaps the diagnoses were broad, they at least allowed men to see a physiological end to the detrimental effects of the practice. Masturbation was not a sign of an inner sinful nature; it was the reason for small genitals. Second, the manufacturers allowed men to dismiss Beard's limited-energy theory, which had long given masturbation its fearful countenance. If masturbation, and by association excessive sex, were problems primarily because they wasted energy-rich semen, electric belts offered the solution. By allowing users to increase their energy reserves, manufacturers effectively neutralized their own scare tactics. One might continue to believe that masturbation was a waste of vital energy, but if wearing a belt in the afternoon could replace the supply lost that morning, it would not be a practice one had to avoid.[46]

With the help of technology, individuals could believe that the days of the sexually limited Victorian body were numbered. It is the power of belief, however, that is here most important. As Lesley Hall reveals, the majority of men who "suffered" from impotence at the turn of the century were those termed "psychically impotent" by physicians. When one considers that it was perhaps the psyche as much as the body that needed treating, the true power of electric belts emerges: belts allowed men to envision a body immune to the either-or choice between sexual pleasure and physical health endemic to the Victorian era. Technology suggested one could have both, and in doing so, it allowed believers to discover an alternative definition of sexual health for the modern era.

Electric Bodies, Superior Glands, and Modern Sex Roles

Electric technology offered users more than restored and improved sexual power. Through subtle iconography and textual suggestions, belt manufacturers positioned their products as devices that could assist men in meeting modern women's sexual needs. In doing so, they presented electricity as force that, once merged with the physical body, allowed men to remain sexually superior to their increasingly assertive partners.

Between 1890 and 1930, "psychic impotence" resulted from more than masturbation. Guilt over past transgressions played a part in the dramatic increase in the number of men who suffered impotence without physiological causes, but it was only one of two elements that made men doubt their sexual capacities. The rise of women's rights in the early twentieth century also played an important role. Scholars have typically focused on the political and social aspects of women's suffrage, elements that were only part of a larger redefinition of the female sex from that of second-class citizens to that of equals. Private activism accompanied this public activism. For some, this meant redesigning the home as a cooperative living space or rethinking the usefulness of marriage.[47] For many others, specifically those of the middle and upper classes, this meant reworking intimate relationships, particularly in the area of sexual satisfaction.

The turn of the century brought marked changes in American women's attitudes about sex. Whereas Victorian women were taught to control sexuality through abstinence, expressing intimate desires in passionate friendships instead, women entering the modern age found license to speak.[48] Karen Lystra refers to this change as women's new "right to say yes" to their own sexual desires. Increasingly, women integrated a satisfying sex life into their very definition of an ideal marriage; in their intimate letters to fiancées, friends, and spouses, twentieth-century women often spoke of sex as a complete bonding between two people.[49]

Katharine Davis's survey of one thousand women of marrying age, most born in the 1890s, supports this change in sexual attitudes. The vast majority of respondents had sex at least once a week, with 40 percent having sex more than twice a week. When asked to rate their sexual urges, 30 percent of the women reported that their desires were at least as strong as those of their spouses. One of the most surprising findings of the Davis survey was that almost half of the respondents admitted to masturbating on a regular basis. Given the taboo against the practice, one can assume that actual figures were much higher. By initiating and fulfilling their own sexual desires, these women challenged traditional sexual roles. No longer waiting for men to initiate sex, nor assuming that their role in the act should be as a passive pleasure giver, many women asserted that the essential element in sex must be mutuality. As one respondent explained, the act should be "no habit at all, but the most sensitive regard of each member of the couple for the personal feeling and desires and health of the other."[50]

Given that women were more willing to discuss the details of their sexual expectations and conduct than were men, it is easier to survey their changing attitudes about intimacy. It would be illogical, however, to conclude that women would have dramatically revised their attitudes about sexuality without impacting men as well. Certainly, many men must have praised their partners' increasing pursuit of sexual pleasure and self-expression. Because one of the tenets of Victorian intimacy was the pursuit of one's ideal self through love, sex, for many couples, may have been regarded primarily as one additional path by which to arrive at the goal.[51] Yet other men, perhaps even a majority, would have found the change confusing at best. According to one expert on the era, the confusion was probably one of the primary reasons for increased psychic impotence. "The male sexual ego, conditioned as it was to always dominate passive female sexual objects, was for a time paralyzed by the new sex roles. . . . [O]f course, not all men became impotent, but the literature on manliness reveals an increasingly anxious preoccupation with the causes of psychic impotence."[52]

Men were not only confused by women's new sexual attitudes; they were also angered. As early as 1901, well-regarded tracts on preventing and treating impotence blamed women's excessive desires for triggering their partners' failings. Victor Vecki, author of the 1901 text *The Pathology and Treatment of Sexual Impotence*, warned men to avoid "over sensual" women who were guilty of "challenging male sexual ability."[53] Earlier advice books for women provided similar admonitions. *Satan in Society*, published in 1871, warned "strongly passionate" women that they could easily "ruin a man of feebler sexual organization." To preserve healthy sexual relations, it counseled, a woman should remember "to await the advances of her companion before she manifests her willingness for his approaches."[54]

Attempts to subvert women's emerging sexuality were not undertaken primarily to keep women in a position of permanent subservience. Instead, they reflected a popular desire to create breathing room in which men might be able to adjust to a series of conflicting cultural demands. Men faced particular challenges in navigating the changing sexual landscape of the early twentieth century. Having grown up under Victorian sexual standards, which preached abstinence but practiced private masturbation and purchased sex, men caught in the wave of women's sexual liberation faced three major redefinitions of sexual intimacy and sexual function. First, men had to begin to consider sexual pleasure as mutual in practice. Even conservative figures suggest that as many as one-third of all men had sex before marriage in 1900.[55] Given that "nice" girls followed popular advice and practiced abstinence before marriage, this left women divided into two groups according to sexual practice: those who did and those who did not. Isabelle Rittenhouse Mayne writes that it was typical to teach boys that "purity is only for women (*some* women) and vice a necessity to them and 'natural.'"[56] Most middle-class men pursued premarital sex through officially unsanctioned but well-developed channels, like prostitution or with working-class girls, known as chippies, who traded material goods for sex.[57] The arrangements allowed men to pursue their own pleasure without an equal concern for their partners, who were, at best, temporary.

The second redefinition came in the body itself. When wives held little expectation of reaching orgasm during sex, husbands could spend little time worrying about the issue. Such a system kept both male sex practices, early experiences with unofficial partners and later experiences with one's wife, equal, at least relative to concern over a partner's climax. Women's changing sexual expectations threw this system out of balance: men suddenly found themselves expected to regulate the sex act according to a woman's needs. Many men found it exceedingly difficult to prolong coitus. And many asked Marie Stopes, a British sex reformer in the early twentieth century, for advice on how to better accommodate their wives' needs. "When my wife desires," one wrote, "I thrill so terrifically that I find I eject before I have been with my wife many seconds."[58] Combined with this insecurity were men's fears that their bodies had been damaged through early sexual encounters. In promotional brochures, many unlicensed impotence "specialists" alluded to the fact that sexually transmitted diseases may have made prospective customers impotent or prone to premature ejaculation. "Someday you will want to get married and have a nice wife," cautioned one, suggesting that only with the help of the maker's pills could a man overcome diseases contracted through indiscreet intimacy.[59]

New expectations combined with a reflection on past transgressions made many men prone to sexual insecurity in the early twentieth century. It was a state exacerbated by a third change in sexual intimacy. Whereas

Victorian partners had increasingly sought to realize one's true self though love, modern partners sought their true selves through sexual pleasure. In 1917, William J. Robinson informed female readers who were not already aware that a new age of sexual mutuality was at hand that "those who believe that sex relations are for racial purposes only" must realize that "the sex instinct has other high purposes . . . and should be indulged in as often as they are conducive to man's and woman's physical, mental and spiritual health."[60] Indulging as often and in a manner in which it was conducive to women provided men with a challenge their fathers had not been advised to undertake. "The hygienic rule in regard to duration," one sex manual advised in 1904, is "the man must adjust himself to the condition of the woman so that they reach the culmination at the same time."[61] For sex to become a means of achieving a higher purpose for its participants, men had to discover way to make these psychological and physiological adjustments.

As late as 1931, men sought advice on this transition. Theodore van de Velde's popular *Sexual Tensions in Marriage* suggested that satisfaction meant more than orgasm: an ideal husband also provided his wife with "sufficient opportunities to develop her sexual feelings and capacities."[62] There is much evidence that this mandate drove many to diagnose their own impotence. As van de Velde recognized, men often found it a tall order to help partners who were capable of multiple orgasms develop their full sexual capacity. "It may be said that her sexual power . . . is much greater than his." As a consequence, "[T]he man may have claims made upon him . . . that he cannot fulfill."[63]

Whether men concluded that they were impotent because their partners told them so, because they feared latent effects from previous sexual activity, or because they compared their own orgasmic capacity to a woman's, many negatively evaluated their virility. One cannot understand the popularity of electric belts without understanding as well this contemporary climate of male sexual confusion. Belt advertisements directly promoted products as capable of returning the energy lost in masturbation and restoring sexual health. The message, however, was not something said outright. Most commonly, the prose skated around the issue by referring to men's difficulties in meeting their "marital requirements." Instead of asking men if they were impotent, Pulvermacher asked if they suffered from an "inability to perform the duties pertaining to married life."[64] Dr. Crystal used similar verbiage while theorizing about what caused that inability. It was common for a man "on account of nervous debility caused by early indiscretion, excessive sensuality, or occasioned by having at some time contacted a loathsome disease," to find that his "sexual organs refuse to respond to the desires of the mind, and . . . [he] is wholly incompetent to perform manly duties, and [he] is entirely incapacitated and unfit for the marital relation."[65]

It is significant that the advertisements did not refer to the problem as one of impotence. Instead, they positioned an invisible woman in the discussion, one with certain expectations necessitated by her status as wife. Given the above advertisement's publication in the 1910s, one can conclude that men would have understood that fulfilling their manly duties meant more than achieving an erection. It meant developing the restraint and stamina necessary to sexually fulfill a female partner.

Advertising iconography further confirms this aspect of electric belts. "The Electric Era," a brochure for the German Electric Agency published in 1901, is unusual in that it features a woman on its cover (fig. 27). One might, at first glance, think of the cover as an appeal to women as consumers. However, positioned as an icon of its era, the image implies something quite different. Its primary actors are the horses, two virile black stallions with muscles taut, harnessed to pull the carriage into the electric age. The female, a figure resembling Columbia, one of the national symbols of the United States commonly used in patriotic iconography, sits passively behind the stallions, her bountiful body carrying a beacon of progress in her right hand, the beam of electric light. Given that German Electric sold products primarily to men, it is logical that readers were meant to identify with the visibly male characters here. It is the stallions that are in control: their pores literally ooze electricity as it radiates from the belts around their necks (perhaps also around an unpictured suspensory sack). The Columbia figure, though in the driver's seat, holds no reins, implying that she has given over her power to the stallion guides. Such iconography can be read as a subtle allegory. Like the stallions, men who wear electric power will experience a dangerous, visible virility. And women who may, through anatomical fate, be sexually superior to men, will relinquish that superiority if satisfied by their stallions. Like Columbia, they will contentedly follow the lead of men and their technology, pleased to share in the electric glow.[66]

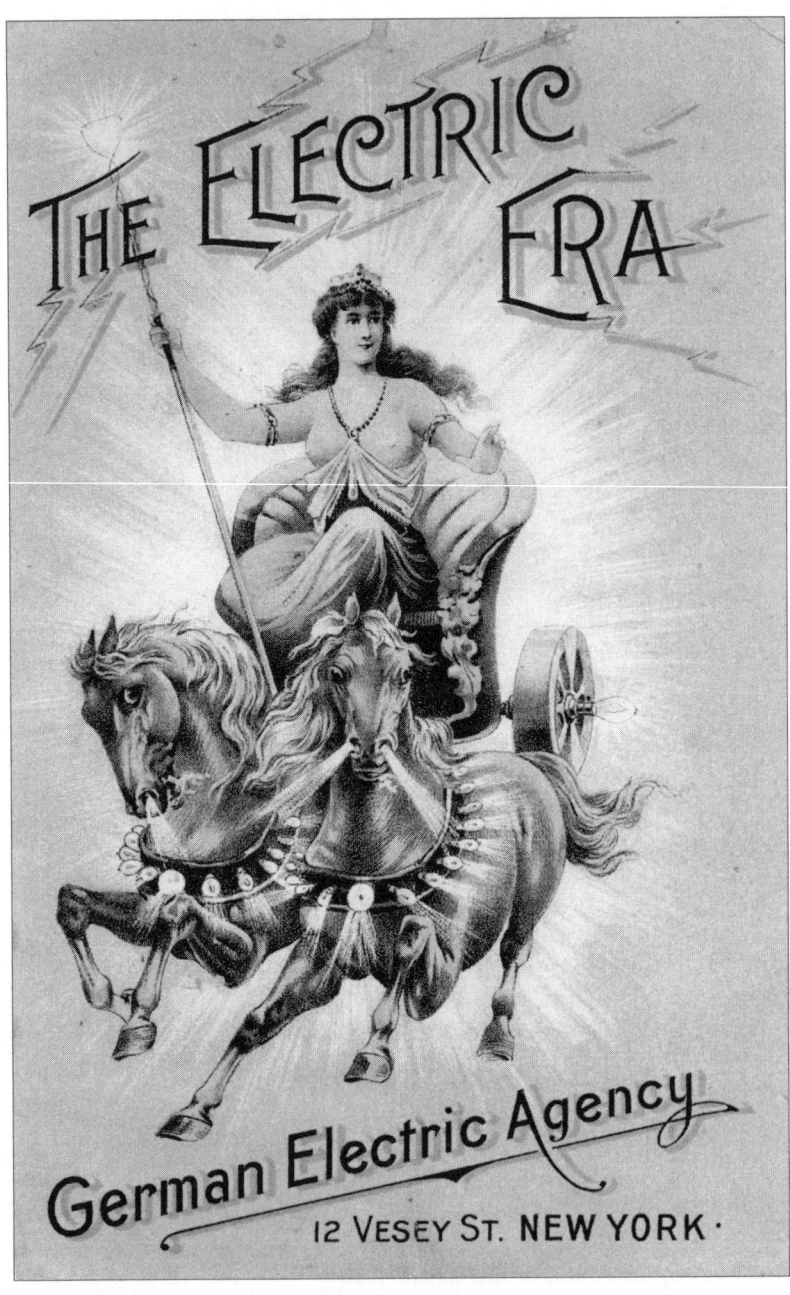

Fig. 27. The electric stallions and the satisfied woman. "The Electric Era,"
German Electric Belt Agency (New York, ca. 1901), ephemera collection.
Courtesy of the Bakken Library and Museum of Electricity in Life, Min-
neapolis.

Beyond Normal: Electric Glands and the Quest for Supervirility

By the 1920s, explorers on the frontier of electric virility treatments had grown impatient with the limitations inherent in earlier "transfer" pursuits. Treating masturbation with electric belts could increase the body's energy beyond that which it possessed prior to the "abuse." It could not, however, maintain the increase indefinitely. Vigor increased, manufacturers suggested, when the genitals were placed in direct contact with electrical power. This might give a man the illusion that an actual physiological change had occurred in his body; should he take off the belt for a few days, however, he would be disabused of that notion. Perhaps connected to such limitations, electric belt sales began to decrease. One can theorize a variety of reasons for the decline: the American Medical Association's litigious efforts to shut down nonlicensed medical practitioners; the public's growing skepticism about miracle cures in general; and the rise of sulfa drugs that could treat and cure sexually transmitted diseases for the first time. Yet to read the demise of electric belts as the end of Americans' belief in the connection between technology and male sexuality is a mistake.

Two electrical products actively marketed between 1920 and 1940 reveal that technology remained a part of definitions of normal male sexuality even as science revealed an increasingly complex male body. The Thermalaid, manufactured by the Electro Thermal Company of Steubenville, Ohio, and its imitator, the GHR Electric Thermitis Dilator, manufactured by the GHR Electric Dilator Company of Grand Rapids, Michigan, both enjoyed market success. The Thermalaid, in fact, was popular enough to be given a good deal of attention by the American Medical Association's legal department, which collected three file boxes of materials on the company in a futile effort to shut it down.[67] The two products offered many of the same remedies as did electric belts: improved vigor and sexual performance, relieved symptoms from varicocele and venereal diseases, and an end to nocturnal emissions.[68] But unlike electric belts, they promised a means of permanently overcoming weakness and increasing sexual power.

Virtually indistinguishable, the Thermalaid and the GHR were narrow metal rods attached to electric power sources (fig. 28). Users first applied a "conducting gel" to the rod and then inserted it into the anus and left it there for several minutes. During this time the rod would warm with the electric current, providing the user with a sensation that could

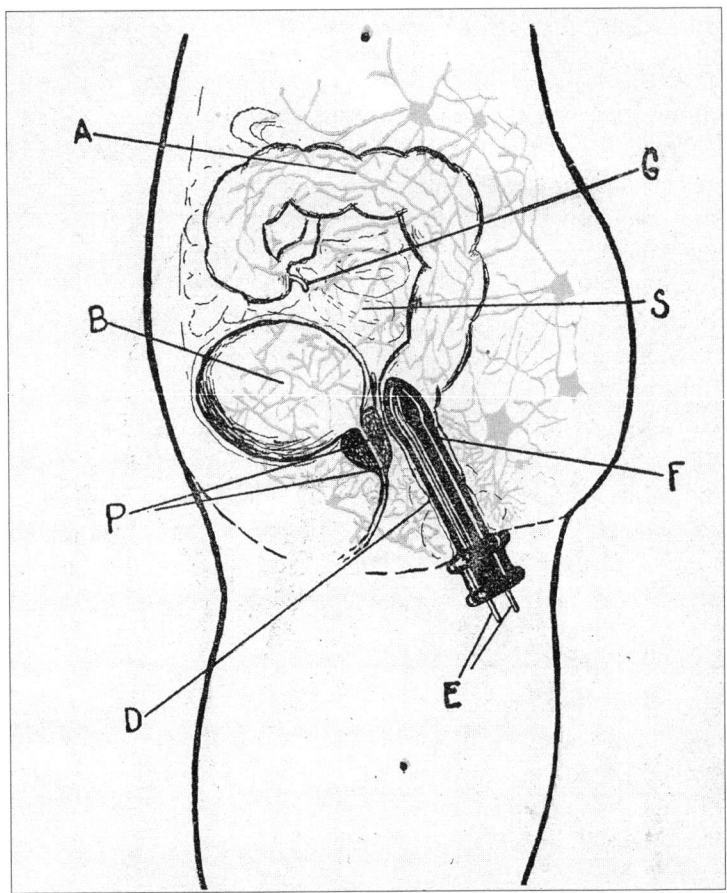

Fig. 28. A diagram of the Thermalaid in use. "Twenty Weeks to Normaltown by Pleasant Travel!" pamphlet, folder 0233-18. Courtesy of the American Medical Association Archives.

be perceived to be electric energy, and would vibrate slightly, which further suggested its efficacy. The anus was not, however, merely a convenient orifice for taking an internal electrical treatment. Central to these products' claims was the relationship between the prostate (labeled "P" in the image), the electric current, and energy for the male body. According to letters sent by GHR to prospective purchasers, the company stressed above all that its product cured because of the "vitalizing influence of continuous electric warmth directly applied to the prostrate [*sic*]."[69]

What these companies may have lacked in anatomical knowledge they made up for in a cogent reading of contemporary American culture. There was nothing new about treating the prostate with electric probes. Surgeon John Butler used the method in the 1880s to reduce enlarged prostates in his patients and advised other physicians to do the same.[70] What was new was the public's interest forty years later in performing the procedure at home. This change was due in large part to a fascination with glands. Numerous products entered the market in the 1920s that played on Americans' nascent understanding of what glands were and how they affected the body. The promoters of Goldglan, one of the most popular products, touted it as a pill of mysterious "double gold chloride" that could ensure a vital sex drive and a long life for both men and women.[71]

Popular gland literature readily mixed the plausible and fantastic; along with diagrams showing the location of pituitaries, thyroids, and sex glands came promises of unlimited sex drives and eternal life. Goldglan offered an illustration of the male and female with fully functioning glands, highlighting the man's muscular physique and the woman's shapeliness, along with bold text proclaiming that "with a perfectly balanced endocrine system one would live forever."[72] For readers exposed only to such hyperbole, it was easy to believe that glands exerted "mastery and control of the entire body," and as such were the singular key to physical, personal, sexual, even spiritual success.[73]

Patent medicine purveyors were not the only promoters of the fantastic-gland theory. Legitimate physicians were equally eager to fulfill Ponce de Leon's quest by exploring the glandular frontier. One of the most dramatic of their attempts was the Steinach operation. Thousands of men, among them such well-known figures as Freud, Yeats, and Harold McCormick (descendant of the McCormick reaper inventor), underwent these drastic operations in the 1920s in Europe and the United States. During the surgery, the vas deferens was cut, separating the testicles from the duct that normally carried semen to the penis. In consequence, a gland that would normally excrete semen instead diffused it into the blood. The operation, described by its proponents as an "eroticization of the nervous system," received mixed reviews. Some physicians reported successes, finding that patients experienced "a return of sexual desire and potency"; some patients, including McCormick, failed to see any perceptible physiological change.[74]

The theory of power through self-insemination allows us to explore more fully the power of wearing an electric belt. We know advertising imagery featured hard bodies, men possessing taut muscles, often in poses where muscles were flexed and arms were raised, as if action were imminent. We also know that the belts and Thermalaids evoked a pleasurable sensation, one that probably caused an erection in more than a few wearers. Together, such imagery and experience suggest that sexual intercourse may not have been the only "consummation" facilitated by electric transfer. It is also possible that wearing the belt, attaining an erection, and then allowing the semen to be reabsorbed into the system, much like the Steinach approach, may have provided a powerful "injaculation" of technology. This was not, of course, part of the products' explicit promotion. Yet in an age where ejaculation still had a lingering connotation of wasted "vital force," it is quite possible that having an erection and not ejaculating could be viewed as a means of increasing vital energy. In this manner, belt wearers may have become embodiments of the vibrators Rachel Maines discusses: requiring neither physician nor partner to enjoy the pleasure and power provided by an intimate technology.

Glands became, for many, a popular religion. According to Morris Fishbein, historian of popular medicine, no method of treating disease had aroused more interest than glandular therapy by the late 1920s.[75] Texts such as *Rest Working*, by Gerald Stanley Lee, urged readers to attribute genius not to genetics but to glands. Lee cited Joseph Conrad to prove his point, asserting that Conrad's success proved "it is the glands . . . pouring or rather suffusing their secretions directly into a man's blood while he writes . . . which alone make literature possible."[76] Yet such pundits did not encourage passive acceptance of one's inherent glandular capacity. At the same time that they attributed human success to gland content, they urged individuals to take control of their inventory. "Be superintendent of your own plant," Lee told readers. The combination of such success sellers, surgeons, and mail-order nostrum providers was a potent one for modern American audiences. To acquire energy one had to do more than build muscle or pursue topical electrical treatments: the key lay in reaching and manipulating the glands themselves.

Thermalaid effectively melded a budding religion of glands with an established electric theology. Its president, John Homan, solidified this connection in 1923 with *Glands of Power and Success*. Free to everyone who ordered the Thermalaid, Homan's book stressed his unique theories of physical and sexual health: healthy glands promoted brain power, leanness, and youth; unhealthy glands prevented those attributes and guaranteed sexual dysfunction.

Homan skillfully incorporated the public's ready fascination with glands into his advertising plan. For individuals hesitant to purchase the imposing Thermalaid, he offered his book as an incentive. This allowed his electrical device to appear as a natural outgrowth of gland research rather than as a foreign device.[77] Thermalaid made conscious attempts to position its product within an accepted repertoire of electric-body devices. An image of it appeared in promotional brochures that bore striking resemblance to some of the earliest home-treatment machines. Instead of showing only the device, Thermalaid placed it within a setting familiar to followers of electrotherapy, the leather case, lined with velvet and cloth, the instruction booklet, and the accompanying battery.

Manufacturers portrayed their product as uniquely capable of fusing two sources of male sexual energy: electricity and the prostate gland. Promotional materials stressed that the device worked without "mysteries," no pills or shocking machines or foreign rays. Instead, it used the "real, positive nature-force" of electrically generated thermic energy, an element that the literature stressed, came directly from the sun. Further, because the force was applied by means of a tool especially designed to reach the prostate, it could be released directly on the gland to improve sex force. Thermalaid emphasized the importance of the prostate, calling it the "sexual brain," which, when swollen, caused the penis to "go to sleep," just as an arm would.[78] The product's claims would have appealed to men who suffered from a prostatic disease as well as those who because of advancing age or psychological factors had diminished sexual capacity. Similar to those for electric belts, Thermalaid advertisements suggested that one needed the product if "the procreative act is often incomplete and premature" or if erections were impossible.[79]

If elements of the earlier devices were familiar to the generation following the electric-belt age, the new devices were still in many ways completely different products. Companies like GHR frequently stressed the miraculous properties of the dilator.[80] It too was advertised to cure prostate inflammation with electric currents. As a bonus, however, users would find the newly energized gland could continually fill them with "new" health, vigor, and vitality. Such a promise went beyond belts, which had been able to assure users only that they would recapture "normal" or slightly better than normal vitality, and only in areas that came into direct contact with the device. The GHR, however, was seemingly unconfined in the power or locality of its treatments. It was a "disease eradicator"; it was a "strength builder" that could simultaneously strengthen erections and eliminate problems with the heart, lungs, brain, and bowels. Further, it held the key to eternal youth.[81] "Why permit yourself to grow old when science has discovered a way out?" one brochure's cover asked in bold letters.[82] The claims went beyond even Gerald Stanley Lee's fantastic gland stories. Given the public appetite for gland promises and its still active fascination with electric power, the GHR found a lucrative home on the American market throughout the 1920s and 1930s.[83]

The dilator and Thermalaid also differed in the way they delivered electricity to the body. Because they were "worn" internally, they removed the equipment that had stood between the body and electricity with belts. With products like German Electric, electricity acted on the body through a visible network of leather, metals, and cords. Even the suspensory sack, which could not be easily seen by its wearers, reminded them of its materiality when they fastened and removed it. With such products, electricity's efficacy came from the wires, leather, and batteries that were apparent on the body; the devices existed as elements apart from the body itself. Prostate massagers dramatically changed this relationship. By applying electricity internally, these devices removed visible barriers between electric currents and the body. Whereas one turned on a belt or plugged in an I-ON-A-CO and fastened it to one's body, one inserted a Thermalaid and plugged oneself in directly. The Thermalaid was literally the physical adaptor that allowed the body to be attached directly to an electrical source. The plug emerging from the anus functions as a prosthetic device, an adaptation that retrofits the body for the physio-electric future envisioned since the earliest days of magnetic machines and static treatments.

Although the dilator and Thermalaid realized the fantasies long promoted by electric invigorating technologists, they pushed the envelope beyond what the public was willing to accept. Users were not going to facilitate limitless erections and halt aging through fifteen-minute daily prostate massages. As more Americans understood the function and limits of glandular systems, such promises seemed preposterous, and perhaps indicative of the "quackery" in lay electrotherapies long charged by regular physicians.[84] The devices' design probably hurt sales as well. After the rise of homophobia in the 1940s and the attendant labeling of homosexuality as an illness, a product meant for anal penetration may have invited unwanted suspicions. Certainly, the devices were used for masturbation for men and women, though this is not discussed anywhere in promotional materials. Curiously, this was not a problem in the 1920s and 1930s; ads almost always featured prominent illustrations of the devices in spite of their phallic appearance. Given that popular health reformer Bernarr MacFadden stressed the "mild-sex-invigorating effect" of prostate massage, it is likely that men did purchase both the Thermalaid and the GHR for sexual stimulation of themselves and their partners, perhaps concluding that the pleasurable sensation proved that the devices were working as promised.[85] Obviously, the American Medical Association believed that they did. In 1925, an AMA investigator concluded that the devices provided "more or less mechanical masturbation."[86] Over time, perhaps people increasingly hesitated to purchase an ostensibly masturbatory product. This may have been compounded by its direct marketing to men.

Electric prosthetic devices allowed users to consummate the relationship between the male body, sexual potential, and electric technology. If they pushed the promises and practice of electrical stimulation too far, they did so only by pursuing to the limits the promises made by Pulvermacher in the 1870s. Glands were not the final frontier of sexual stimulation; electricity was not a technology capable of dramatically pushing the envelope of sexual performance. Yet in German Electric's self-proclaimed "electric era," "where everything is done by electricity," it was only natural that it would be applied to "do" one of the body's most intimate functions. And why not believe that the same power enjoyed by telephones, trains, and electric lights would find its way to procreation, the very essence of human life? In such a world it might be possible to believe that only by fully exploiting electricity, in all of its applications, could life evolve to its fullest potential.

Between 1900 and 1930, Americans experimented with an unprecedented array of energy-expansion strategies. Machines for muscular development infiltrated college gymnasiums and upscale resorts. Electric rejuvenators sold handily through door-to-door salesmen, mail order advertisements, and local physicians. Each enjoyed an expanding market throughout the first decades of the twentieth century as Americans increasingly sought remedies for modern fatigue. It is not an overstatement to say that at least half of middle- or upper-class Americans would have had firsthand or secondhand experience with these products.

Muscular expansion and electric invigoration did not fundamentally alter Americans' understanding of human energy. Both worked well within the three maxims of energy production. First, energy existed in a finite amount and could not be increased. Second, as stated by the second law of thermodynamics, energy was constantly being degraded. Third, physical energy could be expanded through direct contact with external energy sources, but the expansion could not be made permanent. In short, treatments "worked" because they made energy available to the body that it would not otherwise have, either by "unblocking" internal force or by "transferring" force to the body from an external source. Machines and electricity could act as an energy savings account, whereby one could temporarily "withdraw" funds to cover debts, but when the body-mechanism contact ceased, so did the deposits. The close material contact between body and machine kept users aware that the technologies were the source of energy, and that energy could only be as strong as its attendant device. Radium changed these rules entirely.

5

"Radiomania" Limits the Energy Dream

Scientists had been speculating for decades that the universe might contain a reserve of unseen power, but few had imagined that there was so much of it.[1]

—Spencer Weart, *Nuclear Fear*

The idea that new force must be in itself a good is only an animal or vegetable instinct. As Nature developed her hidden energies, they tended to become destructive.[2]

—Henry Adams, *The Education of Henry Adams*

In 1903, dozens of African Americans entered the offices of white scientists, subjected their bodies to radium "therapies," and waited to see their black skin turn white. Over the course of the year, in separate experiments undertaken in Philadelphia and Berkeley, three scientists used African-American bodies as testing grounds to determine the newly discovered element's physical properties. All records indicate that the primarily male subjects came forward willingly for daily "treatment" sessions over a one-month period. One at a time and part by part they exposed their bodies to a scientist whom they did not know and to a substance whose lethal potential they could not imagine. For as long as they could bear, they held their faces, arms, torsos, and legs inches away from vials of radium while X rays were simultaneously shone onto the skin's surface. One can only guess at the discomfort caused by these treatments, which typically lasted fifteen minutes. Yet week after week, many returned for the therapies, even after the dermatological burns appeared and intensified. Each experiment was evaluated with some degree of "success"; Dr. Henry Pancoast of Philadelphia, Dr. Thomas Eldridge of Philadelphia, and senior chemistry student Robert Roos of the University of California all damaged the skin pigmentation of patients to the point where they were deemed partially or completely "white."

We do not yet know who these people were or why they volunteered for these experiments. We know only what newspapers chose to report: that individuals were recruited for their particularly dark skin and that they were "very eager to be made white." Regardless of whether we believe this eagerness or view it as a statement of what scientists and reporters wanted to believe, the fact that dozens of African Americans did, without recorded resistance or remuneration, withstand tremendous pain in pursuit of whiteness testifies to the debilitating effects of racial inequality in the early twentieth century.[3]

The radium treatments offer visceral, material proof of the devaluation and degradation of African-American bodies under a racist cultural system on par with Ida B. Wells's exposés of lynching published in the previous decade.[4] Further, they suggest that the degradation was due not only to direct physical and indirect psychological violence perpetrated against African-American bodies by whites but also to self-inflicted mistreatment by African Americans themselves. Scientists did not force their subjects to expose their bodies to harmful rays. But by supporting a system that legitimized the equating of blackness with inferiority, scientists obliquely participated in the violence. The institutional promotion of white supremacy had yielded a psychological victory and a physiological defeat. Subjects' desires to unmark their bodies may have been an expedient strategy for success within white society, or a coping strategy for an inflicted sense of inferiority. Either way, the volunteers literally burnt their blackness in pursuit of what one report characterized as "a beautiful, soft, creamy white color."[5]

Beyond their implications for early-twentieth-century racial attitudes, these experiments also reveal an exceptional faith in radium's ability to remake the body. By their own speculation that radium could disprove the immutability of racial types, one of the fundamental laws of the nineteenth century, scientists disclosed a belief that radium might rewrite physical laws. Not everyone, however, approved of the revision. Newspaper coverage repeatedly stressed that white skin was not the equivalent of a white soul. According to the *Savannah Press*, in a typical review of the studies, such experiments "would not metamorphose [the African American's] moral or spiritual nature" but would instead "make him a

. . . monster." By 1904, all three scientists had seen their funding cut, and a significant number of their patients were left "partially white," largely because of the overwhelming disapproval of journalists and their readers, particularly in the South.[6]

Attempts to use radium to recast the body as a new type did not end with the 1904 experiments. Instead they underwent a transformation: instead of changing skin tone, the goal became changing energy content. "Radiumizing" the body, it seemed, would finally make good on the promises suggested by theorists including Dudley Allen Sargent, David Butler, George Beard, and Henry Gaylord Wilshire. With radium, it appeared that the body could be fundamentally altered, as long as the product remained within culturally accepted boundaries. Radium would not redefine racial categories; it would, for a brief period, recast human energetic potential.

William Hammer and the "American Radium Discovery," 1902–1907

While experimenting with cathode rays in 1895, William Konrad Röntgen discovered X rays.[7] His work with Röntgen rays dramatically expanded the limits of scientific knowledge, inspiring only months later the French physicist Henri Becquerel to discover the concept of radioactivity. Suddenly, there existed a mysterious force that could pass through the body unimpeded by barriers of flesh and bone. This news traveled quickly. Inspired by Bequerel's work, Marie and Pierre Curie discovered a naturally occurring radium in uranium ore. The Curies embarked on a four-year project to isolate radium particles to collect a sample for measurement and classification. In the often-mythologized tale, the pair went to work in 1898 in a small shed, going through pile after pile of discarded pitchblende ore, a type of uranium ore. After four years and thousands of pounds of pitchblende, they succeeded, and in 1902 announced the new element radium to the scientific world.[8]

Europeans discovered the element, recorded its properties, and hypothesized about its scientific applications. American scientists and physicians learned of the discoveries secondhand. One could argue, however, that there was also an "American" radium discovery, one based more on enthusiasm than experiments. In the United States, radium knowledge evolved from a series of trickle-down information networks, the majority of which were begun by scientists and laymen who had little direct experience with the element. This led to a dramatically different vision of radium than European science could support. Instead of focusing on radium's fragility and volatility, properties that were apparent to those who understood the element scientifically, Americans concentrated on its power and malleability. It was this "discovery" that inspired an American following unparalleled by any previous scientific discovery.

It did not take long after radium's discovery for scientists to envisage fantastic implications for energetic human potential. In actuality, radium's properties did lend themselves to a drastic shift in accepted thinking on the relationship between energy and the body. Even infinitesimally small amounts of the element seemed capable of releasing great quantities of energy during exposure. And due to its extraordinarily long half-life, radium's energy seemed to defy the laws of science: it did not decline in perceptible mass or energy, even over years. In fact, radium seemed not to decrease but rather to increase: its emanations, the gas created when radium dissipated into the atmosphere, created a second element, helium. The conversion effectively stabilized radium's net energy loss, creating an element that posed a profound challenge to contemporary scientific theories.

Radium would have fascinated scientists and engendered impassioned debate had only these principles been true. Yet the element's cultural narrative stretched beyond subjects covered in journals and laboratories. Americans with no scientific training were mesmerized by the possibilities. Between 1900 and 1940, radium inspired thousands of articles, popular songs, fictional stories, "medicinal" fortunes, parlor games, well-heeled parties, and even haute cuisine meals. The attraction was not merely due to the element's newness or even its challenge to entropy. It fascinated because it seemed capable of transforming the body into an system capable of producing its own, limitless energy. Radium's apparent ability to alter cells, killing the damaged and renewing the depleted, challenged American thinking about human energy. Radium entered into and flourished within a popular culture of energy fantasy well established by previous mechanical and electrical energy devices. Yet, unlike machines' and electric devices' measureable limits and inorganic relationships to the body, radium was invisible, ingestible, and seemingly infinite. Many believed that it could power the body by a "technology" as natural as the heart and muscles themselves. Technological energy enhancement would run its final course in the story of radium, a substance that first evoked full physical evolution and ultimately heralded the complete destruction of humankind.

William Hammer brought the first known quantity of radium into the United States. One of the most highly regarded electrical engineers of his day, Hammer's position as Thomas Edison's trusted assistant qualified him as a skilled innovator among his peers. He was also an avid fan of scientific energy advances; in his lifetime his passions included making and marketing arc lamps, experimenting with electric lighting, developing aeronautical efficiency, and discovering practical applications for radium. It was his last interest that brought him notoriety.

In 1902, Hammer had abruptly made a change in profession after first learning of the Curies' radium discovery. He left Edison and headed for Paris, where he joined Pierre Curie in his laboratory. Hammer's intention, as he described it in his writings, was ostensibly pure scientific learning, but it seems clear that from the outset he hoped to return with a sample. After weeks of assisting the Curies with their experiments, poring over their notebooks, and recording his own observations about radium's capabilities, Hammer secured the coveted prize. He returned to the United States nine tubes of radium richer, ready to make his mark on American radium research.[9]

Hammer seems to have divided his time experimenting with radium-derived luminous substances, promoting radium therapy for physicians, and giving paid lectures across the country. Medical historians have primarily concentrated on the second of these endeavors because of their interest in radium's "legitimate" therapeutic history. Most of his contemporaries, however, knew the other two interests best. Hammer was more a showman than a medical professional. Between 1902 and 1907, he was the best known among the hundreds of traveling "radium experts." It was these individuals, among them common charlatans and renowned scientists, who served as primary disseminators of radium knowledge. Although many Americans read newspaper stories on the element, only traveling lecturers enabled people to hear "experts," see images of the element in action, and, in some cases even view a sample of radium with their own eyes. For the lecturers, theirs was a profitable pursuit.[10]

Hammer's brand of radium promotion was part professional expertise and part popular entertainment. He had solid credentials as an expert in science and technology. His work with the Curies had been abundantly publicized; his history with Edison made him one of the technological elite; and in 1903 he had published the first book on radium in the United

States. Promotional bills and newspaper advertisements alerted people to such experience by calling him "the best authority on the radio-active substances there is in the world" and "the most eminent American authority upon radium."[11] Certainly, at a time when Americans could get little firsthand information about radium, Hammer's reputation helped attract crowds. Early in his touring, he easily filled Carnegie Hall with a thousand people.[12] Less than a year later, after the press referred to his "now famous lectures," Hammer gave two talks in Denver; the second had to be moved to the Denver Auditorium when it was realized that some twenty thousand people would try to gain admission.[13]

Hammer had more than powerful oratory to thank for his success and longevity on the lecture circuit. For one thing, big-city and small-town Americans were already primed to be excited about radium. The previous decade had seen enormous X ray enthusiasm. During a single year in the 1890s, more than a thousand papers and fifty books had been published on Röntgen's experiments.[14] It did not take long for scientific interest in X rays to filter down to the general public.

Thomas Edison piqued the curiosity of many outside the scientific community in his 1896 quest to X-ray the human brain. Goaded by William Randolph Hearst's dare (and promised monetary reward), Edison experimented under the watchful eye of numerous reporters encamped outside his West Orange, New Jersey, laboratories. Though he failed, Edison did help create a popular X ray success.[15] During its monthlong monitoring of Edison, the press had plenty of time to publish stories of fantastic X ray speculation. Thus, Edison's failure actually fostered X ray enthusiasm, leaving most Americans believing that X rays would soon unveil the brain through science.

Between 1896 and 1900, the fascination with X rays grew rapidly. And although much of the interest was in such medical implications as disease diagnoses, bone repair, and bullet removal, there was also an element of the fantastic in the attraction. Newspaper cartoons poked fun at those who feared that X ray glasses would soon render people naked at will and that X ray schemes would help pickpockets select better targets.[16] Many people even had their own X ray portraits done, replicating for themselves the well-known image of the hand of William Röntgen's wife, an eerie skeletal finger adorned with a wedding band. According to the *New York Sun*, "[N]o prior scientific discovery . . . had aroused such interest and enthusiasm among American newspapers and their readers."[17] While reporters were feeding popular enthusiasm, American physicians were devoid of firsthand experience. It was not until 1900 that medical schools began training students in Röntgen therapy or X ray techniques.[18] By the time Hammer stepped up to the podium, there was already plenty of excitement about a science that promised to uncover the body's secrets.

It is likely that Hammer was familiar with the unique blend of scientific interest and popular fascination that X rays had stirred up in America, for he entered a space where the rules had not yet been defined and established a strong partnership between radium fact and radium fantasy. Hammer began his tours before experts had thoroughly codified radium's laws. His first lecture in 1902 took place fourteen years before the founding of the American Radium Society and several years prior to the period of major American radium advances. In fact, not until 1913 would a majority of "reputable" American medical institutions explore the use of radium in internal medicine.[19] As a result, few in his audiences were equipped to distinguish radium fact from radium fancy.

Onto this blank slate, then, Hammer painted two vastly disparate pictures. His two-hour talks usually consisted of at least an hour of informative lecturing, including an account of radium's discovery, the tale of his own research with the Curies, and an analysis of what radium was and how it worked. The second hour resembled an old-fashioned tent revival. Perhaps drawing on contemporary fascination with electric marvels, he showed objects altered by radium-containing luminous paint, darkening the lights so that the audience could read glowing watches and clocks and marvel over auto and airplane navigational devices. Hammer also exhibited his own small sample of radium, waiting until the very end to take out the tiny glowing tube for the audience to see. Evidence suggests that the latter half of the lecture was what drew the greatest crowds.

A typical advertisement from 1904 for an upcoming talk stressed that in addition to a "scientific" presentation of the facts on this new element, Hammer would also provide "lantern slides and radium preparations" for those present to examine firsthand.[20] Newspaper advertisements often emphasized that at the end of the talk, Hammer would bring out a satchel containing what was "probably the second biggest individual collection of radium on the planet."[21]

Other lecturers also capitalized on radium's ability to draw a crowd; Professor N. A. Kent often brought a small sample of the element to his unrelated talks on the Louisiana Purchase, most likely to ensure audience satisfaction in spite of the dry subject matter.[22] Like Kent's, Hammer's listeners typically stayed on past his conclusions, waiting in

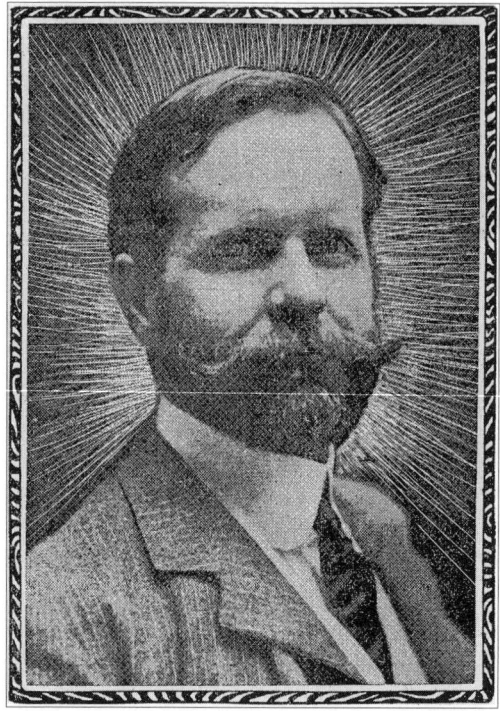

Fig. 29. Image of Hammer with a glowing countenance. "Radium as a Substitute," *New York Journal* (June 21, 1905).

long lines to see the sample and glowing objects up close and to ask questions.[23]

Just what people inquired at these lectures remains a mystery. We can, however, assume that many questions concerned energy, for although Hammer edified with historical information and entertained with illustrative samples, he captivated by declaring that radium would alter energy in the universe. Newspaper accounts of his remarks reveal that Hammer's audiences learned "especially" about what one termed radium's "seemingly exhaustless energy, which almost establishes its claim as a power capable of realizing the dream of perpetual motion."[24] The photographs Hammer used for publicity further reinforced the theme; they portrayed him literally glowing from mysterious electric-radioactive energy waves that encircled his head (fig. 29).

In 1903, the proposition that "exhaustless energy" might be on the horizon bordered on the miraculous. Technological and physiological advances had dramatically increased the amount of energy many people believed was available. For those who believed in the promises of promoters, machines had successfully minimized the body's energy drain and electricity had become an energetic recuperative tool. Yet neither of these was a source of unlimited energy: muscles could be expanded only so far; electricity could be absorbed only for so long. Radium, as Hammer presented it, actually had the ability to grow in energy even as it diminished in quantity. In what seemed to be the first delivery on the ancient alchemic attempt to turn lead into gold, radium actually transmuted as it dissipated: "old" radium became helium, and the gas it emanated became "radon." Both continued to produce usable energy as far into the future as anyone could peer.[25]

Hammer's audience could have interpreted his talks in a variety of ways. Prior to the advent of radio in the 1920s and rise of global media during World War I, public speakers were given considerable attention. The majority of those in attendance would have seen the experience as a source of new information, not simply as an evening's entertainment.[26] What attendees learned, however, depended on what they anticipated hearing. In cities like Denver and Telluride, where Hammer attracted some of his largest crowds, people may have been drawn for economic reasons. Hammer's lecture advertisements touted the properties of a new mysterious element and hence would have attracted those from the local mining industry who hoped to convert popular radium enthusiasm into private economic gain. This scenario is particularly plausible, given that Hammer's lectures coincided with attempts by many counties, including several in Colorado, to uncover their own radium deposits.[27] For those aware of such efforts, limitless wealth rather than "limitless energy" may have captivated their attention.

For the many attendees who had previously read the press' hyperbolic coverage of "exhaustless energy" and "perpetual motion," the experience may have bordered on the religious. Hammer's lectures were not an isolated phenomenon; when he arrived in a town, with flyers highlighting his luminescent profile and mysterious element he entered space primed by forty years of religious revivals. Beginning with Dwight Moody after the Civil War, preachers had focused their efforts on converting urban audiences, often using the same large auditoriums that Hammer used for his presentations. The format of these meetings was similar to that of a radium lecture: an audience would fill seats in a massive auditorium, listen to sermons on the necessity of conversion, and then participate by indicating in response its desire to be saved. Hammer's factual presentations were also saturated with quasi-religious lore. Stories of miracle cures illustrated the medicinal qualities of radium. In one, a blind girl distinguishes light from darkness after having radium applied directly to her optic nerve. Here radium becomes the force of God's energy, literally allowing the modern scientist to perform a "laying on of hands."[28]

If the lecture experience is read as a revival, then coming forward to see radium up close and to touch its luminescent products would have been akin to a conversion experience. Attendees left Hammer's talks with nothing more than information. Yet the fact that his presentations used a revival format, and that they took place in cities, like Brooklyn, that had been inundated with revivals, leaves room to hypothesize that some audience members also took home a sample of belief in the miraculous. This helps explain why Hammer could give the same talk repeatedly in the same city. According to the local Erie paper, townspeople heard three lectures on radium in the 1904 season, and the subject still remained "a name to conjure with" when attracting townspeople's attention.[29] Radium's alchemy of science and salvation would reach a wider audience as it traveled beyond the confines of lecture auditoriums and into the pages of the popular press.

The Rise of "RadioMania": Radium and American Popular Culture, 1900–1915

In February 1904, the *Indianapolis Journal* ran a short account that evoked a far more fanciful view of radium than Hammer had brought to his auditorium crowds. "Cooney Jessap's Overdose of Radium: the Pathetic Love Affair of a Human Lantern," offers a sample of the fiction that formed the basis of "radium knowledge" for many who read the popular press. Cooney Jessap, a hopelessly inept and romantic young man, discovers that his true talent in life is swallowing things. He adopts a rigorous training schedule, graduating from pebbles and rocks to jewelry and tacks. Yet, despite his skills, he fails to attract the favorable attention of even one girl. When a "radium lecturer" comes to town, charging only twenty-five cents admission, Jessap sees his opportunity. While the lecturer isn't looking, and counter to the admonitions that swallowing radium would "sear" one's stomach, Jessap grabs the radium tube and swallows it.[30]

Young Jessap does not become merely another tragic figure in the story of small-town boys with big-city ambitions. Rather, he finds himself physically transformed; finally he is the center of attention that he has always dreamed of becoming. Employers who had turned him away now court him. Offers abound to become the self-lit night watchman, the night-seeing burglar's assistant, the glowing mannequin for window displays, and the scientific subject of college studies. His "glow" extends beyond illumination, drawing numerous young women to his side with what, a generation earlier, would have been called "magnetic attraction." Unfortunately for the young lovers, the girls' peeling lips tell of clandestine kisses and draw parental fury.

Though fiction, Jessap's story bespeaks themes in the relationship between average Americans and radium. First, much of their "information" came, as did Jessap's, from unscientific sources. Second, radium in a tube might be interesting, but radium in your body was the stuff of real excitement. Third, the bodies that might benefit from radium were primarily male. Despite the fact that radium was marketed as a product for the home, its advertising imagery and rhetoric remained a terrain more male than female. And fourth, though "experts" might warn you of radium's physical dangers, those who tried it would find that the benefits outweighed its risks. These themes did not derive simply from one fictional story in one American paper; they appeared repeatedly in fiction, factual reporting, and cartoons in the American popular press over a period of fifteen years. Combined, they told a tale of radium's physical possibilities that was far more inspiring than the factual reporting of regular medical and scientific journals.

When many Americans began to consume radium products in the 1920s, it was largely due to a decade of promotion by the popular press. From the start, most journalists portrayed the new element in a positive light. Radium preoccupied the popular press throughout the first two decades of the twentieth century. As a Sacramento newspaper put it in 1903, "[N]ever, perhaps, was so much ado made over so small a quantity of any substance."[31]

Even as medical professionals increasingly urged restraint and popular experts like Hammer tempered fiction with fact, newspaper reporters remained free from the restrictions of rigor. The radium story they created only amplified the more fantastic features of Hammer's presentations. Their reasons may have been, like Hammer's, at least partly economic; given the public's interest in radium phenomena, the paper that told the tallest radium tale also reaped the biggest readership.[32] Consequently, Americans in towns small and large learned repeatedly that radium was changing the world.

Three principles of postradium life would emerge as truisms by 1910: radium overturned laws of thermodynamics; radium created energy far in excess of anything imaginable; and radium would ultimately create permanent mental and physical power. For many reporters and their readers, the limits of radium were bound by only the limits of the imagination.[33]

Radium demanded a revision of one of the fundamental texts of the nineteenth century, the second law of thermodynamics. Ever since Lord Kelvin's findings had filtered into the United States fifty years earlier, stories had circulated that all energy in the universe was given to dissipation. The jury was still out on how long the earth and its inhabitants had before the sun grew cold and a chill settled across the land, but many Americans read about the inevitability of such a fate. The prediction was an unwelcome reversal of the American progress narrative. Facing such doom, there was little point in expanding the physical and mental limits of human life if one was on a one-way trip to planetary death.

Radium changed the destination entirely. Following the second law of thermodynamics, radium did give off heat and diminish over time, but it also converted its own dissipated energy, creating a constant energy mass. The popular press paraphrased the discovery for its readers. In 1904, a story typical of many, "Most Wonderful Thing in the World," declared that radium, by giving off heat, the equivalent of power, without a loss of substance had fundamentally "upset" the accepted law of the conservation of energy.[34]

For some Americans, radium created a disturbing dissonance between the world they knew and the one being revealed by science. Henry Adams, when confronted with radium at the Paris Exposition of 1900, felt overcome by a new "supersensual world," a place where "he could measure nothing except by chance collisions of movements imperceptible to his senses, perhaps even imperceptible to his instruments."[35] Most Americans appear to have been more eager to celebrate than to contemplate the unknowable element in their midst. In newspapers from Michigan to California stories appeared, touting radium as "the greatest wonder of the new age," one that overturned the laws of limited-energy that had shackled the nineteenth century.[36]

The press wasted little time in concluding that radium must be the long-sought matter that made up the sun. As a result, many people deemed nineteenth-century fears of the sun's demise passé. Articles with titles like "Radium to the Rescue of an Expiring World" reassured Americans that their sweater stockpiling and candle collecting could be brought to an end. A relieved exhalation is nearly audible in a Burlington, Iowa, story from 1903: "What solace to the good people whose waking hours and whose dreams are disturbed by the fear that the supply of heat derived from the sun is diminishing and that the earth is doomed to death through arctic cold."[37]

It might have been enough, in some cultural moments, simply to prove that evolution was not heading toward an eventual heat death. This, however, was the early twentieth century, a time populated by survivors of a neurasthenic age. They exhibited an exceptional appetite for practical applications of radium in daily life. Newspaper coverage often favored radium applications over radium theory. "Radioactivity," explained one chemistry professor in a 1903 article in a popular series, "pointed to 'inexhaustible' power." To illustrate how radium displaced age-old theories of energy dissipation and inert matter, he speculated on its implications. Radium might be the substance to overturn Lord Kelvin's theories and nature's laws, but it was also the substance that if possessed in a pint could "drive an ocean liner from London to Sydney and back."[38]

The American press worried little that knowledge of the element was so nascent that such speculations were questionable at best. Instead of occupying a "safe zone" of admitted conjecture on radium's possibilities, as did most scientists and professors, the press told readers that radium would change the world. With little evidence and less scientific proof, numerous reports in 1903 and 1904 announced the discovery of radium-enabled perpetual motion. In reports of the discovery printed in papers from Kansas to New York, writers stoked the fires of overenthusiasm by declaring that thanks to this miraculous substance, the "dream of the ancients" had at last been realized.[39]

Accounts of how the new energy would change the world, immediately and dramatically, appeared in full force throughout 1904. "It is probable that a few grains might provide energy to drive our locomotives, motor cars, and mechanical engines of every description, and we would cook on radium stoves," Chicago's *Suggestions* wrote. Readers of the popular press were continuously urged to scan the horizon for radium miracles because, as one paper put it, "[D]reams beyond conception may be conjured up as to what radium may do."[40] Visions of radium grains propelling cars and ships around the globe had become commonplace by 1910.[41]

Cartoonists breathed life into such visions, transforming popular ideas into laughter through a complex process that can only be described as alchemy. The humor of cartoon vignettes is more than a form of entertainment. The images can distill opinions, debates, and fantasies to their essence, appearing at once distorted and accurate. The debut in the early 1900s of radium cartoons presupposes that artists and editors assumed an audience already primed for their humor. We can view their stories, then, as glimpses into the radium-powered world of popular imagination. Radium labor was one common theme, demonstrated by a vignette in which a radium tunnel sprayer effortlessly carves a path under the Hudson River, ending the ancient, exhausting, and dangerous job of manual subterranean tunneling. Other cartoons suggest that radium may fight crime; one portrays a man who has inadvertently inhaled radium while stealing a sample. His plan is derailed after his powerful sneezes sink ships, collapse bridges, topple trains, and eventually alert the police to his actions (fig. 30). Still other stories offer more specific, and productive visions of how the substance might alter a user's body. One of these, "Practically Applied," from a 1904 issue of *Harper's Weekly*, depicts eight scenes of individuals whose natural state has been altered (fig. 31). Four of the featured individuals exhibit extraordinary physical power: a messenger delivers in record speed; a woman makes breakfast in an instant; a conductor sweeps people into line; and a creditor is forever preserved. The other four show signs of increased mental ability: children read Greek and Latin and impress visitors with their erudition; a man remembers where he placed a missing shoe; a speaker bowls guests over with his wit. Whether or not readers believed or hoped that radium could bequeath such benefits, the cartoons suggest that the proposition resonated with their understanding of the element's power.

Exposure, in the end, was the most important contribution of the popular press. In towns small and large, daily papers familiarized readers with the folklore of a radium-powered future. Next to accounts of local spelling bees and newsworthy events, stories on radium proliferated. Like the element itself, these stories radiated into the consciousness of their

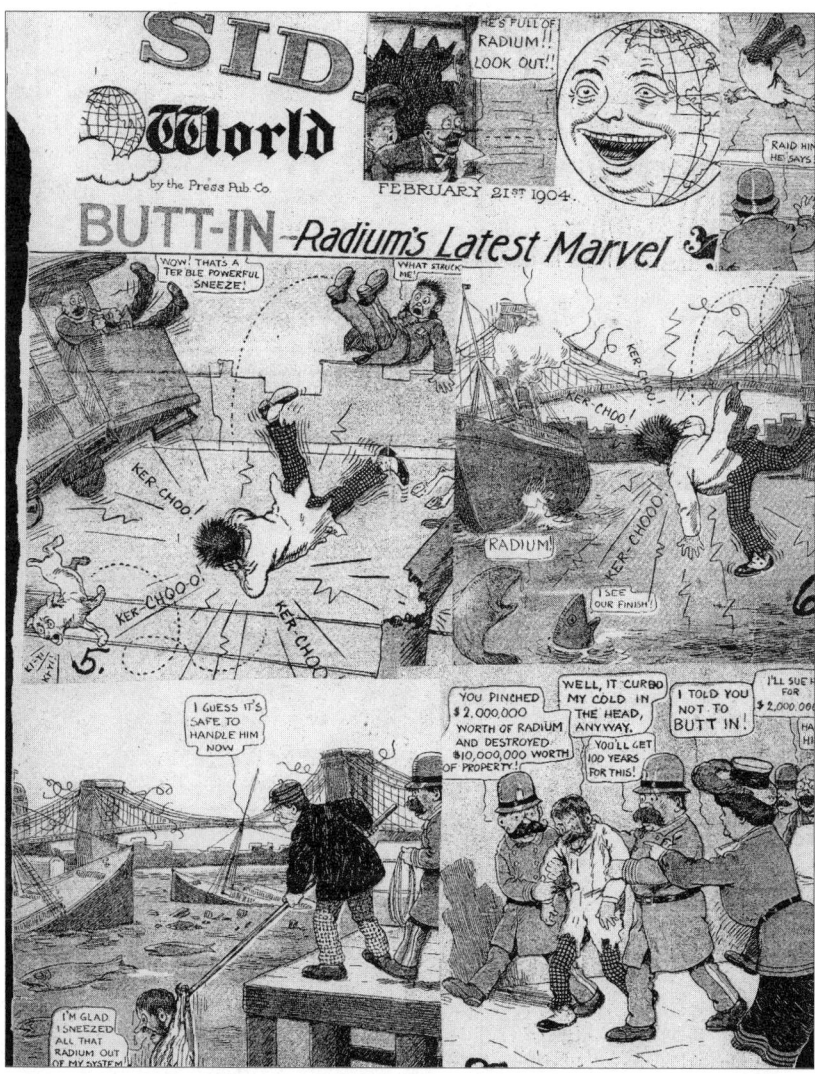

Fig. 30. Radium cartoons. Box 59, folder 2, William J. Hammer Collection, Archives Center. Courtesy of the National Museum of American History, Smithsonian Institution. Originally published in *Harper's Weekly* (February 6, 1904), 199.

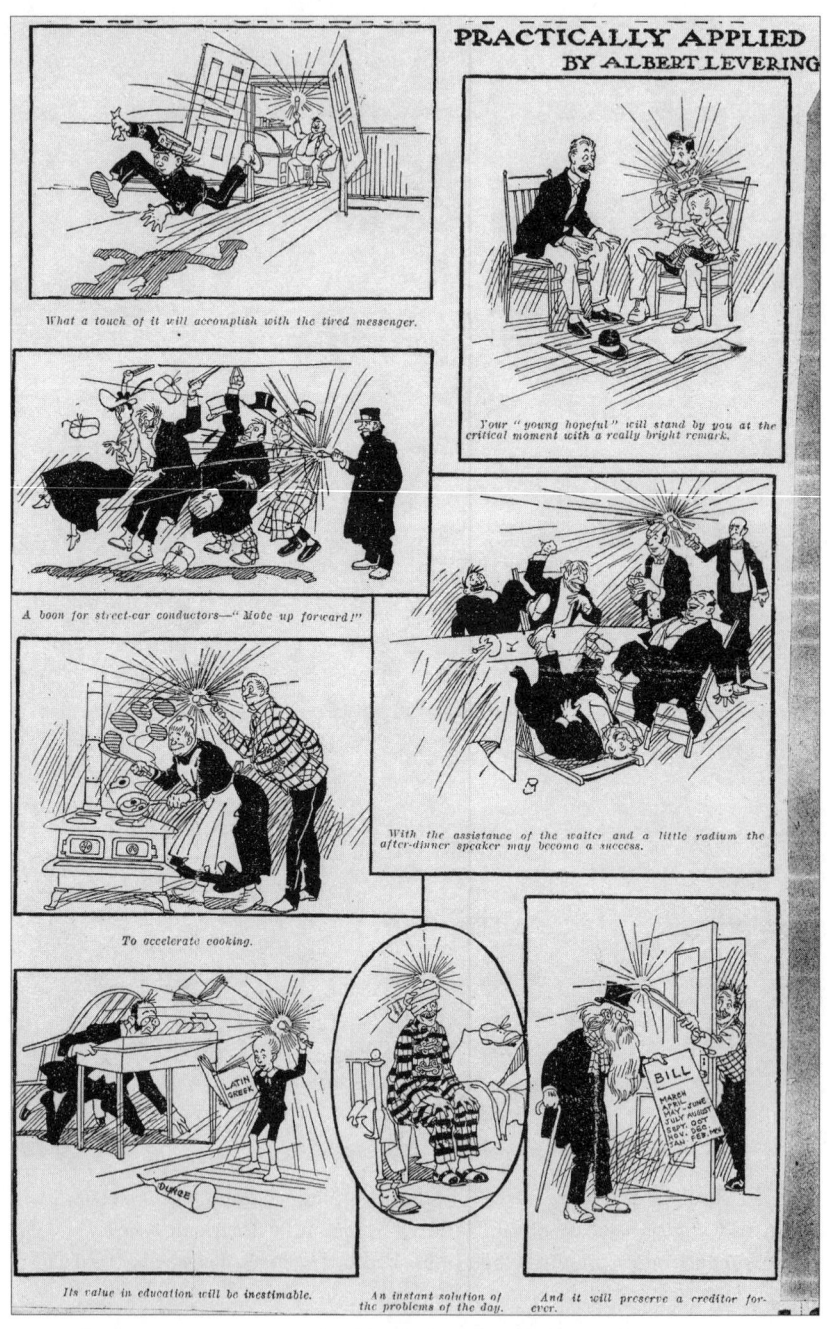

Fig. 31. Radium cartoons. Box 59, folder 2, William J. Hammer Collection, Archives Center. Courtesy of the National Museum of American History, Smithsonian Institution.

readers, and even into those who themselves participated in the myth-making. In a letter to William Hammer in 1904, reporter S. A. Paddock apologized for a recently published mistake-plagued interview. He placed the blame on the linotype man. One could only hope, he told Hammer, that soon radium would become cheap enough that "linotype men and proof readers can buy a little tube of it to be worn about their hats."[42] Paddock's comment may have been meant in jest, but its utterance, like the cartoon's appearance, reveals that the connection between radium and intelligence was already part of the cultural lexicon.

The Parable of Liquid Sunshine: Shedding Light on a Radium Body

Radium stories in the popular press were often neither fact nor fiction. One event in particular, the "Sunshine Dinner" held February 6, 1904, at MIT, reveals that the news that reached newspaper readers was often a composite of the two. The story was repeated frequently in newspapers across the country in the early part of 1904. In brief, it was an account of a dinner and lecture event for eighty students, scholars, and scientists who had gathered to hear several speakers detail recent scientific advances. After the talks concluded, before dinner was served, guests were presented with toasting glasses, each of which contained a tiny tube of radium. The lights were turned off, and guests lifted their glowing glasses and drank.

The facts of the event were not, in themselves, particularly compelling. Neither was the way they were reported in the national press. According to Cleveland Moffett of *Success* magazine, a publication aimed at the emerging white-collar class, the cocktails had been no more powerful, or thrilling, than "half a dozen fireflies."[43] Similar coverage appeared in *Scientific American*, whose readers were professionals and hobbyists. Many of the dinner guests, it reported, declared that any physical benefit resulting from radium would come from playing golf after work with illuminated balls, not from drinking radium-laced liquids.[44]

Most readers, however, read a different version of these events from the popular press, whose reporters eagerly ran with the radium "cocktail story." Throughout February of 1904, versions appeared repeatedly in local papers from New York City to Sioux Falls.[45] Central to the coverage was the notion that drinking radium heightened the body's performance.

Two weeks after the dinner, Sioux Falls readers learned that the scientists who had drunk the cocktails found the effect on their bodies to be identical to "taking a bite out of the sun."[46] Other stories took the comparison between the cocktail's name and its effects even more literally. Downing the "sunshine" cocktail, explained one small-town paper the day of the banquet, left one dinner guest feeling "as if he were lying on a bathing beach inside out"; another guest, as if he were perspiring "sparks."[47]

Reporters had two primary reasons for distorting their "Liquid Sunshine" coverage. The first was economic. Given the proliferation of daily papers in the early twentieth century, reporters knew the importance of telling a good story. Radium's "ability to conjure" made the MIT dinner just that. In this context, attendees' mixed reviews of the cocktail cure may not have been enough to temper coverage of the event itself. With some attendees willing to extol its benefits, and with an imperative to sell papers, editors may have been willing to overlook conflicting accounts and print what many regarded as fiction. Another reason is that reporters may have already believed that the story was true. One *Newark News* reporter, although he himself had not tried the radium cocktail and could not confirm reports of its potent effects, said he had no doubt that it was "a physical rejuvenator not to be sneezed at."[48]

The reporters and their readerships had good reason to think that the Sunshine Dinner had, in fact, created a body that could radiate like the sun. Experiments by a Dr. Morton, covered in newspapers since early January, were said to have employed radium successfully to flood the body with sunshine. Morton believed that his "liquid sunshine" treatment, whereby he used a drinkable radium solution, could produce what he called an internal healing "violet light." And although he had yet to prove that the treatment cured anything, he announced several cases of consumption had already been dramatically improved.[49]

When Morton arrived at MIT on February 6 to set up and introduce the "liquid sunshine" toast, the connection between his unsubstantiated health claims and the "scientists" in attendance legitimized the treatment in the eyes of many reporters. Morton's "liquid sunshine," as the *New York Sun* reported in January 1904, threw "a flood of light upon the internal mechanism of mankind," and "to hear it mentioned or to see it in print is to long to quaff a rainbow tinted beaker of it on the spot . . . a liquid sunshine cocktail! That indeed is a dream worthy to stir the creative genius."[50] Such accounts grew in volume and intensity after the dinner, as

Americans in towns small and large contemplated how they, too, might "sweat sparks" by taking in a bit of radium's "drinkable sun."

"Liquid sunshine" firmly established a relationship between radium's power and the body's potential. Where Dr. Morton may have regarded the event as free publicity and the scientists as novel entertainment, reporters covered it as proof of an ingestible sun. Worshipping the sun as a source of life, heat, and power was a practice as ancient as civilization itself. In 1904, it seemed to many that technology had brought these elemental forces to the human body.

As Americans came into greater contact with radium over the next ten years, they sought ways if not to "perspire sparks," at least to radiate some of the energy suggested by the Sunshine Dinner's promise. Despite charges by a minority of journalists that the theories were products of "radiomania: the disease of the hour," caused by "hazy-mazy ideas about radium among the laity," the physical dreams of 1904 persevered.[51]

Up Close and Personal:
The Radium Fantasy Takes Hold, 1905–1915

By 1904, "radiomania" had escaped from the printed page and taken hold in America's living rooms. Lectures on radium were the latest thing at afternoon teas. Devices called spinthariscopes, magnified viewing tubes containing a miniscule speck of radium, became such popular Christmas gifts that store shelves were emptied. Also popular were radium roulette, an expensive party game played at night with luminous parts, and home-made imitations of "liquid sunshine," called radium punch (usually done with back-lit glasses).[52] Many made vacations out of traveling to stores and exhibitions to see radium samples, which in 1903 would have cost an average of $130,000.[53] Some people might have been fortunate enough to view local displays such as that displayed in a jewel box at Regal Shoes in Milwaukee; most had to travel to larger exhibits such as those at the New York Museum of Natural History or the 1904 St. Louis World's Fair.[54]

Contemporary accounts attest to the excitement of visiting these sites. According to several reports, the twice-daily radium exhibit attracted larger crowds than any other at the World's Fair.[55] The fervor may have been sparked by radium's expanding presence in popular culture.

Whereas "Liquid Sunshine" had previously been reserved for upper-class men, those with access to scientists at places like MIT, its appearance at world's fairs and department stores, spaces frequented equally by men and women of the upper and working classes, represented a shift.[56] This extended to popular performances, as William Hammer's profitable but theoretical lectures found a new competitor in Loie Fuller and her "radium dance" performances. Fuller's costumes illuminated her movements in an eerily darkened theater; the experience, in short, was seeing technology become beauty through the medium of her body.[57] As scientists continued to publish findings on radium's properties, and as experts continued to give public lectures, Americans began increasingly to pursue their own exposures, often through the purchase of purportedly "radium enhanced" consumer products. In 1905, well before medical science offered any "legitimate" equivalents, they created their own radiating bodies using products like "brightening" radium toothpaste, "glowing" radium hair tonic, "invigorating" radium-enriched earth, and "healthful" radium-laced chocolate bars.[58] The efficacy of these products was questionable at best. Their presence, however, suggests that consumers sought connections with radium beyond the analytical. They desired to see the element act on the body, to see its invisibility made visible in the form of topical and ingestible products.

That such products were bought purposefully, even though few contained even a trace of radium, suggests intense desire on the part of Americans to *believe* that radium could safely interact with the body. The desire to merge radium and the body, combined with vestiges of a powerful "liquid sunshine" dream, helps explain the wave of radium water fever that swept the country over the next twenty years.

In Pursuit of "Liquid Sunshine": Radium Waters Away and at Home, 1915–1925

Americans frequented hot springs long before the discovery of radium. Native Americans endowed sites like Hot Springs, Arkansas, and Glen Springs, South Carolina, with spiritual value; early explorers touted their healing capabilities; and, as early as the 1830s, entrepreneurs exploited their profit-making capabilities by building roads and erecting dwellings to draw ill but prosperous Northeasterners.[59] Throughout the nineteenth century, hot springs were seen as Mother Nature's cure for intractable conditions like tuberculosis and syphilis, as well as temporary ailments like neurasthenia. Their popularity had waned by 1915, inspiring several bathhouse owners, such as the Fordyces in Hot Springs, Arkansas, to pour hundreds of thousands of dollars into renovations. They added new mechanized attractions, including Zander machines and electric baths, for people who wanted to combine a recuperative vacation with the latest in scientific gadgetry.[60] Following the renovation, the electric bath facilities did bring in clients, and many spas enjoyed a period of increased profitability after 1915—until the discovery of sulfa drugs in the 1920s rendered mercury and hot water treatments anachronistic treatments for many illnesses.

Renovation and refurbishment, however, are not the whole story. Numerous American spas, including the bathhouses of Hot Springs; Glen Springs, New York; and Williamstown, Massachusetts, "discovered" radium in their waters between 1910 and 1915.[61] There was nothing new about promoting the content of spa water; brochures since the late nineteenth century had regularly contained breakdowns of their minerals. Montvale Springs in Tennessee, for example, listed the amounts of sulfuric acid, lime, and iron in each gallon of its water. Acid Springs in Genesee County, New York, included "silicic acid" and aluminum sulfate in its analysis.[62] Such data helped legitimize resorts' medical claims by connecting specific minerals with specific ailments. High levels of iron could purportedly "feed" unhealthy blood; acids might ameliorate disease. "Regular" medical practitioners typically dismissed the correlation between mineral waters and physical cures. Yet, the data resonated with the public, as evidenced by the ongoing use of the tactic over a period of sixty years.

Radium gave spa minerals a new façade of importance. Following a positive test for radium content in their spring water in 1914, the promoters at Hot Springs, Arkansas, made radium a central element in their promotional materials. In fact, they devoted more attention to radium content than to the costly renovations and machinery. In 1915, a brochure touted the waters as "radioactive to a marked degree." In stressing radium's efficacy, the brochure's writers were willing to sublimate the reputation of their new electrotherapy equipment to make a comparison: "Radio-active substances, unlike any other electro-therapy, are able to carry electrical energy deep into the body." As a result, the substances could subject what were called "the juices, protoplasm, and nuclei of the cells" to electrical bombardment much faster and more thoroughly than even the best electrical treatment could. After a good radium soak, the writers promised, cell activity was stimulated, secretory and excretory organs were aroused, and waste rapidly left the body.[63]

That the owners of the Fordyce would spend an amount four times what it cost to build the average bathhouse, and then give the structure and equipment a back seat to the water speaks volumes about radium's popularity.[64] For Americans trying to decide where to seek relaxation and improved health, radium was at least equally compelling as architecture and machine technology. The Fordyce reinforced in its brochures that electrotherapy, for all of its powerful benefits, had limitations when compared to the power of radium. Whereas at the turn of the century electrical baths and electrical belts had offered the most effective way to infuse the body with energy, radium appeared to go beyond general electrical stimulation to affect the body at a *cellular level.*

For a popular audience who combined ignorance about radium's physical effects on the body with certainty about its practical potential, it seemed reasonable to believe that radium could alter cells and halt decay. It is difficult to find individuals who confirm that this was why they visited Hot Springs, but it is reasonable to assume that marketers would have demoted radium from its central "draw" status had it not been working.[65] It is also likely that places like the Fordyce provided the firsthand experience with radium that so many Americans craved. Regardless of whether people were actually "cured" by the minute amount of radium present in the waters, an unlikely result given that significant exposure usually destroys the body's red blood cells, they may have left feeling that they had gotten a taste of the future, perhaps literally. Their experiences would combine with the old "liquid sunshine" myths, inspiring many who could not make the Hot Springs journey to seek those same rewards at home.

In May 1924, Henry Gaylord Wilshire received a letter from Harry Springdale, the president of Hollywood Radium Laboratories. It was at a critical juncture for Wilshire: he was just beginning to enjoy success from the sales of his electric I-ON-A-CO but still could have abandoned that venture. Springdale presented Wilshire with what must have been an attractive offer: a chance to invest in a new product that he had developed, one that he planned to advertise to twenty million people over the next several years. "Every youth and adult in the United States is a bonafide [*sic*] prospect," he declared, recognizing that it was indeed a fact that "almost surpasses the imagination."[66] The device that Springdale imagined would appeal to virtually every American was a radium-lined dispenser of drinking water. Small enough to fit on a kitchen counter, it offered the first efficient way for people to "take" radium without excessive investment or travel. Wilshire, if he joined quickly, would have the opportunity to bring this "most amazing and mysterious element" to the masses. It would require only a small leap of faith on his part, and an initial investment of several thousand dollars.

The assertion that "every youth and adult in the United States" was a prospective consumer signals a break from previous gender distinctions in energy-product marketing. Machine "unblocking" systems had overtly sought to develop "manhood," whether it was Windship's greater emphasis on men's bodies in his theories and centers or Sargent's greater contact with men's bodies through his careers at Bowdoin and Harvard. Electric "transfer" systems had, until the 1920s, offered to men products to grow active, muscular force and offered to women products to enhance beauty. With the development of radium water systems, a move toward a gender-neutral vision of technological energy emerged. Much as the I-ON-A-CO had combined the female-gendered ethos of beauty and rejuvenation with the male-gendered ethos of strength and force, radium water combined the domestic qualities of water with the scientific qualities of radium. The result was a product that offered women and men vitality that could be consumed together and taken into their respective worlds of business and domestic labor.[67]

Springdale's argument was convincing, though not in the way he intended. By June, Wilshire was attempting to organize his own radium drinking water company, complete with investors and control over product and profit. His archives leave several clues as to why the venture never took off. There was the problem of securing a radium sample, as documented by a 1924 letter from the Belgian embassy denying Wilshire's request for help.[68] Only a day earlier he heard from one R. P. Sherman, explaining that there was already a patent out on such containers, and if Wilshire attempted to market his own, "either ourselves, or some else will certainly bring action."[69] A businessman as resourceful as Wilshire, however, might not have let a shortage of radium and a potential legal entanglement stand in the way of profit. The plan seems finally to have failed because other investors simply would not join. With Wilshire's own capital caught up in electric belts, he probably had little to invest.

The failed venture sheds light on the process by which many of these radium products were deemed effective. In a letter to Williams and

Wilkins, publisher of scientific books, Wilshire asked the firm either to recommend a book proving the effectiveness of radium water dispensers or, if no such book existed, to hire someone to write it.[70] The reply, from a Charles Thomas who had investigated physicians' use of radium for years, must have been disheartening: "I completely failed to find a reputable physician who could give satisfactory evidence that such doses of radium were actually of value," he explained, concluding that although some experiments with large doses of radium had proved fruitful, they had absolutely no correlation to the efficacy of radium water dispensers. Wilshire's request that they simply "hire some" experts suggests that promoters with sufficient funds could buy evidence proving a product's effectiveness, even if scientific evidence was lacking.

It is likely that potential investors had little difficulty deciding not to invest the thousands necessary to purchase radium. Without even a single piece of evidence supporting radium water's efficacy either "scientific" or purchased, many probably felt the whole project was too risky. Yet, in spite of his investors' hesitation, Wilshire had good reason to believe in radium water's promise. Like many Americans, he had read and believed the rhetoric of radium dreams.[71] In a 1923 issue of *Popular Science Monthly* that Wilshire clipped and saved among his personal papers, the question "Will Radium Restore Youth" was answered in the affirmative. The author made little effort to dampen his own enthusiasm for the radium-enriched future on the horizon. "Longer life, new hair on bald heads, a third set of natural teeth, and renewed vigor of youth," he wrote, were just a few of the predictions that "optimistic radium experts" were making. And these experts were not talking about the large doses used in regular medical practice. All of these specific benefits would follow upon using radioactive water alone. The rhetoric is emblematic of the fine line that Americans had to discern between radium fact and radium fantasy. The author admitted that his claims had not yet been "generally accepted" by medical professionals but did not see this as a reason to doubt that the claims were true. There were sufficient experts intrigued enough to experiment, and sufficient success stories circulating that one could easily conclude that some of them must be true. Even without the American Medical Association's endorsement, the author was certain that low-dose radium treatments had "a definite place in medical treatment."[72] For people trying to uncover radium's "real story," there were layers upon layers of conjecture through which to wade.

Wilshire was not alone in setting stock in popular promises over empirical evidence. Radium water dispensers sold rapidly throughout the 1920s. Wilshire's product never made it to the marketplace, but plenty of others did. Mail order pamphlets and newspaper advertisements brought information about the Radium Ore Revigator, the Vitalizer, Thomas's Radium Ore-Lined Jars, the Radiumator, and the VigoRadium into homes nationwide.[73] We can assume from the sheer number of such products that they enjoyed popular acceptance. Further, though Hollywood Radium Laboratories undoubtedly padded its projected success to entice investors like Wilshire, its figure of twenty million potential buyers might not have been too far off. By the 1920s, Americans were ready to see the fifteen-year-old promises of "liquid sunshine" realized. Party novelties and hot springs had kept the dream of perpetual energy and internal sunshine alive but had not provided conclusive results or wide-spread access. Water dispensers were the first inexpensive way to pursue the promise. One could buy a dispenser for an initial investment ranging from eight to fifteen dollars, an amount that a middle-class or working-class couple could save over several months. Further, as with electric belts, sellers typically offered payment options that allowed people to pay as little as a few dollars to have their "radium jar" delivered and set up in the kitchen.

In the 1920s, radium water jars combined improved accessibility with four specific "radium promises" that captured the popular imagination. First, it was "liquid sunshine" for the masses; in form it was almost identical to that which the MIT guests had imbibed fifteen years earlier. Whereas that "liquid sunshine" had been created with tiny tubes of radium put into glasses, radium jars embedded radium in their lining. This created, in essence, a giant glass of "liquid sunshine" that dispensed smaller glasses as frequently as one desired. One could, if one owned a radium dispenser and had access to tap water, enjoy physical radium transformation just as the privileged dinner patrons had. Manufacturers subtly communicated this populist element of their product. In 1927, the Vigoradium corporation, for example, promoted its dispenser in bold letters on its pamphlet covers as putting "health, vigor, vitality within reach of us all."[74] Another manufacturer suggested that consumers might elevate themselves financially and physically to the privileged class by using the product: five glasses daily from the Revigator would "increase your income by keeping you and your family fit . . . with the alertness and vitality possessed only by the people whose bodies are functioning perfectly."[75] Here was a product that not only made "liquid sunshine" possible but suggested to those who might have read about the MIT event that by drinking it they might elevate themselves to MIT-elite status.

Radium jars also borrowed from the rhetoric of liquid sunshine. Morton's cocktail claimed nature as the key to its potency. When one underwent his internal radium therapy, the effect was purportedly similar to placing the internal organs in the direct path of the sun's healing rays. Radium jars, said their proponents, worked by enriching the body with superpowered water. In advertisements, the jars were described as part natural and part scientific in their healing properties. Because their most plentiful product was water, advertisers could say they were offering what was really an age-old cure with only a slightly modern twist. Brochure titles, such as Radiumator's, which carried a description of its dispenser as a "Perpetual Health Spring," stressed that the jars, though created by humans, were not really artificial. "Radio-activity, exactly the same element as is possessed by Revigorated Water," explained the Revigator's manufacturer, "is the element of spring water that reaches every portion of the body and has the peculiar property of ejecting poisons from every organ of the body."[76] This connection to water may have also worked to convince reluctant consumers that in spite of radium's powerful reputation, there was no danger. As the promoter of Thomas's Radium Jars declared in the early 1920s, "[Y]our body is over 75% water. Why not irrigate with Radio-Active Water?"[77]

Radium jars, however, were not portrayed by promoters as exclusively "natural" substances but as essentially "nature's helpers." Water alone, in manufacturers' rhetoric, was not going to get one far in the modern age. Using a strategy similar to that of electrotherapy purveyors, the jar manufacturers stressed that the best kind of "natural cure" was one that added a bit of technological ingenuity. Typical of most sellers, the Revigorated Water Company promoted its brand as able to "normalize" the body's chemistry with radium, the result of which was that "nature" was "again given the strength to help herself."[78] Contextualized as "nature's little helper," radium water jars were able to take on a character that was at once frightening and innocuous. Just as "liquid sunshine" had combined images of internal organs directly exposed to the sun's intense rays with endless bounty and health, radium dispensers fused alpha-ray ingestion to spring water soaking.

Promoters of radium water jars also attempted to educate prospective consumers as to how their products improved health. Earlier schemes, like "liquid sunshine" and even radium springs, had only vaguely hinted at how radium affected the body. Perhaps it was the direct effect of the sun in the case of "liquid sunshine" or the combination of mineral water and radium at places like Hot Springs. Radium water dispenser manufacturers, for the first time, prescribed regimens for treatment and described probable results. Most manufacturers told consumers to drink at least five glasses of the water a day for sixty to ninety days so as to get the "full results." Many warned that their products were not quick fixes; one could enjoy health benefits only by following the plan for an extended period. This strategy, while suggesting that radium jars were not miracle cures, probably established them as legitimate medical regimens for many users.

Theories abounded as to how radium water jars worked and what exactly the treated water did for the body. The promoters of Thomas's Radium Jars said that drinking radium water exposed one's organs and glands to "higher vibrations" that caused the body to resonate properly and eliminated disease.[79] Henry Springdale, in imploring Wilshire to join Hollywood Radium Corporation in 1924, attributed the jars' efficacy to "three elements . . . light, heat and energy," which, when taken together, added "many years to the span of human life."[80] Other companies actually did engage in the mainstream scientific radium discussion by evoking alpha rays, commonly used in physicians' cancer treatments. Although alpha rays could destroy tissue, the Vitalizer's manufacturers conceded, they could also create "healthy stimulation" when emitted in water.[81] Yet exactly how the rays went from agents of cellular destruction to forces of health no one said. Nor did they need to.

Radium jar companies multiplied throughout the 1920s. Vitalizers, Revigators, and Vigoradiums were part of a door-to-door sales boom that proved irresistible to those like Springdale and Wilshire, hungry for an easy profit. And the profit was certainly there for the taking. There is every reason to believe that members of the public, primed by twenty years of popular radium myth making and speculation, simply had faith that five-gallon jugs on their kitchen countertops could remake their bodies. The claims of manufacturers echoed similar ones made by "top scientists" about "liquid sunshine." Robert Young of Wichita, Kansas, for example, said he had gained in "flesh and strength, hope and courage" as a consequence of his five-month Revigator regimen.[82] Likewise, Thomas's radium jar company reported that after several months' regular radium consumption users perceived a new "vigor, . . . joy of living . . . and vanishing of melancholy."[83]

Legitimate scientific research left plenty of space for these extravagant claims to resonate. Of course, there were many, like scientist Paul Boernsen, who after ten years of radium study concluded in 1915 that most of what people were calling "wonderful" about the element was based on ignorance. There probably were no more than six people in all of the United States, he contended, who possessed more than superficial knowledge about radium. The hundreds of others experimenting with it in potions and writing about it in the press were mostly playing around with doses too small to have any effect. Water potions and springs fell into the placebo category, any good they did was because people wanted to believe, not because there was scientific evidence for the cures.[84] Yet between 1900 and 1920, a *Readers' Guide* survey reveals, information on radium's physical benefits was almost always positive.[85] These "inaccuracies and exaggerations," as one reporter called them, were in all likelihood attributable to the cultural moment. Many people who heard about radium's powers were often of the same generation that had once been incredulous about reports of electricity, the telephone, X rays, and the automobile. In each instance, the fantastic had been more rooted in fact than fantasy. As Cleveland Moffett wrote in *Success* magazine, given the precedent, "[W]hy not believe in extending life indefinitely?"[86]

Even the most respected radium scientists held, often against all logic, that radium was, *in all cases,* physically beneficial. Marie Curie, radium's codiscoverer, continued to believe until she died that radium was a benevolent force for the body. Her slow decline, increasing frailty and decreasing bone-marrow density, all suggested that some sort of cancer was consuming her body, yet Curie persisted in denying that radium could have any detrimental effect. Only after her death, when the diagnosis of aplastic pernicious anemia was made, did it become irrefutable that the years of radioactivity exposure had rendered her body's blood cells terminally weakened.[87]

Curie was not alone. Henry Green, a respected radium researcher, believed for years that his ability to work without what he called "appreciable fatigue" was due primarily to radium's stimulating effect. He often bragged about his strength, commenting that unlike most people, going to the office added more energy to his body than it depleted. Even after his skin began to darken and slough off in 1908 and his hands ulcerated, Green continued his research, driven by the notion that if he stopped working with radium his energy level would sink and he would die. Green, like Curie, did eventually succumb to his radium-induced injuries; he never abandoned his adamant belief in radium's physical benefits.[88]

Jar manufacturers legitimized their products by declaring them scientific. Rhetorically, promoters walked a fine line between extolling the natural virtues of their water and stressing the underlying scientific expertise that purportedly created their cures. Water was indeed the primary curative element, Vitalizer's promotion experts explained in 1925, but "all of this has been made possible by the ability of trained chemists and eminent scientists in . . . harnessing [radium's] rays of gas and employing them in medical practice."[89] We know from Wilshire's own investigations that scientists in the 1920s were unable to find evidence that low doses of radium emanations, such as those used in the Vitalizer's treatments, had any beneficial effect on the body whatsoever. Even so, jar manufacturers did not cease equating their miniscule radium dosages and the large dosages given by physicians during office treatments. In an age when irregular practitioners still enjoyed a good amount of influence, jar manufacturers could count on consumer ignorance. Few would differentiate between the proven benefits of radium in "medical practice" and the doubtful claims for radium in water jugs.

Scientific legitimacy was not established through rhetoric alone. Design, iconography, and consumer interaction also played powerful roles. Even in the earliest 1920s models, promotional materials went to great lengths to portray the radium water jars as scientific. One advertisement for the Revigator shows the jar as a vision of modern technology (fig. 32). Its white porcelain finish announces its superior sanitary properties; its rounded edges presage the streamlined designs of the next decades. A lightning-bolt streams downward on its label featuring the product's name, a technique that draws the eye downward to other lightning bolts coming from the water pouring from a gleaming, stainless-steel spigot. The electric imagery is, at first glance, somewhat confusing. First of all, radium did not emit lightning bolts when immersed in water. Second, by the 1920s, electric cures were becoming somewhat passé. The bolts, however, are indicative of the importance of a scientific image to these jars' success. Radium's invisibility necessitated creativity: manufacturers borrowed electricity's cultural cachet, assuming that readers would make the connection.

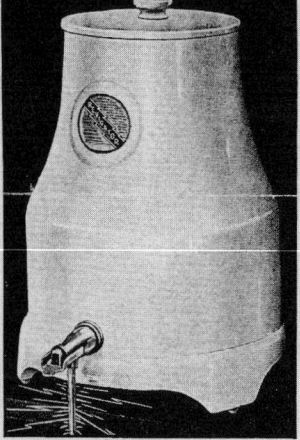

Put One of these in Your HOME!

ENLISTING the help of the Revigator will increase your income by keeping you and your family always fit, always in the pink of good health, with the alertness and vitality possessed only by people whose bodies are functioning perfectly. There is no comparison between the earning power of the man who keeps himself in splendid health and the man who readily falls a victim to those little ailments that sap his vitality, steal his vigor and keep him perpetually "below par." By keeping you always at the pinnacle of glowing health the Revigator will give you new strength to surmount obstacles and reach whatever goal you have set your heart on attaining.

The Revigator

The Revigator is an ornamental porcelain water jar, the interior of which is lined with a patented composition of radio-active ores. This composition actually charges ordinary tap water with the vital radio-active emanation—the potent life giving element that gives spring water its special health giving value. To drink Revigorated water is exactly like drinking water bubbling fresh from the sparkling health springs. No bottled water can have the same effects as the water from the Revigator for the vital radio-active properties of the water as it left the spring are rapidly dissipated upon exposure. For sparkling radiant health—for the wonderful natural properties that only radio activity possesses—drink from the Revigator.

What Revigator Does

Radio-activity, exactly the same as is possessed by Revigorated Water is the element of spring water that reaches every portion of the body and has the peculiar property of ejecting poisons from every organ of the body. The organs, when once relieved of a long storage of accumulated poisons, can naturally act efficiently. Thus, the chemistry of the body becomes normalized—and nature is again given the strength to help herself. It is found for this reason that thousands of chronic sick people everywhere have found relief through the life giving radio-activity of the Revigator, in hundreds of instances where other methods had proved to be without avail.

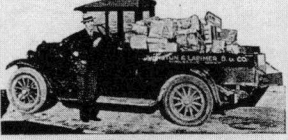

55-Year-Old Man Gains in Flesh, Strength, Hope and Courage

"There is nothing that is too good to say for the Revigator. It has been a wonderful help to me. I bought one and began to drink the water. I gained in flesh and strength, hope and courage. I weighed 138 pounds when I began to drink the water. Now, after drinking it about five months, I weigh 153 pounds. I work every day, and can do as much now as when a young man. I am 55 years old."

(Signed) ROBERT YOUNG,
1712 Mildred Ave., Wichita, Kansas.

NATURE'S HEALTH SPRING

Fig. 32. Advertisement for the Revigator, pamphlet, folder 0723-05. Courtesy of the American Medical Association.

By the late 1920s, this allusion was no longer necessary. New dispensers such as the Radiumator eschewed superficial lightning bolts for a design evocative of a modern chemistry lab (fig. 33). The assemblage of glass tubes, hand pumps, and coils suggested that an elaborate scientific system was at work. The experience of using the device mimicked performing a precise experiment. There were five steps to "radiumizing" water: lifting up the mechanism by pulling on the hand pump; placing a specially designed glass under the base to create an "air tight" connection with the emerging water; pumping the bulb fifteen times to pull the water from the glass; infusing it with radium through the glass tubes; and depositing the finished product back in the glass; and then lifting up the entire contraption once again to release the glass, which had to be drunk "at once" lest any of the infused radium escape.[90] Because the process had to

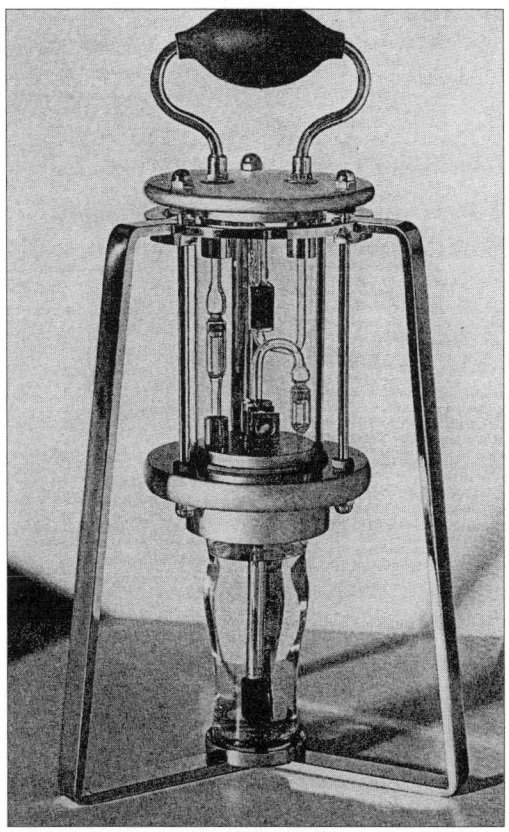

Fig. 33. "Medical Science Harnesses One of Nature's Rarest Forces for Health," The North American Radium Corporation (New York, undated), folder 0719-02. Courtesy of the American Medical Association.

be repeated five times daily, users had ample opportunity to be reminded of the device's scientific precision.

Radium water manufacturers went one step beyond visions of enhanced minds, radiating bodies, and populist science. Vigoradium, a company whose self-proclaimed goal was putting "health—vigor—and vitality within reach of all," illustrated dramatically how its product coordinated the efforts of nature, health, and science to bestow physical perfection upon consumers (fig. 34). Its promotional pamphlet's cover featured a dispensing device similar to that of other companies, but it was overshadowed by a sculpted body. A man stands with the scientific dispenser held high in his left hand while his right hand holds the radium-infused water at groin level. He glances downward, watching the powerful beams of radium's power emanating from his cup as he prepares to drink the contents. Below him, illuminated only by the rays of his beverage, are the undifferentiated masses who reach upward as if hoping to share in his superior power by capturing a part of his radiation beams. It is not the natural water, or the promise of specific cures, or even powerful science that take the center stage in Vigoradium's advertising iconography. The star is the body: tall, muscular, sexualized, confident. Here the accompanying words "health," "vigor," and "vitality" are not merely suggesting that radium will restore one's health to adequate levels. Once connected to the physical image, such words clearly suggest energy transcendence. In Vigoradium's world, the cup of radium water releases unimagined physical power; it is the long-sought source of limitless energy attained.

Realizing Radium's Superman Dreams: The Radithor Controversy, 1925–1932

It would be easy to dismiss Vigoradium's cover image. We could attribute its sculpted male figure to the contemporary art deco vogue of chiseled, physical giants, or declare it one inconclusive pamphlet. Dismissal would be easy, that is, were it not for Radithor. In 1925, "Dr." William J. A. Bailey developed his own brand of "liquid sunshine" with the express goal of creating supermen. His product, Radithor, became the most popular radium cure in American history. The story behind it reveals much about the promises of energy transfer, the relationship between radium and the modern body, and the perils of believing that physical perfection could be achieved by absorbing technological energies.

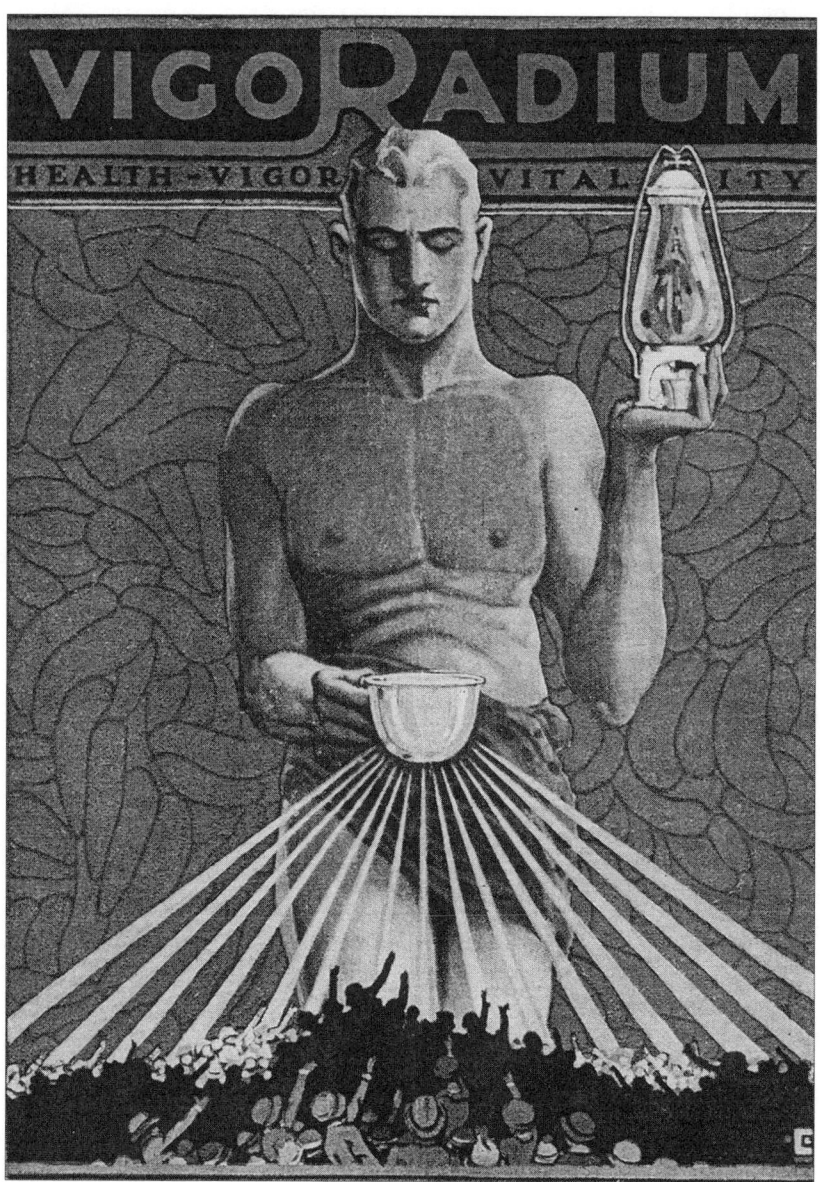

Fig. 34. Advertisement for the Vigoradium water dispenser. "Health, Vigor, Vitality," Vigoradium Corporation (New York, 1927), folder 0721-04. Courtesy of the American Medical Association.

Bailey was born in Boston in 1884. He liked to refer to himself as "Dr." Bailey, although he never made it further in higher education than dropping out of Harvard's class of 1907. Bailey dabbled with importing and exporting in the 1910s before becoming interested in endocrine stimulation and radium in the 1920s. Given his lack of medical background, the sudden career change seems odd. It is possible that he heard Marie Curie during her 1921 tour of the United States. Or perhaps he simply felt the cumulative effect of twenty years of popular radium speculation. In the early twenties Bailey began a New York company called Associated Radium Chemists that turned out products to combat coughs, influenza, and diminished metabolisms.[91] Shortly thereafter, Bailey was shut down for advertising fraud. Undeterred, he began immediately to market the Radioendocrinator, a gold-plated, radium-containing belt that, he argued, could rejuvenate various parts of the body depending on where it was worn: the thyroid if around the neck; the adrenals if around the waist; and the prostate if worn with an included suspensory attachment that fit under the scrotum.[92]

Although Bailey was clearly beholden to his quack progenitors, particularly those like "Dr." Crystal and "Dr." Sanden, he saw radium as a new product that called for new treatments. Bailey's understanding of the body was more sophisticated than that of earlier electric belt and remedy purveyors. He translated Marie Curie's 1910 *Treatise on Radioactivity* from the French, which suggests that he had at least a sophisticated layman's understanding of physiology and how the body reacted to radium exposure.[93] Bailey was certainly never the physician he purported to be, but his self-acquired radium knowledge helped him develop a well-crafted explanation of his products' efficacy. He brought this to Radithor in 1925, a radium-water cure-all that ultimately brought Bailey fame, fortune, and disfavor.

Between 1925 and 1930, more than 400,000 bottles of Radithor were sold worldwide. These half-ounce bottles from Bailey's East Orange factory were a striking commercial success.[94] A great deal of the success could have been attributed to association: Radithor, a liquid radium solution, looked much like the "liquid sunshine" that had driven demand for hot springs treatments and home water jars. It was, in some respects, simply old news in new wrapping. In important ways, however, Bailey set out to differentiate his product from those of his predecessors. In advertising pamphlets and in his promotional book *Modern Rejuvenation*

Methods, written in 1926 by his disciple, Charles Evans Morris, Bailey declared that Radithor was the first effective radium product. Unlike radium water jars, which he called "contraptions . . . of absolutely no therapeutic value" that contained, at best, only a "few cents" of radium, Radithor contained real radium in the form of radium-226 and radium-228.[95] Further, Radithor did not rely exclusively upon radium for its cures; it also contained mesothorium, a secret ingredient that Bailey said he himself had discovered after years of endocrine research. Only mesothorium had "a special affinity for endocrine glands," allowing it to control radium's power.[96] When one drank a bottle of Radithor, Bailey asserted, mesothorium effectively guided the radium toward the endocrine glands, where it could accomplish the most dramatic physical effects.

Bailey was not reticent when it came to Radithor's medicinal benefits. If one took the prescribed daily dosage of one to three bottles, a total of between .5 and 1.5 liquid ounces, one could expect two primary effects. First, in the spirit of "liquid sunshine," Radithor would bathe the body in light energy. *Modern Rejuvenation Methods* related that after one drink of the radium water, "immediately the whole body is flooded with billions and billions of Alpha rays that liberate their energy throughout the entire system like floods of sunshine." In essentially the same language that MIT's dinner guests had used a generation earlier to describe being "turned inside out," here energy dissipation was explained as reaching "every cell, every gland and every nook and corner of the body to revivify and quicken to action every fibre and tissue of the organism."[97] The rhetoric consummated the marriage between Radithor and its forerunners, yet it alone probably would not have created the popular vogue. By including mesothorium, Bailey was able to associate the general claims of "flooding sunshine" with specific bodily effects. His description echoed Butler's for the Health Lift fifty years earlier: as patients drank Radithor, radium and mesothorium went through the stomach and intestines, entered the blood stream, and thence were carried throughout the body. Because of the mesothorium, Bailey argued, the radium then traveled directly to the glands, where it was "greedily attracted" and absorbed.[98]

Bailey used an idiosyncratic combination of mechanical and radium energy theories to explain Radithor's effect. The endocrine system, consisting of the body's major glands, was the "dynamo of the organism."

Here, Bailey borrowed directly from earlier physiologists like Dudley Allen Sargent. Rather than arguing that all energy comes directly from the muscular system, however, Bailey put forward the notion that it emanated from "gland catalysts." Only healthy, powerful glands could stave off diseases like obesity, hypertension, impotence, and even baldness. Bailey wisely avoided fully codifying a system of glandular health, providing few specifics on exactly how certain glands controlled physical traits. Radithor's physical action, however, made such specifics largely unnecessary. By carrying the flood of light energy to each gland in the body, it guaranteed believers that whatever their gland troubles were, the mesothorium "physician" would make sure they were cured. As a result, Radithor seemed a health system that cured particular ailments while increasing the energy and well-being of the body as a whole. According to Morris, Radithor users who had "burned up their energies too rapidly" soon found themselves mentally and physically transformed, a state he described as being fired with "the energy of romantic youth."[99]

Radithor was the only radium cure to explicitly promise to turn external energy into internal energy. As *Modern Rejuvenation Methods* explained, Radithor worked primarily because it was able to bring "new life and energy" to the body through a "transmutation of electronic energy into physical and mental force."[100] The first part of this claim said nothing new: machine, electricity, and radium promoters had long promised to bring new life, new vigor, and new energy into the body's muscular and nerve resources. But Bailey took it a step further, suggesting that Radithor could actually convert radium's "electronic energy" into usable physical force. Given that consumers were already familiar with radium's ability to create perpetual motion and its resistance to decay, such a claim was revolutionary. If radium could actually be absorbed by the body and converted into energy for physical and mental force, then perhaps that force could also be unceasing. Radithor thus became the first permanent solution to the nineteenth-century's "neurasthenic" paradigm. Machines might increase muscles and electricity might energize tired nerves, but only radium could actually transform the glands into continual catalysts for their own rejuvenation.

Bailey saw himself creating a modern American Adam. Disciple Morris called him a "master craftsman for the regeneration of man and woman."[101] The text further makes clear just what Bailey thought he was crafting. Using a quotation in the introduction from Dr. Fritz Haber,

Modern Rejuvenation Methods implies that Radithor is instrumental in the crafting of a new human type: "Science" would soon "bring forth discoveries that [will] produce a race of supermen who may be expected to live as long as a thousand years through elimination of the causes of natural death."[102]

Radithor's vision bears startling similarities to the Vigoradium image. It imagines a body literally on fire with the passions of youth, a body whose every gland is functioning to its energized capacity, staving off illness, impotence, obesity, fatigue, and even death. Bailey clearly believed that his marriage of radium to mesothorium had delivered on the generation-old promise of continual physical renewal. One can see the distinct connection between his claims and the earliest images of radium's promises, such as the illustration accompanying the 1903 article "Radium: Its Possibilities as Seen by its Discoverer," which ran in the *Indianapolis Star* (fig. 35). "It has been stated," explained *Modern Rejuvenation Methods* to prospective buyers, "that there is practically no limit to human life and human energies if the entire chain of endocrine glands can be maintained in full normal functioning power."[103] Here was a way for believers to swallow the promises of radium's continuous rejuvenation and imagine a body more powerful than time itself.

Epilogue: Radium Triumph or Radium Terror?

Radithor should interest us, if only for its theoretical potential. In Bailey we have an American who, like many of his contemporaries, sought to narrow the gap between an enervated nineteenth century and a bountiful twentieth. Born in the 1880s, he came of age at a time rife with doomsday predictions for the human form: from George Beard to Theodore Roosevelt, individuals equated mechanized modernity with physical decline. If we judge by only Radithor's popularity, Bailey successfully offered a way out of this energy paradox.

Yet Bailey did more than theorize; he made a product that worked. Unlike hot springs and water jugs, or even the "liquid sunshine" of 1904, Radithor contained actual radium in doses large enough to affect the body. Its ultimately detrimental effects may have, at their onset, been interpreted by users as signs of improved health. If taken regularly, it decreased the number of red blood cells and increased the pace of glandular

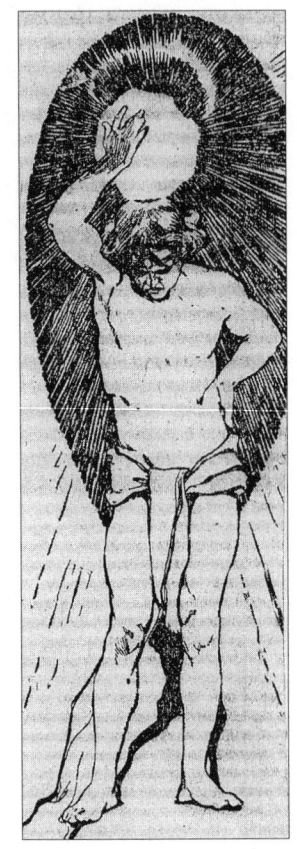

Fig. 35. The radium-powered body. "Radium: Its Possibilities as Seen by Its Discoverer," *Indianapolis Star* (December 29, 1903), 4.

activity; it often lowered blood pressure, reduced weight, and provided a sense of increased energy for users. In this sense, it did "refire" the vigor of youth. Radithor's very success, however, serves as a parable for the ultimate effect of American energy-transfer theories. The product did more than "refire," it literally set the body aflame, creating energy that eventually turned the body upon itself, destroying the supermen it created.

In 1932, Eben M. Byers died slowly and painfully after an eighteen-month bout with a mysterious illness. It did not go unnoticed. As a high-profile industrialist, millionaire sportsman, and prolific socialite, Byers had been characerized as "embodying the spirit of the roaring twenties."[104] He seems to have been afraid of little; he continued to invest in his Pittsburgh Iron Foundry after the 1929 stock market crash, and he was always up to a sportsman's challenge, particularly in trapshooting and golf, at which he was particularly skilled. Above all his accomplishments, however, Byers prided himself on his physique. He was often described as a "broad-chested athlete" of imposing stature. And he was not reluctant to brag about his physical health and his ability to defy the pull of age that was slowing his contemporaries. Yet, it was his turn to Radithor in the late 1920s that accounted for the notoriety of his death.

Byers believed that Radithor was the fountain of youth. Over the years he took daily doses, he frequently sent friends cases as gifts, telling them about the tremendous boost of energy it provided. Byers's conviction in the treatment's effectiveness is clear from his own consumption: soon after starting, he tripled his dosage to two 2.2 ounce bottles each day instead of the .5 to 1.5 ounces recommended by Bailey.[105] Byers was so convinced of Radithor's physical benefits that he continued to take his augmented dosage, even after 1930, when he began to suffer a series of strange ailments.

Over the next year and a half, Byers saw his health gradually deteriorate. First it was repeated bone fractures and skin abscesses. In time, the fractures rendered him immobile and the abscesses progressed to the point of actual holes in his skull. When Byers died in 1932, he weighed ninety-two pounds and all but two teeth of his lower jaw had been surgically removed in a futile effort to stop bone decay. The official cause of death was anemia, brain abscess, and advanced jaw decay.

Byers's death brought the story of physical enhancement full circle. His ninety-two-pound frame resembled those of other self-described weaklings: Butler and Windship. For these machine advocates, technology was a way to build physical strength. Byers's decline from a man of strength to a "weakling" however, was *caused* by his use of technology. His fate represents a consequence unfathomed by early advocates: that technology could actually destroy the bodies it promised to build.

It did not take long after Byers's death for the medical community and press to conclude that Radithor had killed him. The very day after his demise, the *New York Times* front-page headline read, "Eben M. Byers Dies of Radium Poisoning."[106] Physicians joined in the anti-Radithor crusade in letters among themselves, and in pleas to the public.

One doctor, appearing on a radio broadcast following Byers's death, held up what he called a Radithor victim's bones to a Geiger counter in order to demonstrate what he called the "deadly sound of radium."[107] Such public relations efforts soon had the desired effect. By 1933, Bailey had been shut down, his supply of Radithor confiscated as a significant risk to public health.

Byers's dramatic death and the subsequent demise of Bailey's reputation leave one curious as to why it had not happened sooner. Bailey had never attempted to hide the amount of radium in his product. Quite the contrary, he considered it one of Radithor's major selling points, something that differentiated it from "ineffective" cures like radium jars. In a statement startlingly similar to an MIT diner's claim to have "sweated sparks," Bailey declared that if one took a "single drop" of blood or sweat from a Radithor user, you would find it radioactive, even if that person had drunk only one bottle.[108] Despite the admitted radioactivity, Bailey vehemently argued that his solution posed no danger to the body.

In 1926, Morris, speaking on Bailey's behalf, charged that those who said radium could be injurious to the body were talking about far greater doses than he was using. Not once in "millions of treatments" had there been one "single record of harmful effects."[109] Even physicians, contrary to their united front after the Byers incident, had previously given the public reasons to accept Bailey's claims. One doctor who had discovered Radithor while treating neurasthenic patients found that the product worked equally well on himself. Remarking that it was better than the traditional uppers such as opium and alcohol that his colleagues used, F. E. Park urged the *New York Medical Journal*'s readers to consider Radithor: "There are always times in our busy life when the work comes so fast that we are tired out," but the effect of Radithor when one is tired ". . . is simply magical, as I can testify. In my own case I pass, in about twelve hours, from exhaustion to one of perfect well being, and this condition persists."[110]

Radithor survived because its promotional materials told people exactly what they wanted to hear. Bailey's previous attempts at radium elixirs—in cough syrups and impotence belts—had been promptly shut down for advertising fraud. Such items harkened back to the nineteenth century and were thus easily labeled "quackery" and dismissed by professionals and the more educated among the public. Yet Radithor's promise resonated with what laypeople and experts alike had for years hoped possible.

According to Linda Henderson, up through the 1920s any talk of radium's physical hazards was tempered by radium enthusiasm. During the time of Byers's Radithor use, Henderson describes the public's view of radium as "a magical, perpetual source of heat and light—and perhaps even the elixir of life" and asserts that hope "far outweighed concern about its potential perils."[111] A cursory survey of the *Readers' Guide* confirms Henderson's view. Even though radium poisoning had been discovered as early as 1920, positive titles of radium articles outnumbered negative titles two to one. Tellingly, in the 1930s, after the Byers story broke and Bailey found himself out of business, radium (though not Radithor) received even better grades from the press: positive titles outnumbered negative titles three to one.[112]

For a reason that medical figures were at a loss to explain, the American public was not to be easily disabused of its radium dreams. One can sense their frustration in the 1934 comments of physicians Hector Colwell and Sidney Russ, experts on radium injuries and advocates for cautious radium use: "For some reason or other there appears to be a widespread tendency in the public mind to regard everything connected with 'rays' as on that account conducive to health and vitality."[113] Bailey's demise and Byers's death had effectively proven "liquid sunshine" dreams false. There would be no perpetual glandular motion, no permanent transfusion to stave off the effects of age, no technocellular fountain of youth. Yet the dreams did not easily fade. It would take "fallout," the product of an unimaginably powerful "energized" bomb, to turn popular opinion away from radium fantasies and toward radium facts. Only when facing the stark realities of radioactive milk in the refrigerator and radioactive bones in their children did Americans finally abandon radium promises.[114]

As little as five years before Americans confronted the horrors of Hiroshima and Nagasaki, energized radium fantasies persisted. In 1940, Dr. R. M. Langer, a research associate in physics at the California Institute of Technology, told *Colliers* readers what they could expect from the future of atomic power: soon, a world of "unparalleled riches . . . handed from the scientists in their laboratories to the engineers in their factories" would be arriving in the form of atomic power.[115] In language surprisingly similar to that at the onset of radiomania, experts waxed poetic about endless energy produced from reactors. Outdoor grills would burn indefinitely; cars would go around the world on limitless tanks of gas; indoor lights would shine continuously. The vision of unlimited atomic bounty grew hand in hand with visions of unprecedented atomic destruction, for if Americans had learned anything in the past seventy years it was that energy always offered the body more than it took away. One needed merely to trust in the "experts," embrace the technology, and prepare for another round of energy promises that just might deliver on their physical dreams.

Conclusion
The End of an Era?

Just at the time that I was finishing my first draft of this book, a book caught my attention as I was browsing the supermarket aisles. It was a guide to Pilates, the exercise system of stretching and balance founded almost a century ago by Joseph Pilates. I had heard about Pilates from friends who had urged me to come with them to their classes. Up to that point, I had avoided the sessions that had sounded to me like a cross between elementary ballet and medieval torture. Yet I could not help flipping through the book after reading a cover blurb endorsing the "revolutionary new system." Pilates, it seems, is giving us all a better way to train our bodies by bringing us "fitness without machines."

There can be little doubt that the machines of Joseph Butler, Dudley Allen Sargent, and Gustav Zander shaped twentieth-century fitness, for although Dio Lewis's theories of regimented movements remain alive and well in today's jazzercize and aerobics, it is machines that drive modern fitness systems. Many Americans exercise exclusively on machines. And even those who continue to prefer an outdoor jog to an indoor session on the StairMaster frequently use machines to augment their training.

For anyone who has casually looked at his or her local fitness center, it is difficult to argue that these early inventors of machines were inconsequential. Their legacy is that the most popular machines in 2002 still look surprisingly similar to those of 1882. Windship and Butler's Health Lifts can be seen in the heavy-weight section, reflected in back, leg, and calf machines that work by adding or subtracting iron weights. Modern variations on Sargent's rowing machines are requisite in any gym, as are StairMasters and climbers that operate on Sargent's principle of balanced exertion and controlled natural movements. Even the failed "inomotor" lives on in spirit in Cross Trainers, machines that provide elliptical resistance for users' arms and legs and promise a "total body

213

workout" involving "all the major upper and lower body muscle groups."[1] Zanders also continue to influence modern fitness practices, regardless of the fact that passive-resistance machines had fallen out of favor in America by the 1920s. Chest- and leg-press machines, for example, though they use active resistance, are nearly identical in experience and appearance to those of Zander's original design: users still sit on cushioned chairs, place their arms or feet against metal platforms, and measure their muscular success by the progressive motions in the machine.

Machines have become so synonymous with fitness over the past century that systems like Pilates can re-create themselves as "new" and "visionary" merely because they *do not* use them. Yet the machinery's ubiquity does not in itself prove that the energy theories of their creators have had a cultural impact. Certainly it is difficult to find a machine user today who would agree with early inventors' theories about how energy was created in the body. We now understand the circulatory system well enough to realize that energy cannot be held hostage in one portion of the body because of underdeveloped muscles. We also know, as Windship and Butler did not, that lifting tremendous amounts does not force energy through the system; it actually puts a dangerous strain on the heart and joints. And we no longer subscribe to Sargent's belief that physical energy can result only from a perfectly balanced physique. Today, most machine users, if they think about energy at all, regard it as a positive by-product of their workout, not an immediate goal. We no longer live with the fear that our bodies, if unaided, will soon run out of energy and fail to function. Consequently, we appreciate feeling "energized" after a good workout but no longer engage in activities explicitly to get energy. Most gym users are more interested in looking thin and sculpted than in maximizing their energy potential.[2]

One could pose the same doubts about the ultimate effect of electrical energy theories. It is possible to find an occasional electro-magnetic belt, such as the models currently available at Target. The majority of electric health devices, however, are collecting dust in attics. Products such as the Electropoise and the I-ON-A-CO that once inspired fervent letters from true believers had faded from view by midcentury. And although some of their manufacturers' difficulties were due to the persistent efforts of the American Medical Association, a more exact cause of death was simply cultural change. By 1940, mysterious diseases like tuberculosis that might have seemed treatable by "electrified air" had nearly disappeared, thanks to immunizations. Increasingly effective pain relievers dramatically reduced the numbers of arthritis and rheumatism sufferers who had been drawn to inventions like Wilshire's. And a combination of sulfa drugs to treat venereal diseases and a relaxation in the culture's sexual taboos combined to make the need for electric belts far less pressing. Today's electrical therapies have more to do with removing unwanted hair and smoothing wrinkles than with augmenting the body's internal energy in any lasting way.

It is in the area of radium therapy, however, where we have traveled the greatest distance from the beliefs of original promoters. Gone are the days when radium water dispensers made good investments and Eben Byers embodied the promise of radium's limitless physical energy. By 1950, radium was no longer the darling of physicists and entrepreneurs. Byers's well-publicized, gruesome death made many conscious of the real health risks involved in ingesting a substance whose potential remained largely unknown. And once World War II revealed that previously unknown potential to be death itself, one could no longer argue that radium was capable of building a superior body. The greater use of radiation in oncology only further reinforced radium's budding reputation as a destroyer rather than a creator of matter.

Over the course of the 1950s, the enthusiasm that once inspired everything from radium-powered cars to radium-fueled barbecues slowly gave way to fear. This was heightened with the discovery of "fall out," the radioactivity that returned to earth after dissipating into the atmosphere. By the mid 1950s, radium was more likely to be equated with contaminated water, decimated vegetation, and inexplicable birth defects than to be touted as a source of limitless physical potential. It had become, for many, the material that proved what Henry Adams had only intuited: the hidden energies of nature, once revealed, were more likely to be forces of destruction than they were to be forces of good.

One could convincingly argue that technological methods to unblock, transfer, and create human energy were ultimately of little cultural significance. Perhaps in the end, these mechanical, electrical, and radium-based gadgets were merely blips on the cultural radar, interesting fixations of a few savvy capitalists who knew how to milk people's ignorance for a fast buck. There are, however, two problems with that argument. First, we know that millions of individuals, over a period of fifty years, directly experienced what they *believed* was a physical energy enhancement through contact with these technologies. Second, we know that the promise of this energy enhancement has been kept alive in twentieth century popular culture.

Between 1870 and 1930, Americans actively negotiated two separate meanings for industrial, productive energies. On the one hand, machines, electricity, and radium were ominous forces of tremendous productive power and destructive potential. On the other hand, machines, electricity, and radium were advances that cured illnesses, eliminated fatigue, and unclogged the fountain of youth. Even if we acknowledge that many of the foundational principles supporting the latter definition were false, the definition does not become any less resonant for those who believed it a century ago. To understand the context in which Americans accepted these modern energies into their lives, we have to step back into their world of limitless technological possibility.

It is easy to say in retrospect that most of these experiences provided more mental than physical benefits; with the exception of Radithor and health machines, most failed to actually leave bodies with a perceptible change in the quantity or quality of usable energy they had possessed prior to a therapy. Yet in this case, accuracy was not as influential as belief. Realizing that items like the Electropoise, German Electric Belts, and Vigoradium were unable to deliver on their promise of "deposited" usable energy is not the same as neutralizing their effects. If more than a million individuals in our grandparents' generation took I-ON-A-CO treatments, and if even only one-quarter of them actually believed that the I-ON-A-CO deposited electricity into their bodies to improve health, it had an impact on how emergent industrial energies were perceived. This is particularly true, given that many contact centers for energy therapies were in major urban centers, the spaces where people had the most negotiations with energies in their first, ominous context. This is not to say that storefront I-ON-A-CO offices and Butler Health Lift rooms single-handedly created a benevolent context for the potentially threatening energies of urbanizing America. It is to say that these spaces became part of the palimpsest of energy experiences that provided the context in which Americans defined the meanings of mechanized systems, electrical products, and radioactive substances.

Had energy-enhancement strategies been pursued only during this period, it would still be possible to argue for their importance for the twentieth century as a whole. Electropoise systems and Radithor jars may have found their way to trash cans and yard sales by the 1950s, but their effects would have taken longer to disappear. Though it is difficult to prove without ethnographic research, it is within reason to assume that when Americans made decisions about energy, these health products had influence. It would have been easier, perhaps, for individuals to welcome rural electrification in the 1930s, for example, if electricity had been understood as both an agent of health and a source of heat and light. The very vision of Washington state residents, in the depths of the Great Depression, being sold by a government-commissioned Woody Guthrie on technology as the best way to assure their physical and economic health, reveals the success of these early innovators. It was no longer necessary to promote technological devices as capable of "defeating" laboring bodies, as Windship and Sargent once had. Technologically produced energy had become modern energy; it was a power with which individual muscle, produced through productive labor, could not compare. Men who might once have been romanticized for their rugged strength were now the recipients of technological largesse—as Guthrie's "Roll on, Columbia" and "Great Grand Coulee Dam" expressed. It was electric power, not laboring muscles that would ensure survival in the modern age.

Believing in the benevolence of products like Zander trotters, I-ON-A-CO belts, and Radithor waters may have made it more difficult to resist the encroachment of electricity, machines, and even nuclear power in daily life. It is not inconceivable that we became, in the words of David Nye, the leading twentieth-century consumers of energy on the planet partly because we had direct experiences that proved that these energies were creating a national body of perpetual health.[3]

Few of us have "plugged into" electric belts or taken a radium nightcap. Nevertheless, we do use similar products. One needs merely to browse late-night television to see multiple examples of electric health devices. Many are related to "electric transfer" devices in appearance only—the abdominal exercise devices, for instance, are concerned with creating visually sculpted muscles through passive resistance, not adding energy to the body's reserves. Yet some of the most popular alternative electric devices in recent years have been quite similar to those of a century ago. The Brain Tuner, which has sold steadily on the Internet with a price tag of more than two hundred dollars, advertises itself as "an electronic stimulator" that can "rapidly balance and restore the natural energies of your body and mind."[4] A similar product, Microwater, operates much like a radium water dispenser, yet instead of infusing water with radium energy, it purportedly creates "an abundance of electrons that are available as donor(s)" for our depleted bodies. These connections are not limited to late-night infomercials and obscure web sites.

Red Bull, the fastest growing product in energy drinks, itself the fastest growing beverage category, makes promises that would have been familiar to Eben Byers. By ingesting this beverage, manufacturers assure in their promotional materials, consumers receive "extra energy" for their bodies through its "exceptional composition" of ingredients developed by someone "with a lot of scientific know how."[5] In addition to these rhetorical similarities with radium products, Red Bull's packaging—a sleek, silver and blue can shaped like a bullet—evokes the same futuristic spirit as did streamlined dispensers generations ago.

Health machines are no longer placed in a context that stresses the unique power of machines to "unblock" energy, but they still evoke an organic relationship between man and machine. The makers of Nautilus machines, among the first of the complete weight systems with which today we are so familiar, portrayed their machines as extensions of the human body in early fitness guides. Today's popular cybex system suggests, in its very name, that users become cyborgs, or amalgamations of human and machine.

Arguing for similarities between today's energy-enhancement devices and those of a century ago is not the same as arguing that they are identical. In the twenty-first century, we are less likely to believe in fantastic technological elixirs. Yet when we bring these substances next to, or into our bodies, we engage in an act of memory. As George Lipsitz has pointed out, in modern life popular culture displaces traditional forms of memory.[6] Communication channels, media, and technologies have detached us from specific times, spaces, and people, creating realities in which memory is more often an amalgamation of disconnected images than a unified image based on personal experience. By extending this notion to the realm of material culture, it is possible to argue that these things— health machines, enhancing beverages, and electric stimulators—allow consumers to recreate the context in which they originally emerged. This is not to say that we wear an electric device we buy off the Internet as it was worn in 1900. One hundred years has brought us a long way from the worlds of "electric theology" and "liquid sunshine." But as we place electrodes on our bodies, or flip open a can, or climb onto the cybex, we revisit a "groove" worn deep by a generation who believed in technology's unparalleled energetic potential. Whether or not we are conscious of these original products, our physical embrace of their progeny preserves a memory, and embeds in us a sense of limitless technological potential that endures in spite of rational resistance.

It is, in fact, in the realm of popular culture where it becomes clear that our pursuit of a technological "superpower" is a stubborn one. Disneyland's Tomorrow Land emerged in the 1950s as one of the most popular spaces in the Happiest Place on Earth. There one could see fantasies of a futuristic world of happy, healthy people brought to you by technologies. Monsanto's "House of the Future" presented a vision of a germ-free, perennially clean plastic utopia, and GE's "Carousel of Progress" suggested that the best people to inhabit such spaces should be electrically powered human-machines. Visions of healthful technological progress, however, were future powered by more than fantastic diversions for family fun.

According to Lewis L. Strauss, chairman of the U.S. Atomic Energy Commission in 1954, in what he forecasted as a coming great "age of peace," it was "not too much to expect that our children will enjoy in their homes electrical energy too cheap to meter . . . will travel effortlessly over the seas and under them and through the air with a minimum of dangers at great speeds, and will experience a life span longer than ours."[7] Nor was this vision of humans rendered powerful by technology limited to an era of Cold War boosterism and technological optimism. Author Gregg Easterbrook is only one of many to recently propose a future in which technologies forestay death indefinitely, thereby ensuring the perpetual existence of human power: "Suppose as biological life draws towards its inevitable conclusion, a person's patterns of consciousness could be transferred to an electronic support apparatus. The part that matters about you might then exist a very long time, possibly an infinite time. . . . [T]here might someday be something approximately like electronic life."[8]

These techno-body fantasies are powerfully embedded in our mythology, a realm well protected from the probing questions of our rational minds. Rhetorical arguments can be dismissed with words and material artifacts dismissed with disposal. Mythological lessons, however, teach through fantasies that are by very definition impervious to reason. In the 1940s, just as the actual schemes for energy transfer faded, Marvel Comics based characters on the alchemic reaction of inhuman strength, continuous life, and superior intelligence through technology. One need look no further for evidence than Spiderman, an average Joe, who, thanks to the bite of a radioactive spider, is invested with superhuman strength, intuition, and the ability to emerge from danger unscathed.

American popular culture has perpetuated the myth of the technologically powered body, even as reality has pushed it ever further from view. Characters like Flash Gordon, who proudly wears the symbol of his power source in a bolt of lightning on his chest, have made Wilshire's promise of "perpetual energetic health" available to generation after generation. And while the life of any one character is somewhat limited, though Spiderman has enjoyed a recent rejuvenation, new energy heroes continually arise as predecessors fade. Characters like the Six-Million-Dollar Man and the Bionic Woman made real the promise of machine-powered humans in ways that Sargent and Zander could only imagine. Thanks to Jamie Summers, kids of my generation learned that damaging the physical body did not have to mean a loss of power. On the contrary, the most powerful forms of "energy" emerged only when body parts failed and were replaced by machines. Bionic ears, arms, and legs made our heroes human machines. Transformers, popular action figures in the 1980s, carried this to its logical extreme in its men who became machines with several skilled twists of an eight-year-old's hand.

Television and comic books have provided energy-transfer heroes for the past three generations. The promises made by Sargent, Wilshire, and Bailey are alive and well in the stories we tell our children about the "heroic" physical potential of technology. And evidence suggests that the power of these stories is only growing with time. We have traded our electric belts for palm pilots, personal video, and internal Rio soundscapes. And although we may not explicitly state our motivation to "be enhanced by" technological energies, this is in actuality the experience we increasingly create. When one looks to the purest realm for our current techno-physical fantasies, it is clear that we are still looking to technological energies to realize human potential. Cyberspace, which one explorer has referred to as today's "electronic frontier," has opened up an entirely new territory for these century-old narratives.[9] From cult novelist William Gibson's fictional worlds to the very realities of disembodied chat rooms, we are increasingly entering spaces where our very existence depends on merging with technologies. The "fantastic" body that Sargent, Wilshire, and Bailey envisioned is fast becoming antiquated. As Easterbrook reminds us, we have entered a new era, one where technology realizes human potential not by enhancing physical energy but by releasing human energy from its physical confines.

David Nye has recently noted that power systems are easier to create than they are to change. Machines, electricity, and radium did not become the major power sources of the twentieth century because of technological determinism. There exists a traceable history based on the decisions of actual individuals who confronted the complexities of their time. Had neurasthenia not seemed so threatening, it is possible that individuals like George Beard would never have turned to technological sources to augment human energy. Had Joseph Butler not been so impressed by mechanized power, it is possible that he never would have proposed a theory that united man and machine. Had the popular press not made the second law of thermodynamics a public preoccupation, it is possible that radium would have been approached with more caution than enthusiasm. Each of these factors, and countless others, stimulated the desire to unblock, transfer, and create physical energy using technological products. These desires may have in turn cast industrial energies, by their proximity to those that promised physical health, in a benevolent light.

This moment has not yet passed. We dismiss the argument that bodies simply lack the energy to live in the modern world. We dismiss the theories that only machines, electricity, and radium can create a body of sufficient strength. And we dismiss the idea that new energies will bring us a continual improvement in physical health. Yet we continue to live with the inheritance of the techno-body ethic—we regard it as progress to augment human workers with machines, to invest our time in on-line communities, to equate harvesting natural resources for fuel with ensuring national health.

Energy transfer theories created a psychic connection between physical capacity and technological advance. As a result, for the past century, turning against mechanization, electrification, and radiation would have meant denying our full physical potential. By discovering the links between these century-old ambitions and our current mythologies, we recognize the longevity of this strange embrace. Once we have done so, we can more objectively mark the impact of our energy enthusiasms on our bodies and our environment and perhaps, begin to pursue a more healthful separation of physical and technological potentials.

Notes

NOTES TO THE PREFACE

1. See Donna Haraway, "A Manifesto for Cyborgs: Science, Technology, and Socialist Feminism in the 1980s," in *Coming to Terms: Feminism, Theory, Politics*, ed. Elizabeth Weed (New York: Routledge, 1989).

2. See, for example, Judith Waltzer Leavitt, *Brought to Bed: Childbearing in America 1750–1950* (New York: Oxford University Press, 1986), Margarete Sandelowski, *Pain, Pleasure & American Childbirth: From the Twilight Sleep to the Read Method, 1914–1960* (Westport: Greenwood Press, 1984), and Dorthy and Richard Wertz, *Lying-In: A History of Childbirth in America* (New Haven: Yale University Press, 1989).

3. Mythologies about Native American women's "painless" childbirth typically originated with American men who had observed Native American women following the cultural practice of birthing alone and returning to the group with newborn in tow. Rarely did these men themselves actually witness the births to observe birthing women experiencing pain. They concluded that it was the fit, healthy lifestyle of Native American women that rendered the experience painless. In reality, Native American women's active lifestyles likely shortened labors and made them less painful; they did not, however, remove pain entirely. For accounts of Native American births, see George Wharton James, *Indians' Secrets of Health* (Pasadena: Radiant Life Press, 1908), 178, 111; Henry Lyman, *Artificial Anesthesia and Anesthetics* (New York: William Wood & Company, 1881), 68; Samuel Bruckner, "On the Physical Character of the Pain of Parturition," *Galliard's Medical Journal* (January 1900): 799; George Engelmann, *Labor Among Primitive Peoples* (St. Louis: J. H. Chambers & Co., 1982), 5. By 1888, the myth was used to market American products designed to relieve labor pains. Dr. Wrightman's Sovereign Balm of Life's advertisement asserted that because "Indians experience little or no pangs of childbirth due to their simple life in the open . . . it is contrary to all natural laws" that women should suffer in childbirth. See Jackson Lears, *Fables of Abundance: A Cultural History of Advertising in America* (New York: Basic Books, 1994), 148.

4. John Kasson, *Amusing the Million: Coney Island at the Turn of the Century* (New York: Hill and Wang, 1978).

5. Carolyn Marvin finds similar properties in electric products in *When Old Technologies Were New: Thinking About Electric Communication in the Late Nineteenth Century* (New York: Oxford University Press, 1988).

6. Anne Kull sees the cyborg as offering "new metaphors for understanding how science and technologies affect our lives, subjectivities, and concepts." See "The Cyborg as an Interpretation of Culture-Nature," *Zygon* 36, no. 1 (March 2001): 49–56. Stacy Alaimo uses Haraway's theories of the cyborg as a foil for eco feminism in "Cyborg and Ecofeminist Interventions: Challenges for an Environmental Feminism," *Feminist Studies* 20, no. 1 (April 30, 1994): 133. For Haraway's original theories see "A Manifest for Cyborgs."

7. This is something mentioned by both Tom Lutz in *American Nervousness, 1903: An Anecdotal History* (Ithaca: Cornell University Press, 1991) and F. G. Gosling in *Before Freud: Neurasthenia and the Medical Community* (Urbana: University of Illinois Press, 1988). My research affirms that their findings, based on medical data, hold true in the popular realm of "pseudo-science" as well.

8. My own definition of an irregular practitioner is one working outside the accepted, and licensed, medical establishment. For different definitions and explorations of "quack" electric medicine, see Roy Porter, *Health for Sale: Quackery in England, 1660–1850* (Manchester: Manchester University Press, 1989); Arthur J. Cramp, *Miscellaneous Nostrums*, 5th ed., (Chicago: Propaganda Department of the Journal of the American Medical Association Press, 1923); Arthur J. Cramp, *Nostrums and Quackery*, vol. 1–3 (Chicago: American Medical Association Press, 1912, 1921, 1936); Stewart H. Holbrook, *The Golden Age of Quackery* (New York: Macmillan, 1959); Jameson, *The Natural History of Quackery*, 61; David Armstrong, *The Great American Medicine Show: Being an Illustrated History of Hucksters, Healers, Health Evangelists, and Heroes from Plymouth Rock to the Present* (New York: Prentice Hall, 1991).

NOTES TO THE INTRODUCTION

1. According to David Nye, by the end of the twentieth century, the United States had the highest per capita use of energy in the world, roughly 40 percent more than Germany and almost three times as much as Italy or Japan. See Nye, *Consuming Power: A Social History of American Energies* (Cambridge: MIT Press, 1998), 6. Statistics comparing the energy consumption and energy efficiency ratings of forty-seven nations can be found in Benjamin Barber, *Jihad vs. McWorld* (New York: Times Books, 1995), 302–303.

2. See, for example, Paul Israel's *Edison: A Life of Invention* (New York: John Wiley, 1998), and Wayne Lewchuk, "Men and Monotony: Fraternalism as a Managerial Strategy at the Ford Motor Company," *Journal of Economic History* 5, no. 4 (December 1993): 824–856.

3. Cynthia Russett characterizes the period between 1860 and 1900 as one when "health depended upon moderation in the expenditure of energy" and one's achievements in one area necessitated "lesser attainment elsewhere." Tom Lutz explores Beard's theories about a finite "nerve force" that, if overtaxed, could lead to nervous bankruptcy. Both scholars accurately represent Beard's ideas on neurasthenia. If we combine this information with an understanding of Beard's experiments with restorative electric currents, however, his diagnoses appear less dire. See Russett, *Sexual Science: The Victorian Construction of Womanhood* (Cambridge: Harvard University Press, 1989), 112–113, and Lutz, *American Nervousness, 1903: An Anecdotal History* (Ithaca: Cornell University Press, 1991), 3–4.

4. Tim Armstrong, *Modernism, Technology, and the Body: A Cultural Study* (Cambridge: Cambridge University Press, 1998), 6.

5. Cleveland Moffett, "The Sense and the Nonsense about Radium," *Success* (April 1904): 246.

6. Several recent studies suggest that our ability to believe that a drug will work is often a major factor in its effectiveness. According to a recent study at the University of British Columbia, placebos can actually cause a chemical response in the body. Individuals with Parkinson's disease were given either a placebo or apomorphine, a drug that stimulates the body's release of dopamine. Patients were not told whether they were receiving apomorphine or a placebo. After taking the drugs, each of the patients who had received *only* the placebo had a substantial amount of dopamine in his or her system. Researchers concluded that patients' expectations can cause their bodies to simulate the effects of a drug they have not received. Alison Motluk, "Some of the Best Medicines Are All in the Mind," *New Scientist* 171, no. 2304 (August 18, 2001): 19. An additional study has also confirmed that when a condition has a strong psychological component, such as pain, anxiety, and depression, the placebo response rate among patients is frequently high, making it difficult to determine the effectiveness of prescribed drugs. Martin Enserink, "Can the Placebo Be the Cure?" *Science* 284, no. 5412 (April 9, 1999): 238.

7. Pilates, originally developed in the 1920s by Joseph Pilates, has recently enjoyed renewed popularity as a fitness system "without machines." See Brooke Siler, *The Pilates Body: The Ultimate At-Home Guide to Strengthening, Lengthening, and Toning Your Body without Machines* (New York: Bantam Doubleday, 2000).

8. According to Jeffrey Hornstein, the tension between professional and entrepreneurial status marked the twentieth-century American middle class. See

Hornstein, "The Rise of the Realtor®: Professionalism, Gender, and Middle-Class Identity, 1908–1950," in Burton J. Bledstein and Robert D. Johnston, eds., *The Middling Sorts: Explorations in the History of the American Middle Class* (New York: Routledge, 2001), 217–233.

9. See John W. Leavitt, *Exercise a Medicine; or Muscular Action as Related to Organic Life* (New York: J. W. Leavitt, 1890), i–v.

10. Tom Lutz finds that gender conventions shaped treatments for neurasthenia patients in general. Whereas women were prescribed cures of inactivity, men's cures revolved around activity. According to Lutz, "[B]oth cures were represented in terms of a return to traditional values of passive feminity and masculine activity." See Lutz, *American Nervousness*, 34.

11. See, for example, Janice Todd, *Physical Culture and the Body Beautiful: Purposive Exercise in the Lives of American Women, 1800–1870* (Macon: Mercer University Press, 1998), and Frances B. Cogan, *All-American Girl: The Ideal of Real Womanhood in Mid-Nineteenth-Century America* (Athens: University of Georgia Press, 1989).

12. Rachel Maines provides evidence that women were often willing to partake of forbidden technologies, even when the best "experts" told them that devices were unnecessary or dangerous. See Maines, *Technology of Orgasm: Hysteria, the Vibrator and Women's Sexual Satisfaction* (Baltimore: Johns Hopkins University Press, 1994).

13. Gail Bederman makes a cogent argument for this connection in *Manliness and Civilization: A Cultural History of Gender and Race in the United States, 1880–1917* (Chicago: University of Chicago Press, 1995).

14. For work on American masculinity during the modern era, see ibid.; Michael Kimmell, *Manhood in America: A Cultural History* (New York: Free Press, 1996); E. Anthony Rotundo, *American Manhood: Transformations in Masculinity from the Revolution to the Modern Era* (New York: Basic Books, 1993); and John Kasson, *Houdini, Tarzan, and the Perfect Man: The White Male Body and the Challenge of Modernity in America* (New York: Hill & Wang, 2001). For work on technology and the body during this period, see Armstrong, *Modernism, Technology, and the Body*; and Anson Rabinbach, *The Human Motor: Energy, Fatigue, and the Origins of Modernity* (New York: Basic Books, 1990).

NOTES TO CHAPTER 1

1. Debby Applegate describes Beecher's exceptional popularity between 1840 and 1880 in "Henry Ward Beecher and the 'Great Middle Class'": Mass-Marketed Intimacy and Middle-Class Identity," in *The Middling Sorts: Explorations*

in the History of the American Middle Class, eds. Burton J. Bledstein and Robert D. Johnston (New York: Routledge, 2001), 107–124.

2. This was three years before his affair with Elizabeth Tilton led to the sensational 1874 Beecher-Tilton trial and tarnished Beecher's image as a paragon of morality. For more information on the affair and its effect on Beecher's reputation, see Richard Wightman Fox, *Trials of Intimacy: Love and Loss in the Beecher-Tilton Scandal* (Chicago: University of Chicago Press, 1999).

3. The Health Lift Studio was located at 158 Remsen Street. *The Lift: A Journal Designed to Aid in Showing People How to Lift Themselves up in the World* 1, no. 2 (September 1871): 12.

4. Those familiar with what Jackson Lears calls Beecher's "enthusiasm for upper-class pleasures" would have inferred from the endorsement that the Health Lifts were gentlemanly pursuits not terribly taxing on the body. Beecher's own endorsement of leisure and rejection of fasting left little doubt that an activity he praised would be one of limited discomfort and ample reward. See Lears, *No Place of Grace: Antimodernism and the Transformation of American Culture, 1880–1920* (New York: Pantheon Books, 1981), 24.

5. For information on Beecher's sermons, given in what was referred to as "Beecher's theater," see Applegate, "Henry Ward Beecher," 113.

6. We might even see a moral connection between Beecher's vocation and his exercise method of choice: *The Lift* journal and the Health Lift machine suggest a connection between Beecher's religious project of moral uplift and the physical project of "lifting up."

7. Applegate asserts that the contemporary press characterized Beecher's audience as "the great middle class." Her research on individuals who wrote letters to Beecher revealed the occupations that she characterizes as middle class. See Applegate, "Henry Ward Beecher," 111.

8. What has been published on Health Lifts includes Janice Todd, "Strength Is Health: George Barker Windship and the First American Weight Training Boom," *Iron Game History* (September 1993): 3–14. See also Janice Todd, *Physical Culture and the Body Beautiful: Purposive Exercise in the Lives of American Women, 1800–1870* (Macon: Mercer University Press, 1998); Joan Paul, "The Health Reformers: George Barker Windship and Boston's Strength Seekers," *Journal of Sport History* 10, no. 3 (Winter 1983): 41–57; and Harvey Green, *Fit for America: Health, Fitness, Sport and American Society,* 2d ed. (Baltimore: Johns Hopkins University Press, 1988).

9. Terry Smith, *Making the Modern: Industry, Art, and Design in America* (Chicago: University of Chicago Press, 1993), particularly 213–228.

10. John Kasson's work on the Lowell Mills reveals that even in the early nineteenth century, workers understood their interactions with machines as part of their larger cultural experiences, including their rural family backgrounds and

their plans to work in factories for only a limited time. See Kasson, *Civilizing the Machine: Technology and Republican Values in America, 1776–1900* (New York: Grossman, 1976).

11. For more information on nineteenth-century health movements, see Green, *Fit for America*. For more on the uncertainties of middle-class American masculinity that necessitated many of these movements, see Gail Bederman, *Manliness and Civilization: A Cultural History of Gender and Race in the United States, 1880–1917* (Chicago: University of Chicago Press, 1995).

12. See James Whorton, *Crusaders for Fitness: The History of American Health Reformers* (Princeton: Princeton University Press, 1982), 284. By 1900, gymnasiums had so proliferated in the United States that critics weighed in, lamenting the replacement of hard physical labor with "artificial means of contributing to and continuing the physical vigor and virility of the race." See George Ruskin Phoebus, "Civilization, Physical Culture," *Physical Culture* 3 (1900): 21–22, quoted in Michael Kimmel, *Manhood in America: A Cultural History* (New York: Free Press, 1996), 126.

13. A reason for this may have been Luther Gulick, a physician who devised a system of physical training for early YMCAs. A student of Dudley Allen Sargent's, Gulick would have included apparatuses similar to those developed by Sargent at Harvard in each of his YMCAs. Sargent and Gulick are further discussed in chapter 2.

14. For further information on German gymnastics, see Robert K. Barney, "German Turners in America: Their Role in Nineteenth Century Exercise Expression and Physical Education Legislation," in Earle F. Zeigler, ed., *A History of Physical Education and Sport in the United States and Canada* (Champaign: Stipes Publishing, 1975), 111–120.

15. For more information on the connections people made between American gymnastics and the spirit of ancient Greece, see F. L. Oswald, "The Age of Gymnastics," *Popular Science Monthly* 13 (June 1878): 129–139.

16. Alfred Worcester, "Gymnastics," *Popular Science Monthly* 23 (May 1883): 79.

17. The performance was further simplified by being set to rhythmic music. See *Songs for Calisthenics* (Springfield, Ill.: Horace S. Taylor, 1849), and *Songs for Calisthenics* (Northhampton, Mass.: Hopkins, Bridgman & Co., 1857). The exercise method survived well into the late nineteenth century; see *Watson's Manual of Calisthenics: A Systematic Drill-Book Without Apparatus for Schools, Families, and Gymnasiums by J. Madison Watson* (New York: E. Steiger & Co., 1882). To compare calisthenics to the army drills that emerged after the Civil War, see Frank Idone, *US Army Exercises: Rearranged for General Use* (New York: Richard K. Fox, 1904).

18. Dio Lewis, *New Gymnastics for Men, Women, and Children* (Boston: James R. Osgood and Company, 1862). For information on the connection be-

tween balanced physiques and good posture, see David Yosifon and Peter N. Stearns, "The Rise and Fall of American Posture," *American Historical Review* 103 (October 1998): 1057–1095, and C. Dallett Hemphill, *Bowing to Necessities: A History of Manners in America, 1620–1800* (New York: Oxford University Press, 1999).

19. Lewis exemplified the nineteenth-century reformer. Between the 1840s and the late nineteenth century, he supported numerous causes, including health reform, women's rights, temperance, and homeopathy. He developed his system after studying German and Swedish gymnastics abroad in the 1850s. For more information on Lewis, see Todd, *Physical Culture*, chaps. 8–10; Frances Cogan, *All-American Girl: The Ideal of Real Womanhood in Mid-Nineteenth-Century America* (Athens: University of Georgia Press, 1989); and Green, *Fit for America*, 184–199. For more on Lewis's involvement with the Women's Crusade and temperance, see Jack Blocker, *"Give to the Wind Thy Fears": The Women's Temperance Crusade, 1873–1874* (Westport: Greenwood Press, 1985).

20. Lewis, *New Gymnastics* (1873 ed.), 4.

21. For more information, see Green, *Fit for America*, 186.

22. Mary Eastman, *Biography of Dio Lewis, M.D.* (New York: Fowler and Wells Co., 1890), 71–72.

23. Lewis did, however, develop his own machine, the Pangymnastikon. See Lewis, *New Gymnastics*, 124–127, quoted in Green, *Fit for America*, 189. For more information on the Pangymnastikon, see Todd, *Physical Culture*, 244. Todd also argues that Lewis was often more a synthesizer of ideas that he borrowed from others than an originator of those ideas. See ibid., chaps. 8–10.

24. Anson Rabinbach, *The Human Motor: Energy, Fatigue, and the Origins of Modernity* (New York: Basic Books, 1990), 1. For information on how Descartes's ideas were seen by a nineteenth-century audience, see William G. Stevenson, "The Psychological Significance of Vital Force," *Popular Science Monthly* 24 (April 1884): 761.

25. H. H. Sherwood, *The Motive Power of the Human System, With the Symptoms and Treatment of Chronic Diseases* (New York: Jared W. Bell, 1840), 10.

26. See J. M. Stillman, "The Source of Muscular Energy," *Popular Science Monthly* 24 (January 1884): 377–387. For this and other comparisons, see Cecelia Tichi, *Shifting Gears: Technology, Literature and Culture in Modern America* (Chapel Hill: University of North Carolina Press, 1987), 35. It is interesting to note that this was the same time that the mythology of John Henry, the "hammer man" who raced and defeated the steam drill, emerged. Much of the mythology's popularity may have been the comparison of "machines" it evoked. See Brett Williams, *John Henry: A Bio-Bibliography* (Westport, Conn.: Greenwood Press, 1983), 3–13.

27. Stillman, "The Source of Muscular Energy," 187.

28. Tichi offers several examples of this; see Tichi, *Shifting Gears*, 35. For the quotation on disabilities, see Woods Hutchingson, "Our Human Misfits," *Everybody's Magazine* 25 (October 1911): 519.

29. Tichi, *Shifting Gears*, 30. In Robert Herrick, *Together* (New York: Macmillan, 1908), 232, 235.

30. Quotations taken from Jack London, *Call of the Wild* (New York: Macmillan, 1903) and *White Fang* (New York: Macmillan, 1906). For information, as well as machine analogies from Sherwood Anderson's and Edith Wharton's works, see Tichi, *Shifting Gears*, 31.

31. Rabinbach, *The Human Motor*, 2.

32. *Neurasthenia*, a term coined in America, was not a uniquely American phenomenon. European physicians also reported that numerous patients suffered the illness's mysterious symptoms. In 1892, a report on French schoolchildren found a clear state of ill health. It described "muscles without energy painfully support[ing] the body," explaining that with the disease "all of the functions of the organism descend into a characteristic state of decline." See Rabinbach, *The Human Motor*, 6. For more information on the relationship between neurasthenia, exercise, and health, see Patricia Vertinsky, *The Eternally Wounded Woman: Women, Doctors, and Exercise in the Late Nineteenth Century* (New York: St. Martin's Press, 1990).

33. David Armstrong and Elizabeth Metzger Armstrong, *The Great American Medicine Show* (New York: Prentice Hall, 1991), 90. For more information on Beard's specific etiology of the disease and his ideas on nervous force, see Tom Lutz, *American Nervousness, 1903: An Anecdotal History* (Ithaca: Cornell University Press, 1991), particularly 3–7.

34. Beard, quoted in Edward Shorter, *From Paralysis to Fatigue: A History of Psychosomatic Illness in the Modern Era* (New York: Free Press, 1992), 221.

35. For Beard's description of what happened to nerve cells during a neurasthenia episode, see George Beard and A. D. Rockwell, *A Practical Treatise on Nervous Exhaustion*, 3d ed. (New York: E. B. Treat, 1894), 250–251. For more information on Beard and neurasthenia, see Lutz, *American Nervousness*. It is important to note that Europeans also theorized neurasthenia's causes. Philosopher Frederick Nietzche believed the cause was the unreasonable demands made on the body by material progress. For more on neurasthenia in Europe, see Rabinbach, *The Human Motor*, 20.

36. For information on Mitchell and "rough-riding" cures, see Lutz, *American Nervousness*, 32. For Beard's use of electricity, see ibid., 47, and Paul Israel, *Edison: A Life of Invention* (New York: John Wiley & Sons, 1998), 114.

37. John Kasson discusses the connection between the rise of white-collar occupations and the interest in physical culture in *Houdini, Tarzan, and the Perfect Man: The White Male Body and the Rise of Modernity in America* (New York: Hill & Wang, 2001); for quotes from Burroughs, see 166. Kasson also mentions

Theodore Dreiser's *Sister Carrie* and Saul Bellow's *Seize the Day* as examples of fiction that details the malaise of white-collar occupations. For more information on the connection between the new middle class and ill-defined "stresses," see Burton J. Bledstein and Robert D. Johnston, eds., *The Middling Sorts: Explorations in the History of the American Middle Class* (New York: Routledge, 2001).

38. Rabinbach, *The Human Motor*, 20.

39. See, for example, Kasson's analysis of Houdini, Sandow, and Tarzan as rugged foils to the "civilized" world of middle-class labor in *Houdini, Tarzan, and the Perfect Man*. Similar themes are also discussed in Bederman, *Manliness and Civilization*; Robert Ernst, *Weakness Is a Crime: The Life of Bernarr Macfadden* (Syracuse: Syracuse University Press, 1991); and David Chapman, *Sandow the Magnificent: Eugen Sandow and the Beginnings of Bodybuilding* (Urbana: University of Illinois Press, 1994). Further, several exercise programs appeared in the early twentieth century that catered especially to businessmen. Among them, H. Irving Hancock, *Physical Training for Business Men: Basic Rules and Simple Exercises for Gaining Assured Control of the Physical Self* (New York: G. P. Putnam's Sons, 1917), and A. R. T. Winjum, *Manual of Physical Exercises* (Battle Creek: A. R. T. Winjum, 1909).

40. Stephen G. Brush, *The Temperature of History: Phases of Science and Culture in the Nineteenth Century* (New York: Burt Franklin & Co., 1978), 30. Information on Kelvin's paper and the scientific theories behind his second law can be found in Donald S. Cardwell, *From Watt to Clausius: The Rise of Thermodynamics in the Early Industrial Age* (Ithaca: Cornell University Press, 1971), 257. Further information on Clausius's contributions can be found in Rabinbach, *The Human Motor*, 3.

41. What we call the first law of thermodynamics was originally called the universal law of the conservation of energy when presented in 1847 by German physicist and physiologist Hermann von Helmholtz. In it, von Helmholtz asserted that the forces of nature are forms of a single, universal energy or *Kraft* (power), which can be neither added to nor destroyed. See Rabinbach, *The Human Motor*, 3.

42. It was Clausius who stated that the entropy of the universe tends to a maximum, meaning that although the energy of the universe is constant, the amount of energy usable for mechanical processes is constantly diminishing. For information, see Cardwell, *From Watt to Clausius*, 273. For the von Helmholtz quotation, see Brush, *The Temperature of History*, 31.

43. For more information on how "civilization" contributes to neurasthenia, see Beard and Rockwell, *A Practical Treatise*, 253. As Bederman discusses, the term "race suicide" was coined in 1901 by sociologist Edward A. Ross. For more information on the term and Roosevelt's use of it, see Bederman, *Manliness and Civilization*, 200–206.

44. Stevenson, "The Physiological Significance of Vital Force," 760–773; George Iles, "The Dissipation of Energy," *Popular Science Monthly* 12 (April 1878): 701–705; and Sir William Thomson (Lord Kelvin), "The Available Energy of Nature," *Popular Science Monthly* 20 (November 1881): 87–95.

45. Thomson, "The Available Energy," 89.

46. H. F. Walling, "Dissipation of Energy," *Popular Science Monthly* 4 (February 1874): 430.

47. Nikola Tesla, "The Problem of Increasing Human Energy with Special Reference to Harnessing the Sun's Energy," *Century Illustrated Monthly Magazine* 60, no. 2 (June 1900): 175–211.

48. Justus von Liebig discovered in 1842 that the tissues, not the lungs, consume fuel. He believed that "the source of animal heat is really the consumption of the fuel taken in through the stomach and the lungs." He showed that all the activities of life are really the product of energy liberated solely through destructive processes, amounting, broadly speaking, to "combustion occurring in the ultimate cells of the organism." Liebig, "Century's Progress in Anatomy and Physiology," *Harpers* (1898): 632. For more information on Liebig, see William Brock, *Justus von Liebig: The Chemical Gatekeepers* (New York: Cambridge University Press, 1997).

49. Liebig, "Century's Progress," 632.

50. Catharine Beecher, *Physiology and Calisthenics for Schools and Families* (New York: Harper & Bros., 1856), 38.

51. Ibid.

52. Austin Flint, *The Physiology of Man* (New York: D. Appleton and Company, 1868), 215–216. Flint first published *Physiology* in 1867 and found his ideas so readily accepted that a second edition was ordered immediately. For information on Flint, see *Dictionary of American Biography*, 3d ed., 472–473.

53. J. L. Comstock, *Outlines of Physiology, Both Comparative and Human* (New York: Robinson, Pratt & Co., 1836), 227.

54. By 1855, young boys were being explicitly told that the key to being a man was cultivating muscles. Whereas early advice books had concentrated mainly on building young men's minds, later sources believed strong muscular bodies were equally important. "What mud sills are to a building," remarked Daniel Eddy's *Young Man's Friend*, "muscular development is to manhood." See Joseph Kett, *Rites of Passage: Adolescence in America, 1790 to the Present* (New York: Basic Books, 1977), 162–163. My thanks to Anthony Rotundo for initially locating this passage. For Rotundo's analysis of Eddy's phrase, see *American Manhood: Transformations in Masculinity from the Revolution to the Modern Era* (New York: Basic Books, 1993), 223.

55. For the review of Flint's book, see "The Source of Muscular Power," *Popular Science Monthly* 12 (April 1878): 729–736.

56. For this quote see Roberta J. Park, "Healthy, Moral and Strong: Educa-

tional Views of Exercise and Athletics in Nineteenth-Century America," in *Fitness in American Culture: Images of Health, Sport and the Body, 1830–1940*, ed. Kathryn Grover (Amherst: University of Massachusetts Press, 1989), 154.

57. For more information on the history of dumbbells, see Janice Todd, "From Milo to Milo: A History of Barbells, Dumbbells and Indian Clubs," *Iron Game History* 3, no. 6 (April 1995): 4–16.

58. Captain James Chiosso, *The Gymnastic Polymachinon: Instructions for Performing a Systematic Series of Exercises on the Gymnastic & Calisthenic Polymachinon* (London: Walton & Maberly, 1855), 9; in the Todd-McLean Physical Culture Collection at the University of Texas at Austin (TMPC).

59. Universal machines were sold in the 1850s but lacked the promotional effort put out by Chiosso. In one regard, Chiosso's machine would remain distinct from those that followed. One of its selling points, Chiosso believed, was group fitness. It could be used by one person at a time, or "by a number of persons not exceeding ten, acting totally independently of one another." Subsequent machine designers like Windship and Butler did not add the multiple-user option, leading one to assume that group machine fitness was not a desirable American activity. Chiosso, *The Gymnastic Polymachinon*, 13.

60. Chiosso may have been responding to French concerns about energy depletion, even if he was working prior to the naming of "neurasthenia" or the second law of thermodynamics. As early as the 1820s, numerous French medical texts decried the effects of masturbation, which included physical and mental weakness. See Jean Stengers and Anne Van Neck, trans. Kathryn Hoffman, *Masturbation: The History of a Great Terror* (New York: Palgrave, 2001), 3–6.

61. Janice Todd, "Strength Is Health," 3. Windship has usually been remembered for how much he lifted more than for how he lifted. As a result, few historians have focused on the role that machinery played in his philosophy on health. See, as an example, Joan Paul, "The Health Reformers: George Barker Windship and Boston's Strength Seekers," *Journal of Sport History* 10, no. 3 (Winter 1983): 41–57.

62. For more information on strongmen and local theater acts in the mid-nineteenth century, see Todd, "Strength Is Health," 5.

63. Todd has previously discussed Windship's encounter with the lifting machine and his subsequent dedication to designing a machine of his own. See ibid., 5–6.

64. George Barker Windship, "Autobiographical Sketches of a Strength-Seeker," *Atlantic Monthly* (January 1862): 106.

65. Ibid.

66. Todd, "Strength Is Health," 6.

67. For information on the East Coast athletic revival and "Muscular Christianity," see Green, *Fit for America*, 181–215.

68. Todd, "Strength Is Health," 7.

69. Windship quoted from *The Massachusette Teacher,* ibid., 8.

70. An 1863 newspaper article described his office at the Park Street Church Building in Boston as "thronged" with people wanting more information on how to be strong. This private practice was equal parts theory and machines, as evidenced by the "lifting machine" he kept there, a device described as seven feet tall and made of wood with a platform halfway up on which one stood to lift weights that were stored beneath the machine. See ibid.

71. Windship, "Autobiographical Sketches," 106.

72. Windship's father gave him ample reason to determine strength by comparing him to a laboring man. Windship remembered his father's pointing out to him, well after he had acquired "gymnastic" strength, a "large, stout individual" and declaring, "[You] might practice lifting all your life, and never be able to lift as much as that big fellow." This, recalled Windship, was his motivation to build his machine. "Let me construct a lifting-apparatus in the back-yard," he told his father, "and I will soon prove to you that you are mistaken." See Windship, "Autobiographical Sketches," 107.

73. This comparison to laboring bodies was continued in William Blaikie's writings on why men should purchase the Health Lift. In his widely read book of 1879, *How to Get Strong and Stay So,* Blaikie praised Dudley Allen Sargent's machines, similar to Health Lifts, for bestowing strength superior to the "weak farmer." "Scarcely any work in a farm makes one quick of foot," he explained. "All day, while some of the muscles do the work . . . the rest are untaxed, and remain actually weak." The comparisons rendered the yeoman farmer, a symbol of vigorous national health since Jefferson, a delicate figure, weak through the very labor that once evidenced his strength. The switch represents a change from a natural view of physical strength as that which allows one to do work to a technological view of strength as that which allows one to gain measurable, balanced mass. See Blaikie, *How to Get Strong and Stay So* (New York: Harper & Brothers, 1879), 11–12.

74. See Todd, "Strength Is Health," 8. Health Lifts were used at resorts such as the Remedial Institute in Saratoga Springs as early as the 1870s. We can assume that readers of the resorts' brochures would have been familiar with the machines because some included the words "health lift" on their front covers to attract visitors. See "Remedial Institute," brochure, Box 2, Spas and Resorts, Warshaw Collection of Business Americana, National Museum of American History, Smithsonian Institution (WCBA).

75. See S. M. Barnett, *The Gymnasium at Home. Utility and Amusement Combined. Barnett's Patent Parlor Gymnasium and Chest Expander for Schools and Families* (New York: J. Becker & Co., 1871), 74. Readers of magazines like *Popular Science Monthly* had learned by the 1880s that no gymnasium was complete without the Health Lift, which it described as something that "no dyspeptic

should be without." See Felix L. Oswald, "Physical Education," *Popular Science Monthly* 19 (May 1881): 17.

76. Butler quoted in Todd, "Strength Is Health," 9.

77. Ibid.

78. *The Lifting Cure: an Original Scientific Application of the Laws of Motion on Mechanical Action to Physical Culture and the Cure of Disease* (Boston: D. P. Butler, 1868). By 1871, the manual was in its sixtieth edition. Other sources on Butler's system include John W. Leavitt, *Exercise a Medicine; Or Muscular Action as Related to Organic Life* (New York: J. W. Leavitt, 1870), and L. E. Waterman, *A Manual of the Exercise Known as the Butler Health Lift* (New York: Lewis G. Janes & Co., 1871).

79. J. C. Zachos, *The Butler Health Lift: Its Reasons and Its Facts* (New York: Lewis G. Janes & Co., 1871), 9.

80. Ibid.

81. Ibid., 10.

82. Ibid.

83. Zachos's perspective was likely influenced by Butler and his other promoters. Although his ideas were undoubtedly his own, all promotional pamphlets for Butler's system were published by a common publisher, Lewis G. Janes & Company of New York City. Janes was the best known, and most successful, of Butler's students. He managed the principal office of the company in New York and managed all of the company's promotional materials. See the inside front cover of Zachos, *The Butler Health Lift*.

84. Today we would probably call neurasthenia a psychosomatic illness, meaning that the body manifests the symptoms of what is actually a psychological ailment. It was a term unknown in the nineteenth century, a time when disease manifest in the body was believed treatable only in the body itself.

85. Zachos names each of these systems in his critique; see *The Butler Health Lift*, 8.

86. Ibid., 11.

87. *The Lifting Cure*, 16.

88. Ibid.

89. Ibid., 10.

90. Ibid., 11.

91. For more on the elixir craze of the late nineteenth century, see Sarah Stage, *Female Complaints: Lydia Pinkham and the Business of Women's Medicine* (New York: Norton, 1979).

92. *The Lifting Cure*, 11.

93. Ibid.

94. John W. Leavitt, *Exercise a Medicine; or Muscular Action as Related to Organic Life* (New York: J. W. Leavitt, 1890), 13.

95. *The Lifting Cure*, 12.

96. The first successful implantation, in 1982, of the Jarvix-7 artificial heart was, for many, the realization of this promise. For information, see chapter 5, "Desperate Appliance: A Short History of the Jarvix-7 Artificial Heart," in Renée Fox and Judith Swazey, *Spare Parts: Organ Replacement in American Society* (New York: Oxford University Press, 1992).

97. Butler's interest in mechanized fitness extended to other machines he patented, including a pulley machine. It was one of the early versions of a machine that Dudley Allen Sargent of Harvard later became known for; it had a platform and upright post along its back edge. Attached to the post were several wheels placed at differing levels to accommodate users' varying shoulder widths. Pulleys ran across the wheels and connected to adjustable weights on the machine's backside. To operate the machine, one climbed atop the platform, grabbed handles attached to the front end of the pulleys, and bent at the knees. The weight was lifted by the arms; much like our current universal sets, users brought the pulleys in to the chest and released them, bringing the arms and elbows out straight. Butler used this as part of his four-part training method, which also included heavy and light dumbbell work. See Todd, "Strength Is Health," 9–10.

98. It is interesting to note how Chiosso's and Butler's machines reflected the architectural conventions of their eras. The Polymachinon appeared in the 1830s, a decade before structural iron was used in architecture. Like the first buildings to use iron, such as St. Isacc's church in St. Petersburg in 1842 which adopted a stone exterior, the Polymachinon hid its iron components from view. When Butler's machine arrived in the 1860s, structural iron was often expressed architecturally, most famously in Joseph Paxton's 1851 Crystal Palace. In the thirty-year space between machines, European and American architects were increasingly willing to express iron's structural abilities as an element in design. The change may have made consumers more likely to see in the Health Lift's exposed iron an aesthetic expression of strength and beauty. For the use of structural iron see Spiro Kostof, *A History of Architecture, Settings, and Rituals* (New York: Oxford University Press, 1985), 594–604.

99. *The Lifting Cure*, 28. Cecelia Tichi talks about the emphasis nineteenth-century users placed on being able to see how machines worked from the outside. She calls this the "girded" effect by which "onlookers could be involved in a machine's function." This same exposure with the Health Lift machines might have allowed users to see a connection between the girded machines in industry and at expositions with the health machines in Butler's rooms. See Tichi, *Shifting Gears*, xii. It is surely more than coincidence that the leverage system Butler used in his machine closely resembled that of a pulley crane. First introduced in the early nineteenth century, cranes captivated Americans' attention with their ability to hoist enormous mass. According to Linda Henderson, industrial cranes

had become a standard part of manufacturing technology by the end of the century. The Health Lift may have proven, for some users, that this technology could add strength to the body. See Henderson, *Duchamp in Context: Science and Technology in the Large Glass and Related Works* (Princeton: Princeton University Press, 1998), 160.

100. Todd, "Strength Is Health," 10.

101. Michael R. Harris, "Iron Therapy and Tonics," in *Sport and Fitness in America, 1830–1940*, ed. Kathryn Grover (New York: Margaret Woodbury Strong Museum, 1989), 67–85; for specific information, 76.

102. Harris reports that between 1871 and 1900, at the height of American industrialization, there were more than 270 articles on iron in medical journals alone, more than double the number that appeared between 1840 and 1870. Ibid.

103. Kostof, *A History of Architecture*, 594–604.

104. Leavitt, *Exercise a Medicine*, iv.

105. *The Lifting Cure*, 83.

106. Ibid.

107. Ibid., 13.

108. Butler's company headquarters was on the second floor of the Park Bank Building at 120 Broadway. Other known addresses for Butler's fitness centers are 830 Broadway, 348 Broadway, 113 Broadway, 158 Remsen Street in Brooklyn, No. 43 West Street and 784 Washington Street in Boston, No. 24 Post Street in San Francisco, and No. 37 S. Main Street in Providence. See the inside cover listing in Zachos, *The Butler Health Lift*. Other information on locations is found in Todd, *Physical Culture and the Body Beautiful*, 195.

109. Illustrations of midcentury YMCA facilities suggest that health lifts were common equipment for them. One shows a group of middle-class-appearing men exercising with a health lift resembling Butler's wooden model in the foreground. See C. Howard Hopkins, *History of the YMCA in North America* (New York: Association Press, 1951).

110. Dudley Allen Sargent, *An Autobiography* (Philadelphia: Lea and Febiger, 1927), 98. We also know that many Health Lifts marketed for home use were decorated with ornate ironwork and sold for one to two hundred dollars, amounts that only an upper-class income could afford. The fact that these were produced and advertised suggests that manufacturers perceived a demand for these machines as status objects.

111. One of these was the Health Lift Company of New York, which marketed Mann's Reactionary Lifter, a cast-iron lifting machine weighting 130 pounds that worked on air resistance instead of iron weights. The proximity between the Health Lift Company's philosophy of balance and cooperation and Butler's philosophy mirrored their geographical location; the Health Lift Company operated out of 178 Broadway, and the Butler Health Lift room was

located at 120 Broadway. See "The Reactionary Lifter: Its Use in the System of Cumulative Exercise," The Health Lift or Lifting Cure (New York: The Health Lift Company, 1872). For an example of the similarities in pamphlets, see "The Health Lift Reduced to a Science: Cumulative Exercise, A Thorough Gymnastic System in Ten Minutes Once a Day," The Reactionary Lifter (New York: The Health-Lift Company, 1876), 6. For information on how the Reactionary Lifter advertised to women, see Todd, *Physical Culture*, 195.

112. In addition, women were never mentioned in the ubiquitous comparisons made between "developed" health lifters and "secretly weak" laborers. For information on how women trained with Health Lift machines and calisthenics, see Todd, *Physical Culture*, especially chap. 7. For an example of how the Health Lift was reported to ease pregnancies, end miscarriages, and cure pelvic disorders, see "The Health Lift: Reduced to a Science, Cumulative Exercise, a Thorough Gymnastic System in Ten Minutes Once a Day," 17. For Butler's quote, see *The Lifting Cure*, 86.

113. For information on this machine, see Todd, "Strength Is Health," 10.

114. According to Butler's own account, urban professionals constituted most of his clientele; in one publication he estimated he had more than seventy-five bankers, brokers, insurance officers, lawyers, and merchants among "subscribers." See Leavitt, *Exercise a Medicine*, i–v.

115. Ibid.

116. See *The Lift*, 12, 14.

117. Ibid., 12.

118. For more information, see *Sporting Goods: Sports equipment and clothing, novelties, recreative science, firemen's supplies, magic lanterns and slides, plays and joke books, tricks and magic, badges and ornaments* (New York: Peck & Snyder, 1886), reprinted by American Historical Catalog Collection (Princeton: Pyne Press, 1974).

119. *The Lifting Cure*, 12.

NOTES TO CHAPTER 2

1. Bruce Bennett, "The Life of Dudley Allen Sargent and His Contributions to Physical Education" (Ph.D. diss., University of Michigan, 1947), 18. Bowdoin College is in Brunswick, Maine.

2. This was a lesson that, for some students, was also reinforced academically. Under chemistry professor and president Charles Eliot, Harvard improved professional training and recruitment of students in its engineering program. In 1891, what was then called the Lawrence Scientific School received a large donation from Gordon McKray, an industrialist who had made a fortune in shoe-manufacturing machines. The gift made possible dramatic improvements, in-

cluding a postgraduate program. In 1906, Lawrence and its engineering department became part of Harvard College. Thus, many Harvard students would have grappled body and mind with machines. For more information, see the Harvard homepage or Bennett, "The Life of Dudley Allen Sargent," 11.

3. Despite Sargent's impact on physical training and health machines, there is as yet no comprehensive biography of him. One of the best sources remains Bennett, "The Life of Dudley Allen Sargent." Other research on Sargent's contributions include Donald Mrozek, *Sport and American Mentality, 1880–1910* (Knoxville: University of Tennessee Press, 1983), and Deborah Lynn Cottrell, "Women's Minds, Women's Bodies: The Influence of the Sargent School for Physical Education" (Ph.D. diss., University of Texas at Austin, 1993). For the quotation on Sargent's contributions, see Bruce Bennett, *Contributions of Dr. Sargent to Physical Education* (Minot, N.D.: State Teachers College, 1948), 1. Sargent was not the first to bring systematic physical education to the college level. Colleges had hired trained physical educators since the early 1820s. Edward Hitchcock, Jr., is generally credited with being the first formal physical educator at the collegiate level. He was appointed professor of hygiene and physical education at Amherst College in 1861. For more information on Hitchock, see James Whorton, *Crusaders for Fitness: The History of American Health Reform* (Princeton: Princeton University Press, 1982), 282.

4. See Ledyard Sargent, ed., *Dudley Allen Sargent: An Autobiography* (Philadelphia: Lea & Febiger, 1927), 59.

5. For information on the popularity of European strongmen in America, see David Chapman, *Sandow the Magnificent: Eugen Sandow and the Beginnings of Bodybuilding* (Urbana: University of Illinois Press, 1994).

6. They outfitted a local barn with parallel bars, a pommel horse, and rings, and developed a gymnastics routine to showcase their strength and daring. Sargent describes going to neighboring towns like Bangor in his *Autobiography*, edited by Ledyard Sargent, 60–61.

7. Ibid., 82.

8. Sargent was nineteen years old and had not finished high school when he took the job at Bowdoin. See Bennett, "The Life of Dudley Allen Sargent," 16.

9. For a description of Bowdoin's early equipment, see ibid., 18.

10. Sargent blamed Windship's health lift for extending the life of heavy-lifting equipment. He declared them "like mushrooms after the rain," springing up "in parlors and offices and schools everywhere." As a result, we can infer that colleges like Bowdoin, Yale, and Havard kept their own out-of-date heavy equipment because it was similar to Windship's. For information on Sargent's views of Windship, see Sargent, *Autobiography*, 97; for the quote on torturous machines, see 92.

11. Sargent, *Autobiography*, 95.

12. Ibid., 108.

13. Ibid.

14. Ibid., 130.

15. Ibid., 60.

16. Bruce Bennett believes that Blaikie reinforced Sargent's ideas about symmetrical development and mechanized training. It seems almost certain that Sargent's decision to open a gymnasium in New York came as a result of Blaikie's recommendation in *Harper's Magazine*. For Blaikie's call for a New York gymnasium, see William Blaikie, "Free Muscular Development," *Harper's Magazine* 56 (May 1878): 915–924. For information on the connection between Blaikie and Sargent, see Bennett, "The Life of Dudley Allen Sargent," 27.

17. William Blaikie, *How to Get Strong and Stay So* (New York: Harper & Brothers, 1879), 11. Blaikie's characterization of the Health Lift as work suited to a "truck horse" is significant. Eugenicists, or those who advocated a selective breeding program for humans that included "superior" genes and excluded "inferior" ones, often used the term "thoroughbred" to describe those superior individuals. In this context, a "truck horse" would have been assumed to be an individual not merely muscularly deficient but genetically deficient as well. For more information on eugenic thought of the period and its relationship to design, see Christina Cogdell, "Reconsidering the Streamline Style: Evolutionary Thought, Eugenics, and U.S. Industrial Design, 1925–1940" (Ph.D. diss., University of Texas at Austin, 2001). For a useful general survey of eugenics, see Daniel Kevles, *In the Name of Eugenics: Genetics and the Uses of Human Heredity* (New York: Knopf, 1985).

18. Ibid., 74. Unlike Blaikie, Sargent recognized that in rare cases, one could achieve a perfect body without machines. He often praised Eugen Sandow, an Austrian-born strongman, as having the perfect physique. And although Sandow used and sold pulley weights, some even of his own design, he frequently lifted only barbells. Sandow, however, was the exceptional individual born with evenly dispersed musculature. Most students required machines to achieve his measurements. See the following section on anthropometry for more information.

19. According to Sargent, the student body "as a whole" had ignored the Hemenway before he arrived. See Sargent, *Dudley Allen Sargent*, 167.

20. Sargent describes Harvard's old gymnasium as similar to Yale's. For a description of Yale's gymnasium when he arrived there in 1873, see Sargent, *Autobiography*, 138.

21. Edward M. Hartwell, "The Rise of College Gymnastics in the United States," in *Special Report by the Bureau of Education of Educational Exhibits and Conventions at the World's Industrial and Cotton Centennial Exposition at New Orleans, 1884–84*, 670. For a description of the Hemenway's main hall, which measured 125 by 113 feet, and the facilities within it, see Bennett, "The Life of Dudley Allen Sargent," 46. For a contemporary discussion of the gymna-

sium's features, see "Athletics and Gymnastics at Harvard," *The Wheelman* 2 (September 1883): 417–423.

22. At Bowdoin, he built an early exercise machine by using window weights pulled over wooden rollers that students would lift with an iron handle. See Bennett, "The Life of Dudley Allen Sargent," 33. For information on the gym Sargent founded in New York in 1878, experience that was essential in getting him the Harvard job, see ibid., 28.

23. "Athletics and Gymnastics at Harvard," 422. For a complete list of Sargent's "developing appliances" at the Hemenway gymnasium, see Bennett, "The Life of Dudley Allen Sargent," Appendix A, 268–269.

24. "Athletics and Gymnastics at Harvard," 422.

25. Dudley Allen Sargent, "The Apparatus of the Hemenway Gymnasium," *Harvard Register* 1 (February 1880): 45.

26. Corbusier is largely credited for codifying the machine aesthetic in design. See Le Corbusier, *Towards a New Architecture* (New York: Payson & Clarke, 1927).

27. See advertisement for "Professor D. L. Dowd's Home Exerciser," in *Sporting Goods: Sports equipment and clothing, novelties, recreative science, firemen's supplies, magic lanterns and slides, plays and joke books, tricks and magic, badges and ornaments* (New York: Peck and Snyder, 1886). Historical reprint from the American Historical Catalog Collection (Princeton: Pine Press, 1976).

28. Narragansett of Rhode Island later became Sargent's official machine producer. Bennett argues that Sargent's no-patent agreement with Harvard prevented him from ever making significant money from his machine designs. For a discussion of this, see Bennett, "The Life of Dudley Allen Sargent," 140–145.

29. Sargent, *Autobiography*, 151.

30. For information on Sargent's prescribed exercises, see ibid. Archibald Maclaren from Oxford said that exercises should mimic natural movements in his 1869 book, *A System of Physical Education: Theoretical and Practical* (Oxford: Clarendon Press, 1869). For more information on Maclaren's ideas in relation to Sargent's, see Bennett, "The Life of Dudley Allen Sargent," 34–35.

31. D. A. Sargent, "The Inomotor: A Fundamental Mechanism for a New System of Motor Vehicles, Testing Apparatus and Developing Appliances," *American Physical Education Review* 5 (December 1900): 312. Sargent explained in 1890 that actual labor produced "good physical results in certain directions," but only a system of exercises that resembled actual labor could "supplement the deficiencies of one's occupation" and "develop him where he is weak." Sargent, "The System of Physical Training at the Hemenway Gymnasium," in *Physical Training: A Full Report of the Papers and Discussions of the*

Conference Held in Boston in November, 1889, ed. Isabel C. Barrows (Boston: Press of George H. Ellis, 1890), 63.

32. "Athletics and Gymnastics at Harvard," 421. For the praise concerning the abdominal machine, 422.

33. For information on Sargent's battle with the faculty over Inomotor training, see the letter from Sargent to the President and Fellows of Harvard College dated March 25, 1905, in the Harvard archives. Letter quoted in Bennett, "The Life of Dudley Allen Sargent," 147.

34. Sargent described one young bicyclist who won several competitions but nonetheless died of consumption after graduation. Sargent attributed the death to the student's unwillingness to train his arms and chest, for the student had once told him that "arms and chests do not win bicycle races." See Sargent, "The Inomotor," 315.

35. Ibid., 314.

36. Speakers who came to the Hemenway also echoed the message that machines could positively impact nerve force. Dr. Walter Channing of Boston gave a lecture at the Hemenway, "The Relation of Physical Training to the Nervous System," in which he described the perfect operation of the "nervous mechanism." Although man has a tendency toward degeneracy, he explained, it could be corrected by systematic physical training. One assumes he meant the kind of systems available at the Hemenway. See his "Value of Physical Training," article from unspecified source in the Sargent archives, Harvard University.

37. Sargent described this by saying that "the momentum acquired by the rapid revolution of these wheels will flex and extend the arms, trunk and legs for a considerable time without any active efforts, thus improving the returning circulation of the blood and removing the cause of fatigue when it has been produced." See Sargent, "The Inomotor," 323.

38. For more information on Spencer's basic theories, see Ronald Martin, *American Literature and the Universe of Force* (Durham: Duke University Press, 1981), especially xiii–xiv.

39. See Rick Rylance, *Victorian Psychology and British Culture, 1850–1880* (New York: Oxford University Press, 2000), 220.

40. Spencer's own background as a railroad engineer, as well as his background in math and natural sciences and his birth during the height of the British industrial revolution, probably contributed to his desire to view human systems through a mechanical framework.

41. For more on this "universe of force," see Martin, *American Literature and the Universe of Force*, xiii.

42. *Harvard Catalog*, 1880–1881. 216. Harvard faculty and staff could also use the Hemenway's facilities without charge, except for a small locker fee. See Bennett, "The Life of Dudley Allen Sargent," 48. Harvard did not require physi-

cal education for freshmen until after Sargent retired in 1919. *Athletic Committee Minutes* 1, 69.

43. From 1879 to 1885, there were roughly one thousand students enrolled in Harvard each year. This number had increased to two thousand by 1904. See Bennett, "The Life of Dudley Allen Sargent," 78.

44. By the late 1880s, these exhibitions had been discontinued. See ibid., 49.

45. *Annual Reports of the President and Treasurer of Harvard College*, 1883–1884, 31. Quoted in Bennett, "The Life of Dudley Allen Sargent," 50.

46. Letter from Edward E. Allen, instructor at the Perkins Institution for the Blind, in "Dudley Allen Sargent, Fiftieth Anniversary, 1869–1919," 79. This tribute pamphlet is in the Sargent archives, Harvard University.

47. Barrett Wendell, "Social Life at Harvard," *Lippincott's Monthly Magazine* 39 (January 1887): 157.

48. For information on Sargent's work with women, see Cottrell, "Women's Minds, Women's Bodies," and Bennett, "The Life of Dudley Allen Sargent," chap. 9, 98–117.

49. Sargent developed his machines at Bowdoin, an all-male college. In addition, even his New York gymnasium, where he admitted women and children, was geared primarily toward men. He had more hours for men to use the facilities, reserving the morning hours for business and professional men who came on the way to work. Women used the facility in late morning; after a break at the gymnasium for consultations, children came from 2:00 to 5:00. Before supper was a time reserved for businessmen, and a young men's group exercised from 8:00 to 10:00 in the evening. This meant that men had at least five hours on the equipment; women, about two. Women did not have access to exercise equipment at Harvard until 1943 and at Bowdoin until 1971, the years they were first allowed admission. See Bennett, "The Life of Dudley Allen Sargent," 29. Further, even women who did learn the Sargent system seemed to have difficulty implementing machine-training programs for other women. Helen Putnam, physician and director of Vassar's gymnasium, trained with Sargent in the late 1880s. Photographs of Vassar's gymnasium in the years following show rings, clubs, a trapeze, and balance beam but no machines. Correspondence with Dean Roberts, special collections assistant, Vassar College, August 26, 2002.

50. Sargent first used this measuring system in 1873 at Yale when he used chins and dips to test the efficiency of students in handling their weight, a preliminary test for heavy gymnastics work. See Sargent, "Twenty Years' Progress in Efficiency Tests," *American Physical Education Review* 63 (October 1913): 454.

51. See Bennett, *Contributions of Dr. Sargent*, 3.

52. There is little written about Sargent's measuring machines. One of the best accounts is Roberta Park's in her survey of physical educators. See Park, "Physiologists, Physicans and Physical Educators," in Jack Berryman, ed., *Sport*

and Exercise Science: Essays in the History of Sports Medicine (Urbana: University of Illinois Press, 1992), 153.

53. These three machines are described in one of Sargent's popular articles in addition to his regular medical texts. See D. A. Sargent, "The Physical Proportions of the Typical Man," *Scribner's Magazine* 2, no. 1 (July 1887): 7. For a more specialized description of the equipment, see D. A. Sargent, "Anthropometric Apparatus with Directions for Measuring and Testing the Principal Physical Characteristics of the Human Body" (Dudley Allen Sargent, 1887).

54. For more information on these three machines, see Sargent, "Anthropometric Apparatus," 12–14.

55. Dr. Edward Hitchcock at Amherst measured students weight, height, finger reach, chest girth, lung capacity, and strength in 1869. According to Bruce Bennett, Hitchcock's system had little influence on other schools. See Bennett, "The Life of Dudley Allen Sargent," 6.

56. Carl Linnaeus, author of the 1735 text, *Systemanatural*, is credited as the first anthropometrist. For more information, see John S. Haller, *Outcasts from Evolution: Scientific Attitudes of Racial Inferiority, 1859–1900* (Urbana: University of Illinois Press, 1971), 4. Anthropometry first became popular in the United States during the Civil War, when the U.S. Sanitary Commission measured soldiers to determine their fitness for service. This early research was similar in motivation to Sargent's; the commission wanted to learn what made some individuals succeed and others fail. It looked for an answer in physique and physical strength. Not incidentally, the first large-scale anthropometric endeavor during the war happened after Union troops lost at Bull Run. Many of these studies were sponsored by insurance companies through agencies like the Sanitary Commission in order to predict health risks by creating statistics on "average" Americans' health. See Haller, *Outcasts from Evolution*, 19–20. After the Civil War, the commission distributed its devices to colleges and institutions across the country, with the hope that their instructors would continue to compile statistics on Americans' height, weight, and physical performance.

57. Anthropology inherited much anthropometric equipment in 1865 after the U.S. Sanitary Commission's studies as academics set out to posit their own arguments about racial superiority or equality, depending on their views. Franz Boas's study of immigrants used anthropometry, for example, to prove that they did not remain distinct "unamerican types." By proving that immigrants' and their children's bodies took on more average national measurements, Boas could argue that there were no permanent racial separations between old and new Americans. See Immigration Commission, Mr. Dillingham, "Changes in Bodily Form from Descendents of Immigrants," 61st Cong., 2d sess., 1910, S. Doc. 208 (Washington, D.C.: Government Printing Office).

58. During the Civil War, Army doctors were asked to measure and compare black and white soldiers in intelligence, physical performance, and military abil-

ity. Most of the doctors responded that the soldiers performed equally; some declared blacks inferior, based on physical measurements. Even recruits marked having "good physical endowment[s]" could fail to measure up, given the standard. Flatter feet or longer torsos than the average, taken from mainly white soldiers, were among traits used to mark them inferior. See Haller, *Outcasts from Evolution*, 30.

59. According to Roberta Park, Sargent was the most prolific anthropometry promoter between 1880 and 1900. He published charts and directions for taking measurements and promoted his "developing appliances." In addition, the "Sargent system" was one of only three that were extensively discussed at the 1889 Boston Conference on Physical Training. See Park, "Healthy, Moral, and Strong: Educational Views of Exercise and Athletics in Nineteenth-Century America," in Kathryn Grover, ed., *Fitness in American Culture: Images of Health, Sport, and the Body, 1830–1940* (New York: Margaret Woodbury Strong Museum, 1989), 123–168, especially 150–152. Sargent's neglect reflects the larger neglect of sports history in surveys of the era. Excellent work has been done within the field of sports history. More of this work, however, should be integrated into general historical, sociological, and anthropological texts. For a survey text on sports history, see Richard Swanson and Betsy Spears, *History of Sport and Physical Education in the United States*, 4th ed. (New York: McGraw-Hill, 1995). See pp. 183–184 for a perspective on "missing" sports scholarship.

60. Sargent did his studies between 1880 and 1900, a time that historians have defined as "the golden age of anthropometric measurements." See Bennett, "The Life of Dudley Allen Sargent," 174.

61. Other fitness promoters also applied theories of strengthening equally across racial groups. Sandow, the nineteenth-century Austrian strongman, often declared that his physical training system could be used by whites and non-whites to achieve physical perfection. In his popular magazine, he used images of himself and other white teachers along with their muscular, dark-skinned students, accompanied by text wherein he proudly discussed their physiques. In 1905, he traveled to Dutch Java, Japan, and British India and covered the story for his own *Sandow's Magazine* 117 (September 1905): 343–344. He also discussed Indian fitness programs in the *Daily News* 19 (September 1905). For more information, see Michael Budd, *The Sculpture Machine: Physical Culture and Body Politics in the Age of Empire* (Houndsmills: Macmillan, 1997), 83. There is evidence that Sandow may have thought that dark-skinned people, in fact, possessed superior bodies. According to one historian, in 1903 Sandow compared British to Indian peoples and preferred the latter. Sandow reported that he "often watched crowds bathe . . . with a critical eye, and always came to the conclusion that they were less shapely than many of the dark-colored peoples whom I have seen." See *Sandow's Magazine* (October 1903): 168. Also see Eugen Sandow, *Physical Development for Men* (London: published by author,

no date), 11, in the Todd-McLean Physical Culture Collection (TMPC). Other physical culture promoters would use measurement studies to promote eugenics. The popular American promoter Bernarr Macfadden told his magazine readers in 1921 to read Madison Grant's eugenic text *The Passing of the Great Race*. See Tim Armstrong, *Modernism, Technology and the Body: A Cultural Study* (Cambridge: Cambridge University Press, 1998), 106.

62. Washington is listed among Sargent's students in the *Harvard Catalog*, 1887–1888.

63. For more information on Taylor and his program, see Martha Banta, *Taylored Lives: Narrative Productions in the Age of Taylor, Veblen, and Ford* (Chicago: University of Chicago Press, 1993).

64. One of Taylor's early studies involved workers at Bethlehem Steel who were trained to load three times as much pig iron in a single day, thanks to Taylor's scientific management system. See Frederick Winslow Taylor, *Principles of Scientific Management* (New York: Harper and Brothers, 1911); part 2 discusses his actual experiments.

65. Anson Rabinbach, *The Human Motor: Energy, Fatigue and the Origins of Modernity* (New York, Basic Books, 1990), 23.

66. For information on "scientific eating," see James C. Whorton, "Eating to Win: Popular Concepts of Diet, Strength, and Energy in the Early Twentieth Century," in Grover, *Fitness in American Culture*, 95.

67. In the 1880s, the Frenchman Etienne-Jules Marey experimented with photography, inventing a portable inscriptor to measure the way body parts moved in accomplishing a task. He was able to analyze the time it took a nerve impulse to travel to a muscle and get a reaction, thereby recommending ways to make movements more efficient. For more on Marey, see Rabinbach, *The Human Motor*, 93–94.

68. Taking pictures at 1/500 of a second allowed Muybridge to remove the mystery behind physical movement. Along with Thomas Eakins at the University of Pennsylvania, Muybridge made 100,000 negatives of bodies running, weight lifting, and doing the high jump to discover the secret behind fluid motions. For more information see Mrozek, *Sport and American Mentality*. Also see Rabinbach, *The Human Motor*, 101. Some of the researchers gave bleak forecasts for the modern body, based on their measurements. Marey's view was especially troubling: he believed humans were unable to learn efficient means of movement and, as a result, would suffer inescapable energy loss. See Rabinbach, *The Human Motor*, 118.

69. Sargent explains the symmetry ideal in "The Sargent Anthropometric Charts: Descriptive Circular," Sargent archive, Harvard University.

70. One newspaper article that appeared after Sandow's 1893 Trocadero performance commented, "[W]hat a wretched, scrawny creature the usual well-built gentleman is compared with a perfect man. Sandow, posing in various stat-

uesque attitudes, is not only inspiring because of his enormous strength, but absolutely beautiful as a work of art as well." In addition, Professor R. Lankester, director of the Natural History branch of the British Museum, made a plaster Sandow for the museum's exhibit on the "perfect type of European man." For information, see Kenneth R. Dutton, *The Perfectible Body: The Western Ideal of Male Physical Development* (New York: Continuum Publishing Company, 1995), 124. We can assume from its representational ubiquity that Sandow's musculature enjoyed wide popularity. One anatomy book used it as an illustration, labeling it merely "Sandow's arm," on the assumption that readers would know just who Sandow was. See F. A. Schmidt and Eustace H. Miles, *The Training of the Body for Games* (New York: E. P. Dutton & Co., 1901), 157. For more information on Sandow, see Chapman, *Sandow the Magnificent*. For reference to his "machined figure" see Budd, *The Sculpture Machine*, 116.

71. Linda Dalrymple Henderson, *Duchamp in Context: Science and Technology in the Large Glass and Related Works* (Princeton: Princeton University Press, 1998), 160.

72. For more on Sargent's measurement session with Sandow, see John Kasson, *Houdini, Tarzan, and the Perfect Man: The White Male Body and the Challenge of Modernity* (New York: Hill & Wang, 2001), 44–46; quote from p. 45.

73. It is likely that students learned from their interactions with Sargent's dynamometers. John Harvey Kellogg used the dynamometer in the early 1900s and commented that "the procedure is a fascinating one, and the machine itself, with its mode of operation, often proves more absorbing to the newcomer than his own performance." We can assume that Sargent students would have reacted similarly to the process. Kellogg, "The Battle Creek Sanitarium Book" (Battle Creek: no publishing data), 105.

74. Attila's name was actually Ludwig Durlacher. See ibid., 33–35.

75. Ibid., 45.

76. Sandow may also have reinforced this connection. Those who read Sandow's opinions would have known that he did not see mail-order devices, including his own, as constituting a complete muscle-building system. In an interview in 1902, with perhaps a subtle nod to Sargent's system, Sandow stressed that machines were only as good as the intelligence behind them:

> I approve of every apparatus that aids the mind in its dominion over the body. But if a man thinks that eight shillings will buy an apparatus that will make him strong he will be disappointed . . . the test of muscle is that when relaxed it is as soft as a babe's, and when contracted hard as steel. It is only intelligence that can do that. No mere mechanical appliance alone will ever achieve it.

Given that Sandow knew Sargent at this time, and that a cast of his body was already on display at the Hemenway, it is likely that this comment endorses

Sargent: ". . . A chain is only as strong as its weakest link . . . the secret is to 'know thyself' . . . and knowing one's weakness, to concentrate the mind and energies upon that weakness with a view of correcting it." "Sandow Interviewed in America," *Sandow's Magazine* (1902): 56–57. Sargent's review of Sandow ran in the *New York World*, June 25, 1893, 4. According to John Kasson, a similar verdict was reached by a physician in San Francisco in 1894. See "Sandow Examined," *San Francisco Examiner*, May 6, 1894, 4. Both articles cited in Kasson, *Houdini, Tarzan*, 45. Sandow also included Sargent's anthropometric chart in his own 1894 book on strength training, captioned "Dr. Sargent's chart showing Mr. Sandow's measurements and the variations from the normal." See G. Mercer Adam, ed., *Sandow on Physical Training* (New York: J. Selin Tart & Sons, 1894), 241. Sandow's balanced physique was also alluded to in reviews of his shows that compared him to a "work of art." One reporter declared in 1902 that "as Mr. Sandow stood upon the stage, he indeed looked the embodiment of perfect manhood." Quoted in Dutton, *The Perfectible Body*, 124.

77. Sandow actively sought to portray himself as both an expert on anatomy and as an impressive strength performer. His book, edited by Mercer Adam, includes detailed lists of the proper names of all muscle groups and physical diagrams showing their placement. It also contains numerous illustrations of Sandow performing his most popular feats, including lifting concrete blocks and balancing a horse and rider on his body. See Adam, *Sandow on Physical Training*, 183, 235. *Sandow's Magazine* served a similar function. The 1902 combined issue presented an image of Sandow in suit and tie surrounded by classical statues and lions on the cover. An article on "practical anatomy," accompanied by a copy of the Sandow cast then on display in Harvard's Gymnasium, made it clear that Sandow made Harvard's endorsement of his body a major part of his "brand" value. See "Practical Anatomy," *Sandow's Magazine: Physical Hygiene, Culture, Recreation* (January 1902): cover and 51–54.

78. Ladd and Putnam directed the gymnasiums at Bryn Mawr and Vassar, respectively. Each attended Sargent's school of physical education and received medical degrees from the University of Pennsylvania. Putnam also served as the vice president of the American Association for the Advancement of Physical Education in 1895. The student list is from *Harvard Catalog, 1887–1888*, quoted in Bennett, "The Life of Dudley Allen Sargent, 86. For a detailed list of Sargent's student enrollment, see Sargent, *Autobiography*, 212.

79. McKenzie carried on Sargent's traditions. He explained in 1905 that his physical education department was not there to create athletes: "A strong, healthy, symmetrical body for the mass of our students has been our primary object." See "The Physical Side of College Men," *Illustrated Sporting News* 5 (August 12, 1905): 4. Mrozek says McKenzie had a "virtual obsession with the symmetry of the whole figure." See Mrozek, *Sport and American Mentality*, 72–73.

80. Whorton, *Crusaders for Fitness*, 284. For more information on the

YMCAs' use of Sargent's system, see J. Gardner Smith, "History of Physical Training in New York City and Vicinity in the Young Men's Christian Associations," *American Physical Education Review* 4 (September 1899): 306.

81. Sargent, "The Physical Proportions of the Typical Man," 3–17.

82. *Official Catalogue of Exhibits and Descriptive Catalogue, World's Columbian Exposition, Department M. Anthropological Building, Midway Plaisance and Isolated Exhibits* (Chicago: W. B. Conkey Company, 1893), 20–22.

83. Park, "Healthy, Moral, and Strong," 152.

84. Sargent, "The System of Physical Training at the Hemenway Gymnasium," 65.

85. Sargent, "The Physical Proportions of the Typical Man," 15.

86. For information on the Corliss engine, see John Kasson, *Civilizing the Machine: Technology and Republican Values in America, 1776–1900* (New York: Grossman, 1976), 161–165.

87. For information on the Swedish exhibit, see Frank Norton, ed., *Frank Leslie's Historical Register of the United States Centennial Exposition, 1876* (New York: Frank Leslie, 1877).

88. For a copy of the brochure accompanying Zander's exhibit, see Dr. Elis Sidenblah, "Swedish Catalogue. I. Statistics, International Exhibition, 1876. Philadelphia" (Philadelphia: Hallowell & Company, 1876), 70–71.

89. Ibid.

90. For more information on Zander's early years, see Marian Fournier, *The Medico-Mechanical Equipment of Dr. Zander* (Leiden: Museum Boerhaave, 1989), 1–5.

91. Zander had institutes in Germany, Austria, Sweden, the Netherlands, Hungary, and South America. For a complete list from 1906, see A. Levertin, "A Short Review of Dr. G. Zander's Medico-Mechanical Gymnastics Method," in A. Levertin, F. Heiligenthal, G. Schuetz, and G. Zander, *The Leading Features of Dr. G. Zander's Medico-Mechanical Gymnastic Method and Its Use in Four Separate Treaties* (Wiesbaden: Rossel, Schwartz & Co., 1906), 13.

92. Further evidence that Zander often trained injured workers is found in a description of how to guide patients; it advised doctors to test those who "pretended that [they were] not able to lift anything" by putting them on the arm-flexion apparatus that measured arm strength. Feigning weakness might have been a way for employees to avoid returning to jobs they did not enjoy. For more information, see Levertin et al., *The Leading Features*, 12.

93. For more information on the relationship between state rehabilitative support and Zander's success, see ibid., 11.

94. See John K. Mitchell's description of the Zanders. He describes them as having "not much vogue" here but attaining "a place of sufficient importance abroad to call for some description." Mitchell, *A System of Physiologic*

Therapeutics: A Practical Exposition of the Methods, other than Drug-Giving, Useful for the Prevention of Disease and in the Treatment of the Sick (Philadelphia: P. Blakiston's Son & Co., 1904), 12.

95. European therapy treatments declined in the 1920s, largely due to the high costs of rehabilitative programs. This, combined with the advent of cheap pulleys that could do what Zander's expensive equipment had, brought about their demise. For information, see Fournier, *The Medico-Mechanical Equipment*, 9 and 12.

96. For a list of Zander machines in the United States and Europe, see Levertin et al., *The Leading Features*, 13–14.

97. See "The Dr. Savage Health Studio," in the Warshaw Collection of Business Americana, National Museum of American History (hereafter NMAH), Smithsonian Institution.

98. For information on Kny-Scheerer's role in producing Zander machines, see the accession files, Division of Medical Sciences, Department of Science and Technology, NMAH, Smithsonian Institution. According to its files, "by 1894 there were units in New York and St. Louis. These units have disappeared as has the importer KNY-Scheerer."

99. Historian John Hoover estimates that between 1911 and 1930, 62,000 people a year visited the Homestead, where Zanders were included in the price of treatments. Interview with John Hoover, historian, Homestead Resort, Hot Springs, Va., August 22, 1999. The Greenbriar reportedly saw 20,000 patients a year when Zander treatments were popular. Interview with Bob Conte, historian, Greenbriar Hotel, White Sulphur Springs, W. Va., September 1, 1999.

100. Fournier, *The Medico-Mechanical Equipment*, 11.

101. According to John Hoover, by 1890, all explicit references to cures and illness had been taken out of the resort's brochure. Interview with John Hoover, historian, Homestead Resort, Hot Springs, Va., August 22, 1999.

102. For information on the Fordyce Bathhouse's modernization efforts in 1915, see Carolyn Thomas de la Peña, "Recharging at the Fordyce: Confronting Nature and Technology in the Modern Bath," *Technology and Culture* 40, no. 4 (October 1999): 750–755.

103. Accession memos, Division of Medical Sciences, NMAH. For information on the cost of other resort facilities, see Thomas de la Peña, "Recharging at the Fordyce," 750.

104. See Dr. Michael Cohen, "The Homestead Zander Collection," unpublished report in the accession files, NMAH. According to John Hoover, many of these machines remained in working order through the 1970s. Interview with author.

105. Levertin et al., *The Leading Features*, 9.

106. For detailed descriptions of the Zander equipment, see *Kinesotherapy* (New York: The Kny-Scheerer Company, 1914).

107. Fournier, *The Medico-Mechanical Equipment*, 7.

108. Levertin et al., *The Leading Features*, 9.

109. Gustaf Zander, L. Wischnewetzky, ed., "Mechanical-Electrotherapeutics and Orthopedics by Means of Apparatus," in Alfred Levertin, Dr. *Zander's Medico-Mechanische Gymnastik, ihre Methode, Bedeutung und Anwendung* (Stockholm: Königl. Buchdruckerei, P. A. Norstedt & Söner, 1892), 180.

110. Kellogg, *The Battle Creek Sanitarium Book*, 168. Kellogg also used anthropometric measurements similar to Sargent's at Battle Creek. For more information, see 31.

111. John Harvey Kellogg, *The Art of Massage: Its Physiological Effects and Therapeutic Applications* (Battle Creek: Modern Medicine Publishing Co., 1895), 23.

112. Ibid., 24. Kellogg told his readers that ample massage could result in an actual increase in height. He reported that chiefs among the South Sea Islanders who were massaged daily were "very much larger than the average of people." See 38.

113. Kellogg patented his own machines, but their similarities to Gustav Zander's suggest that Kellogg may have had more than a general sense of Zander's machines in mind during the design process. For an example of this, see Kellogg's vibrating chair and apparatus for kneading the abdomen, which he calls "similar to Zander's," in Kellogg, *The Art of Massage*, fig. 115, p. 164, and fig. 122, p. 173, respectively.

114. Dr. G. Schütz, "On Medico-Mechanical Treatment of Injuries," in Levertin et al., *The Leading Features*, 20. For information on how Zander machines were part of a larger repertoire of vibratory appliances in the early twentieth century, see Mitchell, *A System of Physiologic Therapeutics*, 188.

115. Mesmerism taught believers that one person's energy could be channeled into another person's in order to improve health. For a clear description of the philosophy behind mesmerism and a description of a mesmerism session, see anonymous, *The History and Philosophy of Animal Magnetism with Practical Instructions for the Exercise of This Power* (Boston: J. N. Bradley & Co., 1843), 10–15.

116. Mitchell, *A System of Physiologic Therapeutics*, 136.

117. Levertin, "A Short Review," 20.

118. Kellogg, *The Battle Creek Sanitarium Book*, 30. Members of the general public that did not attend Kellogg's Sanitarium also had a chance to learn the energy-enhancing effects of these machines. In 1904, Kellogg had an exhibit on the sanitarium at the St. Louis World's Fair. His vibrating chair was reported so popular for relieving exhaustion that "the exhibit was thronged daily by hundreds inquiring for the 'rest chair.'" See ibid., 22.

119. For more information on the Fordyce's natural symbols, see Thomas de la Peña, "Recharging at the Fordyce," 760–764.

120. Fournier, *The Medico-Mechanical Equipment*, 14.

121. The description is based on the author's observations of a Zander "horse" machine in storage in the summer of 1999 at the National Museum of American History, Smithsonian Institution.

122. The machine moved at a rate of three movements per second; Fournier, *The Medico-Mechanical Equipment*, 26.

123. *Sentinel-Record* (February 28, 1915): 1. Source quoted in Carol Petravage, *The Fordyce Bathhouse, Hot Springs National Park, Arkansas* (Harpers Ferry, W. Va.: National Park Service, 1988), 185.

124. Fournier, *The Medico-Mechanical Equipment*, 5.

125. Viewing machines as nature's helpers would not have struck bathers as entirely new. In the fifty years prior to the Fordyce's opening, physicians and laymen often recommended electricity as a way to restore "natural" energy. In advertisements for electrical belts, wigs, and "invigorating" chairs, promoters rarely stressed the equipment's mechanics, instead saying that it worked by harnessing unused power within the body, "restoring impaired vigor . . . and renew[ing] vital energy." For examples of such questionable medical devices, see Carolyn Marvin, *When Old Technologies Were New: Thinking about Electric Communication in the Late Nineteenth Century* (New York: Oxford University Press, 1988), 131.

126. It is interesting that these machines enjoyed a renaissance of sorts in the late 1970s and early 1980s as mechanical bulls gained popularity in bars around the country. One could argue that the same fears of mechanization and human obsolescence reappeared in this time of economic recession, encouraging people to seek the same dominance over mechanics that the Zanders offered sixty years earlier.

127. In "Taking the Waters: The Humbug of Hot Springs," Dr. Woods Hutchingson blames bathhouses like the Fordyce for trying to cure what he called "the overdissipation" of businessmen by subjecting them to five weeks of the "intellectual life of a jellyfish." He makes no mention of the intellectual life of female patrons. See *Everybody's Magazine* (February 1913): 167.

128. Petravage, *The Fordyce Bathhouse*, 143; see also fig. 94, p. 493 for an image of the women's baths.

129. Comparing the Fordyce to the New York Downtown Athletic Club (DAC), which opened in 1931, reveals similarities in what one might call "male-driven" design. Like the Fordyce, the DAC advertised itself as having the latest in mechanical fitness and water therapy. It, too, offered bathing facilities, massage equipment, and artificial sunbathing in a modern facility devoid of ornament. Because the DAC catered only to men, the similarities between it and the Fordyce suggest that the design elements in the latter did appeal especially to male patrons. See Rem Koolhaas, *Delirious New York: A Retroactive Manifesto for Manhattan* (New York: Monacelli Press, 1994).

130. According to the *Journal of the Arkansas Medical Society*, even men of "slender means" could stay in Hot Springs. See "Why Not Try Our Home Spas?" *Journal of the Arkansas Medical Society* 11 (1914): 144. The price of a week at the Fordyce would have been well within the budget of a typical middle-class clerk. According to Olivier Zunz, the typical salary for even low-level white-collar workers in the 1910s was $800 a year, or $67 a month. See Zunz, *Making America Corporate, 1870–1920* (Chicago: University of Chicago Press, 1990), 130.

131. "The Lost World of the Great Spas," 204, accession files, NMAH.

132. Levertin et al., *The Leading Features*, 10.

133. Sidenblah, "Swedish Catalogue," 70–71.

134. Cohen, "The Homestead Zander Collection," 6.

135. Levertin et al., *The Leading Features*, 12.

136. Fournier, *The Medico-Mechanical Equipment*, 11.

137. Ibid., 24.

138. For this characterization of the era see Cecelia Tichi, *Shifting Gears: Technology, Literature and Culture in Modernist America* (Chapel Hill: University of North Carolina Press, 1987), 19, 100–105.

139. Between 1900 and 1910, the number of white-collar clerks increased by 127 percent. By 1950, 37 percent of American workers held white-collar jobs, a figure up from 3 percent in 1900. Zunz, *Making America Corporate,* 126. In one such company, New York's Metropolitan Life, 3,600 employees fielded calls from more than 15,000 visitors a day in an organization that, according to Zunz functioned as "an enormous machine dedicated to processing insurance claims." See ibid., 116.

140. Mitchell, *A System of Physiologic Therapeutics*, 135.

141. The Fordyce's machines would also have appealed to the muscular business aesthetic developed at the turn of the century by men like Bernarr Macfadden. In his magazine *Physical Culture*, Macfadden frequently made the connection between a muscular physique and a successful business career for men of the aspiring middle class. The muscle-bound professional was eventually replaced by the "brain-worker" as the ideal in the 1920s, but when the Fordyce opened, there was a clear connection between a strong body and a profitable career. One advertisement in the early 1920s suggested that only by taking a muscle control course could readers find happiness because, it declared, "success depends on upon health and strength." Earlier ads were less ambiguous; one stated that only an electrical invigorator (similar to the oscillator used at the Fordyce) could return one's "dissipated manhood" by giving "new courage, increased vigor, more pep." Harvey Green, *Fit for America: Health, Fitness, Sport, and American Society* (New York: Pantheon Books, 1986), 252.

142. In other words, if tumbling down a coal chute and "crashing" into another train could be enjoyable, then it was easier to cope with such fears in real

life. See John Kasson, *Amusing the Million: Coney Island at the Turn of the Century* (New York: Hill & Wang, 1978). John Sears also discusses the fascination that turn-of-the-century Americans had with technology both in industry and entertainment; see Sears, *Sacred Places: American Tourist Attractions in the Nineteenth Century* (New York: Oxford University Press, 1989), 189.

143. Carroll Pursell, *The Machine in America: A Social History of Technology* (Baltimore: Johns Hopkins University Press, 1995), 203.

144. Sandow, *Physical Development for Men*, 9.

NOTES TO CHAPTER 3

1. "An Electric Treat," *Electric Review* (February 26, 1887): 13. Quoted in Carolyn Marvin, *When Old Technologies Were New: Thinking about Electric Communication in the Late-Nineteenth Century* (New York: Oxford University Press, 1988), 130–131.

2. The Leyden jar was a glass jar lined two-thirds of its height on the inside and outside with tin foil. For more information on the Leyden jar and the discovery of static electricity, see Sanford Bordeau, *Volts to Hertz: The Rise of Electricity: From the Compass to the Radio through the Works of Sixteen Great Men of Science Whose Names Are Used in Measuring Electricity and Magnetism* (Minneapolis: Burgess Publishing Co., 1982). The subject was also often covered in electrotherapy texts. See, for example, *Electrotherapy in the United States* (Minneapolis: Medtronic, 1977), 1. Tim Armstrong provides a brief summary of early experiments with electricity in Europe; see Armstrong, *Modernism, Technology and the Body: A Cultural Study* (Cambridge: Cambridge University Press, 1998), 15.

3. For a description of the Leyden jar applied, see Margaret Rowbottom and Charles Susskind, *Electricity and Medicine: History of Their Interaction* (San Francisco: San Francisco Press, 1984), 30.

4. For a description of Galvani's experiments as viewed through late-nineteenth-century eyes, see Edwin Jouston and A. E. Kennelly, *Electricity in Electro-Therapeutics* (New York: W. J. Johnston Company, 1896), 1–5. See also Marcello Pera, *The Ambiguous Frog: The Galvanni-Volta Controversy on Animal Electricity*, trans. Johnathan Mandelbaum (Princeton: Princeton University Press, 1992), and Brenda Himrich and Stew Thornley, *Electrifying Medicine: How Electricity Sparked a Medical Revolution* (Minneapolis: Lerner Publications Company, 1995), 20.

5. Pera, *The Ambiguous Frog*, 139–145, 160.

6. More information on Paige's practice is available in Dr. A. Paige, *The Electropathic Guide Devoted to Electricity and Its Medical Applications* (Boston:

Damrell & Moore, 1849). For more information on the persistence of the belief that electricity was the vital force, see Eric Jameson, *The Natural History of Quackery*, (Springfield, Ill.: Charles C. Thomas, 1961), 133.

7. A. Paige, *Mental and Physical Electropathy, or Electricity; Its Physiological Relations and Medical Applications* (Philadelphia: Browns' Steam Power Book and Job Printing Office, 1852), 20–21.

8. The United States government commissioned the Flexner report, released in 1910, to survey the state of American medical education. Abraham Flexner, its author, found that the vast majority of American medical schools provided substandard educations and that an alarming number of American physicians received their degrees through correspondence courses, often completing the M.D. degree work in less than a year. For information on the Flexner report and the state of American medical education at the turn of the century, see John Duffy, *The Healers: A History of American Medicine* (Urbana: University of Illinois Press, 1979), 260–266.

9. For more information on Louis Pasteur and his discovery of germ theory in the 1860s, see Patrice Debre, *Louis Pasteur* (Baltimore: Johns Hopkins University Press, 1998).

10. Dr. E. J. Fraser, *Medical Electricity: A Treatise on the Nature of Vital Electricity in Health and Disease with Plain Instructions in the Uses of Artificial Electricity as a Curative Agent* (Chicago: C. S. Halsey, 1863), 11. See also John Ives, *Electricity as a Medicine and Its Mode of Application* (New York: John T. Ives, 1879).

11. Fraser, *Medical Electricity*, 13. Electrotherapists followed the gender patterns of nineteenth-century American medicine in that most practitioners were male. There were, however, some prominent female practitioners. The Bakken Library's electrotherapy files feature postcards from a Virginia K. Orvis, medical electrician in Williamsport, Pennsylvania, and an unnamed woman photographed in her electrotherapy office in Butte, Montana, in 1914. See Bakken Library and Museum of Electricity in Life, Minneapolis, Ephemera Collection (hereafter BLEC).

12. Fraser, *Medical Electricity*, 21.

13. For information on mesmerism in America and the ways in which mesmerism and magnetism were conflated, see Alan Gauld, *A History of Hypnotism* (Cambridge: Cambridge University Press, 1992), 179–194; and *Electrotherapy in the United States* (Minneapolis: Medtronic, 1977), 8.

14. There is some debate about whether mesmerism enjoyed more popularity in America than in Europe. Alan Gauld, in *A History of Hypnotism*, argues that mesmerists concentrated on American audiences in the 1830s after falling into disfavor in Europe. Medtronic's more self-serving historiography argues that Americans resisted mesmerist claims; its reliance on evidence from Benjamin

Franklin and Thomas Jefferson's publicized dismissal of the practice rather than on popular culture, however, makes its findings suspect. See *Electrotherapy in the United States*, 9.

15. For a sample of mesmerist Charles Poyen's writings, see Poyen, *Progress of Animal Magnetism in New England* (Boston: Weeks & Jordan, 1837).

16. J. H. Bagg, *Bagg on Magnetism or the Doctrine of Equilibrium* (Detroit: Bagg and Harmon, 1845), 109.

17. As Bagg explained it, the only substance driving the body was "magnetic fluids, and that Galvanism, Electricity, Light, Caloric and oxygen with hydrogen gasses are but different effects upon the corresponding five senses of the body, produced by one principle, the Magnetic fluids, and are therefore identical." See ibid., 1.

18. Ibid., 116.

19. Ibid., 243. Magnetists and mesmerists typically referred to an electrical or magnetic force that emanated from them and cured patients. S. B. Brittan, a magnetizer in the 1860s, cured patients with "appropriate manipulations in all directions from the supposed point of electrical convergence." See Brittan, *Man and His Relations: Illustrating the Influence of the Mind on the Body* (New York: W. A. Townsend, 1864), 242. Such ideas seem illogical to modern readers, but they were actually part of electric therapies that inspired ardent admirers for more than a generation. As early as 1790, Elisha Perkins marketed his "magnetic tractors" to an eager audience. Despite the fact that the tractors were only pieces of metal with little magnetic force and no curative powers, Perkins enjoyed success for a number of years in door-to-door sales. For more on Perkins and on physicians' rejection of electrotherapy because of his fantastic claims, see Rowbottom and Susskind, *Electricity and Medicine*, 60–64. For information on the connection between "animal electricity" and his tractors, see John Vaughan, *Observations on Animal Electricity in Explanation of the Metallic Operation of Doctor Perkins* (Wilmington, Del.: W. C. Smyth, 1787).

20. As late as 1899, authors still published texts on magnetism, presumably because they found others wanting to purchase them. For example, see Albert Chavannes, *Magnetation* (Knoxville: Albert Chavannes, 1899). It also crept into the American lexicon through phrases like "magnetic personalities" and "sexual magnetism." For examples of the terms used in the early twentieth century, see Edmund Shaftesbury, *Private Lessons in the Cultivation of Magnetism of the Sexes* (Cleveland: Ralston Society, 1934), and, by the same author, *Instantaneous Personal Magnetism* (Meriden, Conn.: Ralston University Press, 1926), as well as pamphlets like "New Secrets of Personal Magnetism" (c. 1930), from the Todd-McLean Physical Culture Collection, University of Texas at Austin (hereafter TMPC).

21. There are numerous similarities between the energy that "mind cure" advocates like Quimby and Baker advocated and the energy that regular and irregular electrotherapists advocated. In both cases, the argument was that humans had reserves of energy that could be accessed for health and well-being. The difference was that mind-cure believers were trying to access only internal energy, in a fashion similar to machine theorists like Butler and Sargent; irregular electrotherapists were trying to incorporate external electric energy into the body. Interestingly, this difference may have contributed to the fact that far more women directed mind cures than electric cures. As I argue in the introduction, it was acceptable for women to uncover the body's "natural" power, as mind-cure practitioners said they were doing, but it was not acceptable for women to infuse the body with more power than it had to begin with. For more on the mind cure, see Donald Meyer, *The Positive Thinkers: A Study of the American Quest for Health, Wealth and Personal Power from Mary Baker Eddy to Norman Vincent Peale* (New York: Doubleday & Company, 1965).

22. Price figures are from the *McIntosh Battery and Optical Company: Electro-Therapeutical Catalogue* (Chicago: McIntosh, 1881) and the *Partnick, Bunnell & Co. Catalogue and Price List of Telegraphical and Electrical Instruments and Supplies* (Philadelphia: Rue & Jones, 1873). Jerome Kidder also sold a basic galvanic-faradic machine for $24 in 1882; see S. E. Morrill, *A Treatise of Practical Instructions in the Medical and Surgical Uses of Electricity* (Kalamazoo: Kalamazoo Publishing Company, 1882), 74. Drescher's sold seventeen different electrotherapy machines in 1873 at prices ranging from $10 to $250. See *Drescher's Illustrated Catalogue and Price List of Electro-Therapeutic Apparatus* (New York: self published, 1873). The inexpensive devices, weighing between six and twenty-two pounds, would have been portable for physicians practicing alone. See *McIntosh Catalogue*, 16. For more on the development of portable electrotherapy equipment in France and Great Britain see Rowbottom and Susskind, *Electricity and Medicine*, 59.

23. For sources on nineteenth-century electrotherapy see "Electrotherapy," *A System of Electrotherapeutics as Taught by the International Correspondence Schools*, vol. 4 (Scranton: International Textbook Co., 1902); *McIntosh Battery and Optical Company: Electro-Therapeutical Catalogue;* Morrill, *A Treatise of Practical Instructions;* and Alan McLane Hamilton, *Clinical Electro-Therapeutics, Medical and Surgical: A Hand-Book for Physicians in the Treatment of Nervous and Other Diseases* (New York: D. Appleton and Company, 1873).

24. In cases of localized pain, direct electrical stimulation for brief periods of time can relieve discomfort and improve blood flow. Electrical treatments, most often given by small electrodes applied to or inserted under the skin, have also been proven to cure chronic conditions such as tendonitis. For information, see T. Manual et al., "High Intensity Electrical Stimulation for Pain Management," *Physical Therapy* 80, no. 5 (May 2000): S62; J. A. Chiu et al., "Transcutaneous

Electrical Nerve Stimulation (TENS) Helps Manage Pain," *Essential Information on Alternative Health Care 5*, no. 7 (November 1999): 6; Nigel Harris et al., "The Microvascular Effects of Electrical Spinal Cord Stimulation in Painful Diabetic Neuropathy and Other Painful Conditions," *Diabetes* 49, no. 5 (May 2000): A164.

25. By the late nineteenth century, however, irregular electrotherapists were far more likely to treat sexual dysfunction than were regular electrotherapists, if the surviving advertising material is to be believed. See chapter 4 for more information.

26. For example, Dr. G. C. Craig wrote to battery manufacturer Otto Flemming in 1887 thanking him for his help in selecting a battery for Craig's new electrotherapy practice. Like many physicians in the 1880s, Craig was new to the field; he had studied electrotherapy for only four months. He had asked Flemming for advice on how to choose and use a battery, admitting that he "knew absolutely nothing about the selection of a battery." See Craig to Flemming, "Copy of Appreciation," January 17, 1887. Copy included in the Bakken Library copy of *Illustrated Catalogue of Flemming's Electro-Therapeutic Apparatus, Electro-Surgical Apparatus, Electrodes, Etc.* (Philadelphia: Press of Wm. H. Bartholomew, 1886), Bakken Museum and Library on the History of Electricity in Life (hereafter BLEL).

27. Just how one would self-administer internal treatments with the rather torturous-looking devices is a question that Wells did not address. S. M. Wells, *The Electropathic Guide: Prepared with Particular Reference to Home Practice* (Chicago: S. M. Wells, 1888), 13–16.

28. For more information on American medicine in the pre-Flexner era, see Duffy, *The Healers*, 260–266.

29. *Moorhead's Graduated Magnetic Machine* (New York: D. C. Moorhead, 1847), 2.

30. Ibid., 3.

31. Ibid., 5. Other magnetic products also found eager buyers. Dr. George Scott sold magnetic belts and corsets in the 1880s, primarily by telling buyers that magnets could improve digestive flow and cure constipation. See *The Doctor's Story: A Treatise on Electricity and Electro Magnetism* (New York: Pall Mall Electric Company, 1888). The Chicago Magnetic Shield Company sold shoe insoles and garments with the same idea: "Electricity . . . is derived from Magnetism," assuring consumers that shoe magnets could provide the body with electricity's power. See *Our Answer to Numerous Correspondents Pointing Out a Plain Road to Health Without the Use of Medicine* (Chicago: ca. 1885), 8–9. For more information on the Chicago Magnetic Shield Company, see *Health and Wealth*, U.S. Insole Co. (Chicago: 1886). One could also buy magnetic pills from H. H. Sherwood, author of *The Motive Power of the Human System, with the Symptoms and Treatment of Chronic Diseases* (New York: Jared W. Bell, 1840).

32. Albert J. Steele, *Theory and Practice of Electrical Therapeutics, or Electricity as a Curative Agent* (New York: American News Company, 1871), 1.

33. For examples, see William Channing, *The Medical Application of Electricity* (Boston: Thomas Hall, 1865), 11, and A. W. Tipson, *A Revised and Enlarged Edition of Clark's New System of Electrical Medication* (Chicago: Chas. J. Johnson, 1882), 41. Additionally, neurologists used electrical metaphors to explain neural pathways while charting them in the 1860s and 1870s. See Armstrong, *Modernism, Technology and the Body*, 15.

34. See, for example, *Electrotherapy in the United States*, 3.

35. Lauren Belfer, in a historical novel about Buffalo's electrification, discusses the enthusiasm evoked among the middle class by the switch from gas lamps to electric lighting in private homes. See Belfer, *City of Light* (New York: Dial Press, 1999).

36. In Muncie, Indiana, only twenty-two homes had electricity in 1899. By 1907, there were one thousand. According to David Nye, between 1880 and 1910, only 5 percent of American homes had electricity. Large-scale domestic electrification did not happen until after the end of World War I. See Nye, *Electrifying America: Social Meanings of a New Technology* (Cambridge: MIT Press, 1990), 239 and 260.

37. Ibid., 382.

38. In 1907, electrical appliances were so new that Edison hired trucks to drive moving displays of various household appliances through towns to familiarize Americans with items such as sewing machines and electric fans. See photograph, "Moving Display of Electrical Household Appliances," *Western Electrician* (August 3, 1907): 83.

39. Americans accepted more electricity in their urban spaces than did Europeans. According to David Nye, although electric outdoor signs were embraced in the United States, they met with criticism in England and Scotland. Nye, *Electrifying America*, 49.

40. The Paris Plan is discussed ibid., 29. Cities nationwide installed these electric lamps in downtown areas. In some cities, like Austin, Texas, the light towers remain in older neighborhoods.

41. For more on the lights at Luna Park and Dreamland, see John Kasson, *Amusing the Million: Coney Island at the Turn of the Century* (New York: Hill & Wang, 1978), 66, 85.

42. Albert Bigelow Paine, "The New Coney Island," *Century* 68 (August 1904): 538. Originally cited in Kasson, *Amusing the Million*, 66. For similar descriptions of the 1893 Columbia Exposition's electric display, see Marvin, *When Old Technologies Were New*, 172–173.

43. According to David Nye, roughly one-third of America's population, or fifty-five million individuals, passed through the three World's Fairs held in this country between 1893 and 1904. See Nye, *Electrifying America*, 34.

44. Suggestively, Disneyland keeps alive the connection between human energy and fantastic electric displays in its nightly Electric Light Parade. Between the early 1970s and 1996, as electrically synthesized music played, illuminated mechanical characters danced through the park, often accompanied by humans dressed in excessive electrical garb. Even the way the parade began, with complete darkness throughout Main Street and staggered lights that traveled from one end of the street to the other, replicated Luna's display. After a five-year hiatus, the Electric Light Parade began running again on July 4, 2001, at Disney's California Adventure.

45. Even Edison, one of the most famous scientists of the era, regularly blurred the lines between human and electrical force. See Paul Israel, *Edison: A Life of Invention* (New York: John Wiley & Sons, 1998), 100. See also Thomas Hughes, *American Genesis: A Century of Invention and Technological Enthusiasm, 1870–1970* (New York: Viking, 1989).

46. Lewis Mumford, *Sketches from Life: The Autobiography of Lewis Mumford: The Early Years* (New York: Dial Press, 1982), 129–130. Mumford cited in Nye, *Electrifying America*, 74.

47. For information on Whitman's belief in the "Romance of Technology" as expressed in his "I Sing the Body Electric," see Jonathan Benthall, *The Body Electric: Patterns of Western Industrial Culture* (London: Thames and Hudson, 1976), 165.

48. Donald Meyer was the first to study Beard. His 1960 text remains a useful source for understanding Beard's impact on his contemporaries. See Meyer, *The Positive Thinkers*. More recent sources on Beard include Tom Lutz, *American Nervousness, 1903* (Ithaca: Cornell University Press, 1991); Anson Rabinbach, *The Human Motor: Energy, Fatigue and the Origins of Modernity* (New York: Basic Books, 1990), 153–155; John Haller and Robin Haller, *The Physician and Sexuality in Victorian America* (Urbana: University of Illinois Press, 1974); Helen Lefkowitz Horowitz, *Alma Mater: Design and Experience in the Women's Colleges from Their Nineteenth-Century Beginnings to the 1930s* (New York: Knopf, 1984); Cynthia Eagle Russett, *Sexual Science: The Victorian Construction of Womanhood* (Cambridge: Harvard University Press, 1989); Charles Rosenberg, *No Other Gods: On Science and American Social Thought* (Baltimore: Johns Hopkins University Press, 1978); Janet Oppenheim, *"Shattered Nerves": Doctors, Patients, and Depression in Victorian England* (New York: Oxford University Press, 1991); Peter Gay, *The Tender Passion* (New York: Oxford University Press, 1986); and George Drinka, *The Birth of Neurosis: Myth, Malady, and the Victorians* (New York: Simon & Schuster, 1984).

49. For more on Beard's theories, see George M. Beard, *A Practical Treatise on Nervous Exhaustion* (New York: E. B. Treat, 1869), and Beard, *American Nervousness: Its Causes and Consequences* (New York: G. Putnam's, 1881).

50. George Beard, "American Nervousness: Its Philosophy and Treatment," *Virginia Medical Monthly* 6, no. 4 (July 1879): 258.

51. Ibid.

52. Beard quoted in Nye, *Electrifying America*, 164. Beard, *American Nervousness*.

53. Beard, "American Nervousness," 259.

54. See Nye, *Electrifying America*, 164. In 1890, there were 1,261 miles of railroad track in the United States; by 1902, 21,290 miles. See Stephen Kern, *The Culture of Time and Space, 1880–1918* (Cambridge: Harvard University Press, 1983), 114.

55. For more information on the relationship between Beard and Edison, see Nye, *Electrifying America*, 164. Beard's indictment of Edison for indirectly causing physical decline is discussed in Armstrong, *Modernism, Technology and the Body*, 18.

56. An example of this is Edison's experiments with "etheric force." For example, to determine the properties of this "new force," which he believed he had discovered by touching wire to a magnet and producing sparks, Edison used his body as a conductor and emerged unscathed. See Neil Baldwin, *Edison: Inventing the Century* (Chicago: University of Chicago Press, 1995; 2001 ed.), 62.

57. Edison reportedly sold more than one hundred of the devices within two months of its appearing on the market. For more information on Edison's fascination with electricity as a novel device and as a medical treatment, see Israel, *Edison: A Life*, 100. Edison's son, Tom, would become known as a promoter of pseudomedical electric devices. He designed the medically questionable Magno-Electric Vitalizer in the early 1900s and promoted it as an energy-enhancing device. For more on the context in which this device appeared, see chapter 4.

58. Baldwin, *Edison*, 64.

59. Alphonso Rockwell, *The Medical and Surgical Uses of Electricity* (New York: W. Wood, 1896).

60. Beard, "American Nervousness," 260. Beard believed that the urban environments and climates unique to this country made neurasthenia an American disease. "Although it is found in England and on the Continent," he argued, "it was first here systematically described, and here exists in greater variety and frequency than in all other countries combined." He suggested the disease might properly be called "Neurasthenia Americana." See ibid., 263. His treatments focused particularly on American sufferers. At the same time that "brain workers" absorbed increasing amounts of electrically generated information, Beard believed, the country's climate made it impossible to release the electricity into the atmosphere. "Dry air also prevents the electricity of the body from being conducted away, and thus we become excessively charged with that force, and excessively stimulated by its confinement in the body." Their moist air protected Europeans from epidemic levels of neurasthenia. See Rowbottom and Susskind,

Electricity and Medicine, 113. Ibid., 113–114. Janet Oppenheim talks about British doctors who used electricity to treat nervous ailments in the mid-nineteenth century. See Oppenheim, *"Shattered Nerves."* S. Weir Mitchell, the infamous "rest-cure" physician, also used electrical treatments in his practice. See Thomas Stretch Dowse, *Lectures on Massage and Electricity in the Treatment of Disease* (New York: E. B. Treat & Co., 1906), 145–164, and Ernest Earnest, *S. Weir Mitchell, Novelist and Physician* (Philadelphia: University of Pennsylvania Press, 1950).

61. Beard's basic approach was similar to the way that electrical currents are used today in medical practice. To treat tendonitis, for example, electrodes are placed on affected areas for fifteen to twenty minutes a treatment. The primary difference is that today electricity is applied to specific, localized areas for pain relief only. See Manual et al., "High Intensity Electrical Stimulation." It is possible that this close contact also influenced Beard's theories; he often used his own hand to impart the electric current to patients, acting as a conduit for electricity in order to judge the strength of the current. See Herbert Tibbits, *How to Use a Galvanic Battery in Medicine and Surgery* (London: J. & A. Churchill, 1879), 30–31.

62. According to Tom Lutz, Beard told patients that electrical treatments could replenish nerve force by sending new currents coursing through the system if their current stock had been depleted. See Lutz, *American Nervousness,* 47.

63. *Scrapbook,* Alphonso Rockwell, c. 1865–1900, Bakken Library and Museum of Electricity in Life. It is interesting that Rockwell, although an ardent proponent of electricity's healing power, did not fully understand its properties. He declared that the tree-branch pattern embedded in the skin of lightning victims was due to displaced tree particles picked up from the atmosphere and transferred to the body in the shock. See Sinclair Tousey, *Medical Electricity, Röntgen Rays and Radium* (Philadelphia: W. B. Saunders Co., 1921), 355. Seals's pain may, in fact, have been relieved; Rockwell's treatment is similar to those used today for chronic pain. See Manual et al., "High Intensity Electrical Stimulation."

64. J. Emmett O'Brien, *The Identity of Nerve Force and Electricity* (Chicago: AMA Press, 1903). Information on O'Brien can be found in the American Medical Association's *Directory of Deceased American Physicians, 1804–1929* (Chicago: American Medical Association, 1993), 1162.

65. O'Brien, *The Identity of Nerve Force and Electricity,* 13–14.

66. Beard enjoyed popularity as a speaker for twenty years, and his book went through fourteen editions.

67. Beard cited in Nye, *Electrifying America,* 164, and in Meyer, *The Positive Thinkers,* 26. For more information on Beard's idea that the nervous system was similar to Edison's electric light, see Russett, *Sexual Science,* 112–113.

68. Popular light therapy by the 1920s and 1930s had become a mixture of

scientific knowledge and popular speculation. Finsen's phototherapy is evoked in titles like "Light and Health," a layman's guide to light therapy. Its text explaining "light and gland personalities," however, went beyond Finsen's specific application to skin diseases by asserting that light therapy could remake the body and psyche. See M. Luckiesh and A. J. Pacini, *Light and Health: A Discussion of Light and Other Radiations in Relation to Life and to Health* (Baltimore: Williams and Wilkins, 1926).

69. For more information on the concept, see Marvin, *When Old Technologies Were New*, 125–126. According to David Nye, by World War I, electricity was being referred to in the popular press as "white magic" that promised an "electrical millennium." See Nye, *Electrifying America*, 66.

70. For information on Fuller, see Elizabeth Coffman, "Women in Motion: Dance, Gesture and Spectacle in Film, 1900–1935" (Ph.D. diss., University of Florida, 1995), chap. 1.

71. For information on the spectacle of women dressing as electricity in the late nineteenth century, see Marvin, *When Old Technologies Were New*, 138–139, and unnumbered images.

72. "The Use of Illuminated Girls," *Electrical World* (February 6, 1886): 56. Quoted, ibid., 138.

73. "At Last! An Electric Light for the Necktie," *Ohio Electric Works Illustrated Catalogue* (c. 1890), 4, BLEL. Suggestively, men might also dress in electricity by performing magic tricks. By the mid-nineteenth century, magic books were telling readers how to perform a number of electrical tricks, each of which involved the magician's body somehow electrifying an object. See descriptions of the electrified paper, electric feather, electrical cat, electrical kiss, and galvanic tongue in the anonymously published *The Magicians Own Book* (New York: Dick & Fitzgerald, 1857).

74. "Future of Electrical Development," Amos Dolbear interview, *Western Electrician* (January 9, 1897): 24. As quoted in Marvin, *When Old Technologies Were New*, 127.

75. John D. Huber, "Arrhenius and Electric Children," *Scientific American* (April 13, 1912): 334. As quoted in Kern, *The Culture of Time and Space*, 114.

76. Trowbridge was a physics professor at the time that he wrote. John Trowbridge, *The Electrical Boy or the Career of Greatmen and Greatthings* (Boston: Roberts Brothers, 1891), and L. Frank Baum, *The Master Key: An Electrical Fairy Tale* (Indianapolis: Bowen-Merrill Company, 1901). Both Trowbridge's and Baum's texts can be found at the Bakken Library. David Nye talks about similar issues in the Tom Swift books; see Nye, *Electrifying America*, 147. Electricity was also functioning as both plot and metaphor by the twentieth century. For examples of electricity in modern literature, see Tim Armstrong, *Modernism, Technology and the Body*, 19–24.

77. Marvin, *When Old Technologies Were New*, 141.

78. "The Electric Boy," *Electrical Review* (October 8, 1887): 7.

79. *Electrical Review* (October 30, 1886): 5. Marvin refers to these stories of electric absorption as "electric miracles." They bestowed power upon the individuals who experienced electrical enhancement and those who promoted their stories by elevating both parties, in popular culture, to an expert status above even that of electrical engineers. See Marvin, *When Old Technologies Were New*, 134.

80. This desire went beyond scientists to popular fiction. In Baum, *The Master Key*, the young boy asks for electric pills as one of his three electric wishes from the Demon so that he could ingest pure energy instead of having to eat food.

81. John Harvey Kellogg discussed how electricity promoted plant growth. He believed it also enhanced human growth, particularly nail and hair growth. See John Harvey Kellogg, *Light Therapeutics: A Practical Manual of Phototherapy for the Student and the Practitioner* (Battle Creek: Good Health Publishing Company, 1910), 20.

82. *Electrical Review* (September 24, 1887): 4. Originally quoted in Marvin, *When Old Technologies Were New*, 123. The cocktail bears a striking resemblance to "liquid sunshine," a radium beverage drunk at an MIT party and reported in newspapers across the country. See chapter 5 for more information.

83. For more on electrical speech in the twentieth century, see Nye, *Electrifying America*, 155.

84. M. Allen Starr, "Electricity in Relation to the Human Body," *Scribner's Magazine* (pamphlet, c. 1890): 589–603 (BLEC). Starr's article was one in a series on electricity, parts of which seem to have countered his attempts to tone down electricity's image as a modern elixir. See, for example, C. F. Brackett, "Electricity in the Service of Man," *Scribner's Magazine* (June 1889): 643–659.

85. Morrill, *A Treatise of Practical Instructions in the Medical and Surgical Uses of Electricity*, 27.

86. For information on the American Medical Association employee Arthur Cramp's thirty-year campaign to discredit "illegitimate" products and practitioners, see the AMA's Historical Health Fraud Collection (hereafter AMAH-HFC), Chicago.

87. Margaret Talbot, "The Placebo Effect," *New York Times Sunday Magazine* (January 9, 2000): 34–39. For further information on scientific studies involving the placebo effect, see Mitchell J. Noon, "Placebo to Credebo: The Missing Link in the Healing Process," *Pain Reviews* 6, no. 2 (July 1999): 133–142; and Allison Motluck, "Some of the Best Medicines Are All in the Mind," *New Scientist* 171, no. 2304 (August 18, 2001): 19.

88. Pulvermacher worked on telegraph machines and telegraphing techniques before electric belts. See J. L. Pulvermacher, *Galvanic Electricity: Its Pre-*

Eminent Power and Effects in Preserving and Restoring Health Made Plain and Useful (London: Galvanic Establishment, 1875), 37.

89. Ibid., 47.

90. For more information on these companies, see the BLEC: Dr. Al Owen (Chicago: The Owen Electric Belt and Appliance Company, ca. 1890); Pulvermacher Galvanic Company, "Electricity: Nature's Chief Restorer" (Cincinnati: Pulvermacher Galvanic Company, 1876); "The Electric Era" (New York: German Electric Agency, ca. 1901); and John L. Greenway, "Nervous Disease and Electric Medicine," in *Pseudo-Science and Society in Nineteenth-Century America*, ed. Arthur Wrobel (Lexington: University Press of Kentucky, 1987), 46–73. For information on Thomas Edison's son's electric belt efforts, see Israel, *Edison: A Life*, 391.

91. A sampling of advertisements in the BLEL reveals belt ads in *Harper's, Frank Leslie's Illustrated Newspaper*, *The New Voice*, and *The Graphic*.

92. Direct mail offers were used as early as 1848 in New York, when Moorhead's Graduated Magnetic Machines encouraged prospective consumers to improve the "principle of vitality of life."

93. David Nye explains that electric appliance manufacturers often used door-to-door sales. See Nye, *Electrifying America*, 265.

94. Arthur Cramp, *Nostrums and Quackery and Pseudo-Medicine*, vol. 3 (Chicago: AMA Press, 1936), 116.

95. This represented $105,905.67 in gross sales and an average of 489 sold per month. See public accountant to Mr. Gaylord Wilshire, I-ON-A-CO financial records, June 22, 1926, box 7, Henry Gaylord Wilshire Collection (hereafter HGWC).

96. The Electric Appliance Company, makers of Addison's Electric Belt, advertised in *Billboard* around 1910, suggesting that men in the industry were "losing some nice easy money if you fail to work our high grade electric belts, appliances, body batteries. Also a nice sideline for performers making one to six days' stands, 500–1,000 per cent profit." See advertisement reprinted in Cramp, *Nostrums and Quackery*, vol. 2, 689.

97. Advertisement seen on-line at eBay, Internet auction site, for Addison's Electric Belt.

98. Jameson, *The Natural History of Quackery*, 137.

99. "The Electric Era," German Electric Belt Agency, ca. 1890, BLEC.

100. Dr. Bell Electro Appliance Company to Myrtle M. Kesten, February 3, 1915, box 0029-15, AMAHHFC.

101. Marvin asserts that this feeling went beyond the Court of Appeals: "In the public perception, electrical accidents were an increasing risk of urban life." See Marvin, *When Old Technologies Were New*, 121.

102. *Electric World* (June 5, 1886): 257. Quoted, ibid., 120.

103. *Electric Review* (October 9, 1888): 4. Quoted, ibid.

104. Kemmler died at Auburn prison on August 6, 1890. See Marvin, 149. The fatal force of electric currents fascinated electric experts. In 1903, Edison produced a short film, *Electrocuting an Elephant*, illustrating how the current might be used to do just that. See Armstrong, *Modernism, Technology and the Body*, 40.

105. This theory is further supported by manufacturers' textual claims. The names alone, in many cases, suggests that manufacturers intended that prospective customers associate their belts with excessive amounts of electric power. The 1900 Sears, Roebuck and Co. home catalogue did this quite literally by offering readers the Giant Power Electric Belt from Heidelberg Belts. Not only does the belt emit electrical charges from each of its five conductors, the text reminds readers in boldface headings that the "80-gauge current" contains three times the power of any other belt. Sears, Roebuck and Co., *Consumer's Guide* (Fall 1900), 39.

106. "As Wonderful as the Telephone and Electric Light," *Frank Leslie's Illustrated Newspaper* (March 26, 1881). London Electric did not go so far as to use Edison's name to promote its product. Thomas A. Edison, Jr., the inventor's son, did. He began the Thomas A. Edison, Jr., Chemical Company, sellers of the Magno-Electric Vitalizer, a nerve tonic to be worn around the neck to revitalize the body. The product contained nothing electrical. The junior Edison's conviction of postal fraud is covered in the *New York Times* (October 5, 1904): 1.

107. "The Electric Era," German Electric Belt Agency, ca. 1890, BLEC.

108. Even a company like Pulvermacher, which had originally produced belts in Europe, had moved its headquarters from London to Cincinnati by the 1880s in search of the greater profits available in the United States.

109. Jameson, *The Natural History of Quackery*, 138.

110. German Electric sent out a letter offering a $5.00 belt for $2.00. Letter from the German Electric Belt Agency, 329 Livingston St., Brooklyn, New York, ca. 1890, BLEC. The price could decrease dramatically, depending on how long one took to answer solicitation letters. Dr. Bell Electro Appliance Company of Vancouver wrote to Myrtle M. Kesten of Chicago repeatedly over a five-month period after she had written asking for information in Feburary 1915. In March, it offered her credit or wholesale: "[W]e stand ready to meet you half way" on belts that cost $16.50 for basic models and $49.00 for fancy models. In May, its offer was to give her $5.00 off any item she wanted. In July, it wrote to say it had lost money on her and would sell her the cheapest belt, a $20.00 model, for $10.00. See correspondence, Dr. Bell Electro Appliance Co., electrotherapeutics 0029-15, AMAHHFC.

111. See the ad for Heidelberg Electric Belt in Lutz, *American Nervousness*, 48.

112. Advertisement in *The New Voice* 2, no. 49 (November 26, 1903).

113. See "Ionaco Operating Instructions," box 11, folder 21, HGWC. The connection between electric belts and Chinese medicine, never discussed in promoters' marketing materials, was probably not lost on Chinese readers. Belt promoters typically suggested that their products be worn on traditional acupressure and acupuncture sites, including the ankle, the neck, and the waist, a particularly important region for promoting vitality in Eastern medicine. Work needs to be done exploring the influence an Eastern understanding of the body had on Western electrotherapy practitioners, ranging from the "regular" George Beard to the "irregular" Henry Gaylord Wilshire. For an example of a Western medical diagram that probably borrowed from texts on acupuncture, see Maurice F. Pilgrim, *Mechanical Vibratory Stimulation: Its Theory and Application in the Treatment of Disease* (New York: Metropolitan Publishing, 1903).

114. The popularity of electric belts among the working class also suggests that neurasthenia research has focused too narrowly on the disease as a middle- or upper-class malaise. Certainly most who purchased an electric belt felt themselves victims of some sort of modern depletion, given the advertising documents.

115. See Pulvermacher, *Galvanic Electricity.*

116. Electric belts were eclipsed in the 1920s by innovations like the I-ON-A-CO. However, products that shot sparks and applied visible electric force to the body remained popular well into the 1920s. For a similar product, see the Electreat home electric system. "Electreat Relieves Pain" (Peoria: Electreat Manufacturing Company, ca. 1920), BLEC.

117. "Electropoise: An Oxygen Home Remedy System," undated advertisement from *McClure's Magazine*, BLEC.

118. For information on how violet rays worked, see "Violet Rays: The Scientific Treatment" (Vi-Rex Company, ca. 1915), BLEC; "Master Violet Rays," undated brochure, BLEC; and Noble M. Eberhart, "Physician's Directions for Renulife Treatments" (Renulife Electric Company, 1926), BLEC.

119. I have come across no scholarship on violet rays, and the only historical account of Hercules Sanche and his Electropoise or ozone purifiers dismisses the products as evidence of consumer gullibility and ingenious quack promotion. See Holbrook, *The Golden Age of Quackery*, and Jameson, *The Natural History of Quackery.*

120. The product is the Oxypathor produced by E. L. Moses of Buffalo. Cramp, *Nostrums and Quackery*, vol. 2, 710. Interestingly, the company's sales manager was a Clarence E. Edson. Given the similarities between Edson's Electric Garter and the Oxypathor, it is likely that this is the same Edson.

121. Ibid., 709.

122. For information on the Oxypathor, the Oxydonor, and the Oxybon, all products sold around 1915, see ibid., 707–717. For reference to the polarizer and conducting cord, see "Electropoise." The Electropoise offers us rare proof

that companies actively combated physicians' attempts to discredit their products. On August 2, 1895, J. E. Dubois, vice president and general manager of Electropoise, wrote to Mr. H. R. Chadeayne of Cornwall, New York, responding to his order and to what must have been an inquiry about the product's legitimacy. "You must be mistaken in regard to 'a N.Y. Daily Paper saying the electropoise was a humbug,' aren't you?" he asked. "The majority of papers are better posted on the improved methods of the age." Chadeayne seems to have written to numerous electrotherapy manufacturers during this period, perhaps testing the legitimacy of their products. Sales receipts for his purchase of battery devices can also be found with this letter. J. E. DuBois to H. F. Chadeayne, August 2, 1895, BLEC.

123. Advertisement quoted in Cramp, *Nostrums and Quackery*, vol. 2, 296.

124. Sanche had changed the name of the Electropoise to the Oxydonor by 1900 and eliminated all references to direct electrical properties in advertising materials. We can assume, however, that this was more to safeguard himself against lawsuits than to drop the connection with electricity. By 1900, it had become difficult to declare that a product was electrical if it was not, given the tenacity with which the AMA was pursuing its postal fraud campaigns against irregular practitioners. By then, oxygen remedies had long been associated with electricity; Sanche could remove the electrical references without losing the implied electrical effect on prospective consumers. For information on how easy it was to prosecute Sanche for electrical claims, see Cramp, *Nostrums and Quackery*, vol. 2, 303. We also know Sanche still considered the Oxydonor an electrical device from the language in his patent: "Our invention relates to improvements in medical instruments such as are used for supplying electric currents to the human body." See ibid.

125. Jameson, *The Natural History of Quackery*, 142.

126. Sanche was a savvy promoter and protector. He not only safeguarded his advertising claims against fraud charges, he also began a fraternal organization committed to arguing against naysayers wherever they might be. Although it is difficult to ascertain whether it had any members, the earnest effort Sanche put into the group suggests he was indeed serious in its formation. His Fraternity of Duxanimus, defined as a "Cosmopolitan Organization of the Beneficiaries of the New Method of Curing Disease," took as part of its oath a promise to protect the Electropoise/Oxydonor against all charges questioning its efficacy. See Holbrook, *The Golden Age of Quackery*, 126.

127. Katherine Ott, *Fevered Lives: Tuberculosis in American Culture Since 1870* (Cambridge: Harvard University Press, 1996), 46; for the discussion of treatments involving carbolic acid and creosote, see 45. See also Sheila Rothman, *Living in the Shadow of Death: Tuberculosis and the Social Experience of Illness in America* (New York: Basic Books, 1994).

128. Ott, *Fevered Lives*, 48.

129. Ott, *Fevered Lives*, 9–16. The product's advertisements regularly featured beautiful women called "Gibson Girls" referring to the famous sketches by Charles Dana Gibson for *Life* magazine. See Holbrook, *The Golden Age of Quackery*, 124. For more on death as a design motif and general fascination of the Victorians, see Kenneth Ames, *Death in the Dining Room and Other Tales of Victorian Culture* (Philadelphia: Temple University Press, 1992).

130. See *Cosmopolitan* (October 1895).

131. Ott, *Fevered Lives*, 1. For comments on the product's popularity, see Cramp, *Nostrums and Quackery*, vol. 2, 297. The company's success is also apparent from its expansion to two headquarters in Chicago by 1914. Ibid., 706. Although the Electropoise/Oxygenator was not sold long after 1915, products like the Electrozone from the Electrozone Corporation of New York carried into the 1930s the idea that electric air could purify air and kill disease. Electrozone claimed to generate a "silent electrical discharge" to restore the germ-killing, electrical ozone that nature supplies but had been used up in "thickly populated districts." Electrozone systems were installed in civic centers and schools; in 1918, all St. Louis schools were equipped with Electrozone Ventilating Ozonators. This made electricity an important weapon in the war against air-borne illnesses that historian Nancy Tomes locates in the first half of the twentieth century. For information on Electrozone and the St. Louis program, see "Pure Air and Pure Water by Scientific Methods," (New York: Electrozone Corporation of New York, 1927). See also the AMA campaign against Electrozone in Arthur Cramp, *Miscellaneous Nostrums*, 141. Electricity was also used to put ozone into water for a healthful beverage in the 1930s. See, for example, "Electrovita, 'The Key to Health,'" salesman's guide, ca. 1932, BLEC. For more on the fear of germs, see Nancy Tomes, *The Gospel of Germs: Men, Women and the Microbe in American Life* (Cambridge: Harvard University Press, 1998). Suellen Hoy discusses the germ reformers in *Chasing Dirt: The American Pursuit of Cleanliness* (Oxford: Oxford University Press, 1995).

132. This use of electricity to power a woman's beauty is also evident in vibration products, such as the Vit-O-Net vibrating bed blanket that purportedly soothed the body and enhanced circulation. An image used to sell the product featured women in a bedroom, one making herself attractive at a makeup area and another lounging in bed. The former, "Miss Has-Used-It," says, "Hurry up, Grace; we'll be late." Grace, or "Miss Using-It," replies, "Please don't hurry me, Lorraine; it's SO restful." Their youth, attractiveness, and sexuality as suggested by their placements in the three photos are attributed to their electric vibrational blanket. See "Awake the Greater Health Within You: A Message of Hope" (Chicago: Vit-O-Net Corporation, 1928).

133. Image in box 7, folder 9, HGWC.

134. Cramp, *Nostrums and Quackery and Pseudo-Medicine*, vol. 3, 114. Other manufacturers used similar strategies to prove to consumers that electric

products were really working. Gravity-powered gas pumps originally used glass cylinders at the top through which people watched the gas supply diminish as they pumped. When manufacturers replaced these with electric pumps in the 1920s, they kept a small window, but it had no function other than to assure users that electricity was flowing.

135. Henry Gaylord Wilshire to the Council on Pharmacy and Chemistry, 12/16/25, 0403-11, AMAHHFC. For a list of agents, which includes one doctor among the individuals, see box 7, folder 9, HGWC. Donald Davis Jr. has located forty-one distributors in southern California in 1926 alone, suggesting that the total number of agents may in fact exceed 200. See Davis, "The Ionaco of Gaylord Wilshire," *The Historical Society of Southern California* (December 1967): 432.

136. Some of the cities in which Wilshire advertised: Pittsburgh, Detroit, San Francisco, Cincinnati, Newark, Spokane, San Diego, Salt Lake City, Cleveland, and Omaha. See attachment to letter from Arthur Cramp to Dr. Fishbein, 10/22/28, 0913-10, AMAHHFC.

137. Even after Wilshire's death, radio stations continued to broadcast his shows. Allen Shoenfield talks about radio broadcasts in March 1928 in a letter to Morris Fishbein, Wilshire correspondence, 0914-04, AMAHHFC.

138. The Theroid was a direct descendant of the I-ON-A-CO; it was created in 1928 by Philip Isley, who had worked in Wilshire's Cleveland office. For information on later versions of the I-ON-A-CO, see "Electromagnetism and Your Health" (Minneapolis: Thernoid of Minneapolis, ca. 1930); Electronet advertising letter, 7/13/25, Electrotherapeutics folders, 0229-08, AMAHHFC; letter on the Magnecoil from M. G. Ripley to N. B. Salerni, 3/23/28, ibid.; the report on the Restoro from the Chicago Better Business Bureau, 8/31/28, ibid., 0232-17; and miscellaneous materials on Iona-tone and Master Circletone, ibid.

139. The I-ON-A-CO sold for $58.40 cash and $65.00 credit when it first went on the market. See Cramp, *Nostrums and Quackery and Pseudo-Medicine*, vol. 3, 114.

140. The only published records of Wilshire's life and his belt business are the Duraind biography and an article published nearly forty years ago;, see Donald G. Davis, Jr., "The Ionaco of Gaylord Wilshire," *Southern California Quarterly* (December 1967): 425–453, reprinted copy in box 13, folder 9, HGWC.

141. Holbrook, *The Golden Age of Quackery*, 135. See also Wilshire's thin official biography, George J. Duraind, *Gaylord Wilshire and His Amazing Discovery* (Los Angeles: The Iona Company, 1927), available in HGWC. One can also find information on Wilshire's real estate speculations, including the founding of the city of Fullerton in Mike Davis, *City of Quartz: Excavating the Future in Los Angeles* (New York: Verso, 1990).

142. Duraind, *Gaylord Wilshire*.

143. See "A Delightful Road to Health," *Liberty* (January 15, 1927): 82.

144. Duraind, *Gaylord Wilshire*, 9.

145. Wilshire's archival letters make it possible to argue that he knowingly promoted a fraudulent product. After receiving a copy of Wilshire's "Iona" promotion booklet in 1925, Allan McIntyre, a reporter whom Wilshire knew well, wrote to thank him for "giving me the biggest laugh I've had in a long time" and congratulating him because "every dam [*sic*] boob in the country will want one of these" after he hears of it. McIntyre speculated that Wilshire would easily "get a half a million out of it." Wilshire then wrote a friend, the writer George Sterling, repeating McIntyre's reaction and hoping that "you will get as much of a laugh out of my circular." Sterling's response, however, suggests that both he and Wilshire were I-ON-A-CO believers who could appreciate other people's reactions while lamenting their disbelief. "Profuse thanks for the invaluable information supplied by your circular," replied Sterling, who noted "with grief the skeptical attitude of your misguided friend, McIntyre . . . he will prove forever opaque to the truth." See McIntyre to Wilshire, February 21, 1925; Wilshire to Sterling, February 25, 1925; and Sterling to Wilshire, February 28, 1925, all in box 7, folder 1, HGWC.

146. For information on Sinclair's endorsement, see Robert Ernst, *Weakness Is a Crime: The Life of Bernarr Macfadden* (Syracuse: Syracuse University Press, 1991), 53. For further information on Sinclair, see Leon Harris, *Upton Sinclair, American Rebel* (New York: Crowell, 1975). For information on Sterling, see Holbrook, *The Golden Age of Quackery*, 141–142.

147. For example, see the report on Wilshire's lecture at San Diego's Masonic Hall before the San Diego I-ON-A-CO office opened, 9/27/26, Wilshire, Gaylord correspondence, 0913-07, AMAHHFC. See also John Sillman's letter to the AMA propaganda department, reporting Wilshire's demonstrations in Palo Alto, 11/16/26, Wilshire, Gaylord correspondence, 1925–26, 0913-13, AMAHHFC.

148. "A Delightful Road to Health," 82.

149. For information on his lecture at the Fairmont, see Wilshire to K. E. Vankuran, May 20, 1926, box 7, folder 12, HGWC.

150. Wilshire to Mollie Price Cook of New York, April 25, 1925, box 7, folder 1, HGWC. Wilshire also extended his advertising efforts to immigrants. Several brochures in his archives are printed in Mandarin. Unfortunately, his sales records contain no demographic information and there are no existent letters from self-identified immigrants. For the brochures, see box 10, folder 21, HGWC.

151. It is highly likely that there were treatment centers other than these three. Wilshire's records do not contain a master list of all of his facilities, but they do contain letters that refer to offices in Florida and Boston as well. See business records and correspondence, box 7, folders 6–11, HGWC.

152. In November 1926, Wilshire reported selling more than eight thousand

belts. During this same period, Wilshire was making roughly $100,000 a year in profits. See business records, box 7, folder 10, HGWC.

153. In addition, 125 people were classified as "callers" during the same period, suggesting that the total number of people who interacted with the belts at the center is closer to 700. See business records, box 7, folder 11, HGWC.

154. In addition to these centers, there were numerous other informal "centers" that offered I-ON-A-CO treatments. One of these, as reported by the head of Wilshire's Portland, Oregon, office in 1927, was a gas station owner who, to draw new customers, advertised a free I-ON-A-CO treatment with the purchase of a tank of gas or an oil change. Carl L. Wernicke to Wilshire, January 22, 1927, box 10, folder 18, HGWC.

155. See Dr. Arthur Wolford to AMA, 1/10/26, correspondence, 0913-07, Wilshire Gaylord, Advertisements and Testimonials 1927, 0913-06, AMAH-HFC.

156. See Wilshire Gaylord, Advertisements and Testimonials 1927, 0913-06, and Dr. A. Davidson to the AMA Bureau of Investigation 7/31/25, Ionaco-Gaylord Wilshire, Correspondence, 1925–26, 0403-11, AMAHHFC.

157. Margorie Speed to *Hygeia*, 2/4/27, Gaylord Wilshire, advertisements and testimonials 1927, 0913-14, AMAHHFC. Speed's opinons seem to have been shared by Thomas "Bert" Fisher, who, when dying of cancer at the age of 24 in 1928, purchased the I-ON-A-CO after seeing it advertised. According to a website chronicling the Fisher family, "Tom used it some and always said it seemed to soothe his aches and pains." The author of the web text disagrees, stating that it "was of no value to Bert." See http://www.Oklahoma.net/~king-fish/Places/places.htm. It is difficult to determine whether the individuals who sold the I-ON-A-CO were equally convinced of its efficacy. Most seem to have primarily utilitarian motives in becoming its sellers. One Dr. A. G. Emerson, who said he was the chief of staff at a Las Vegas tuberculosis facility, asked Wilshire for a sales position; he could sell many because he was "generally trusted" as a physician and frequent health lecturer. He also commented that he thought the device was "great." Others stressed financial need over product faith. Adolph Linsenbarth, a sixty-six-year-old former foreign languages editor, asked for a position in Florida or Boston because he had not "seen much work since the war" and needed income. The same impulse drove Adelaide Fenton Coronado, who sought work after her attorney made it clear that there was "little prospect of getting much" out of her husband. For Emerson's letter, see Emerson to Wilshire, 1926, box 11, folder 17; for Linsenbarth's letter, see Linsenbarth to H. R. Learns, January 11, 1926, box 7, folder 10; for Coronado's letter, see Coronado to Wilshire, January 27, 1926, box 7, folder 10, all in HGWC.

158. Anna Lyle to Arthur Cramp, December 1, 1926. Correspondence in folder 0403-11, AMAHHFC. Lyle seems to have converted to Wilshire's method. In a quotation that I have been unable to verify, Lyle reportedly later en-

dorsed the I-ON-A-CO in the *Ionaco News*. According to Stuart Holbrook, Lyle wrote that she had "fallen for the I-ON-A-CO strongly" and found it effective in treating David Starr Jordan, president emeritus of Stanford University. Holbrook, *The Golden Age of Quackery*, 141–142.

159. The two best, if brief, cultural histories of popular electric therapy devices can be found in larger studies of electrification: Marvin, *When Old Technologies Were New*, and Nye, *Electrifying America*. Additionally, Harvey Green provides an overview of several electric devices in *Fit for America: Health, Fitness, Sport and American Society* (Baltimore: Johns Hopkins University Press, 1986). Among the more typical dismissals of "quack" electric devices are Himrich and Thornley, *Electrifying Medicine*; "Electrotherapy in the United States" (Minneapolis: Medtronic, 1977); Rowbottom and Susskind, *Electricity and Medicine*; Jameson, *The Natural History of Quackery*; and Holbrook, *The Golden Age of Quackery*.

160. See Emerson to Wilshire, 1926, box 11, folder 17, HGWC.

161. See, for instance, Manual et al., "High Intensity Electrical Stimulation," Harris et al., "The Microvascular Effects," and Chiu et al., "Transcutaneous Electrical Nerve Stimulation."

162. See Talbot, "Placebo Effect"; Motluk, "Some of the Best Medicines"; and Martin Enserlink, "Can Placebos Be the Cure?" *Science* 284, no. 5412 (April 19, 1999): 238.

163. Wilshire promotional brochure, box 10, folder 21, HGWC.

164. For more on McReynolds Wilshire see Davis, "The Ionaco of Gaylord Wilshire," 441.

NOTES TO CHAPTER 4

1. In fact, Carolyn Marvin describes numerous electrical gadgets sold at the turn of the century that were designed specifically to control women's sexuality rather than create sexual pleasure. Among these were electric corsets that emitted a whistle when pressed. See Marvin, *When Old Technologies Were New: Thinking about Electric Communication in the Nineteenth Century* (Cambridge: Harvard University Press, 1988), 131. For evidence on women's use of vibrators see Maines, *The Technology of Orgasm: "Hysteria," the Vibrator, and Women's Sexual Satisfaction* (Baltimore: Johns Hopkins University Press, 1999).

2. Eric Jameson, *The Natural History of Quackery* (Springfield, Ill.: Charles C. Thomas, 1961), 137.

3. For examples of these, see The Robut-Man, The Monster Auto-Man, and the corresponding pump developers advertised by Presto Products in the early 1900s in its newsletter "Good News," folder 0204-05, American Medical Association Historical Health Fraud Collection (hereafter AMAHHFC). Many men

were interested enough in these products to propose their own inventions. One wrote the American Medical Association with a sketch of his design, with parts, including the rubber diaphragm, glass tube, flexible rubber tube, and air pump, carefully labeled. He hoped to find out if something like this could be purchased or perhaps manufactured, but it is unlikely that he received any assistance from the AMA, given Arthur Cramp's stance against medical fraud and quackery. See letter to Cramp, Roanoke, Virginia, September 26, 1925, folder 0204-03, AMAHHFC.

4. Pulvermacher Galvanic Company, "Electricity Nature's Chief Restorer" (Cincinnati: Pulvermacher Galvanic Company, 1876), 27, Bakken Library Ephemera Collection (hereafter BLEC).

5. See Morris Fishbein, *The New Medical Follies: An Encyclopedia of Cultism and Quackery in These United States* (New York: Boni and Liverright, 1927), 100.

6. Brochures appeared in the early twentieth century suggesting that men had begun to tire of strenuous exercise and were looking for quick ways to build muscle. See Luther Gulick, "Ten Minutes' Exercise for Busy Men" (New York: American Sports Publishing Company, 1902) and Gulick, "Muscle Building: Practical Points for Practical People" (New York: American Sports Publishing Company, 1905).

7. Cynthia Eagle Russett, *Sexual Science: The Victorian Construction of Womanhood* (Cambridge: Harvard University Press, 1989).

8. See Lesley Hall, *Hidden Anxieties: Male Sexuality, 1900–1950* (Cambridge, Mass.: Polity Press, 1991), 116.

9. Physicians quoted, ibid., 115.

10. Sir James Paget quoted, ibid.

11. For information on Todd's book and Gardner's response, see G. J. Barker-Benfield, *The Horrors of the Half-Known Life: Male Attitudes toward Women and Sexuality in Nineteenth-Century America* (New York: Routledge, 2000; originally published in 1971), 136.

12. For more on how scarcity helped create the wilderness preservation movement in America, see Roderick Nash, *Wilderness and the American Mind* (New Haven: Yale University Press, 1967), 148–149. Gail Bederman provides a more critical interpretation of the movement's advocacy of rugged manhood and noble savagery. See Bederman, *Manliness and Civilization: A Cultural History of Gender and Race in the United States, 1880–1917* (Chicago: University of Chicago Press, 1995).

13. Frederick Hollick, *Popular Treatise on Venereal Disease* (New York: 1852), 69.

14. For information on Graham's belief that masturbation caused physical decline, see John Haller and Robin Haller, *The Physician and Sexuality in Victo-*

rian America (Urbana: University of Illinois Press, 1974), 97. E. Anthony Rotundo discusses Beecher's sermons against the "solitary vice" that led, inevitably, to insanity and death. See *American Manhood: Transformations in Masculinity from the Revolution to the Modern Era* (New York: Basic Books, 1993), 72–73.

15. John Humphrey Noyes agreed and forbade his male followers at Oneida to engage in either masturbation or coitus interruptus on the grounds that they wasted a precious fluid better retained until required for procreation. See Spencer Klaw, *Without Sin: The Life and Death of the Oneida Community* (New York: Penguin Press, 1993), 179.

16. Rotundo, *American Manhood*, 72.

17. Alfred G. Garratt, *Electro-Physiology and Electro-Therapeutics: Showing the Best Methods of the Medical Uses of Electricity* (Boston: Ticknor and Fields, 1860).

18. George M. Schweig, *The Electric Bath: Its Medical Uses, Effects and Appliance* (New York: G. P. Putnam's Sons, 1877), 111. The electric bath first became popular in Europe and America in the 1850s. For more information on methods of healing with currents in water, see J. Chaplin, *The Origin and Use of the Electro-Chemical Bath for the Extraction of Mercury and Other Metallic Substances from the Human Body and Its Curative Agency in Other Diseases* (London: William Freeman, 1856).

19. A. E. Rockwell, *Electrotherapeutics of the Male Genital Organs* (New York: William Wood & Co., 1874).

20. George Beard, "Nervous Exhaustion (Neurasthenia), with Cases of Sexual Neurasthenia," undated pamphlet, New York Academy of Medicine, ca. 1880, 6. For a secondary account on how galvanic therapies were used to combat fatigue, see Stephen Kern, *The Culture of Time and Space, 1880–1918* (Cambridge: Harvard University Press, 1983), 107.

21. Haller and Haller offer a brief discussion of this general theory in nineteenth-century medicine. See *The Physician and Sexuality*, 23.

22. C. L. Dana, "On the Pathology and Treatment of Certain Forms of Nerve Weakness," *Medical Record* 24 (1883): 61.

23. M. J. Grier, *The Treatment of Some Forms of Sexual Debility by Electricity* (Philadelphia: Medical Press Company, 1891), 1.

24. Ibid., 2.

25. "The Great Nerve Stimulant Zardon" (Toronto, Ohio: Elenita Company, ca. 1901), box 9, folder 8, Warshaw Collection of Business Americana (hereafter WCBA), National Museum of American History (NMAH), Smithsonian Institution.

26. German Electric Belt Agency, "The Electric Era" (New York: 1901), 15, BLEC.

27. "Electricity: Nature's Chief Restorer," 15–23.

28. "The Electric Era," 14.

29. A. Crystal, "Professor Crystal's Electric Belts and Appliances," 15, folder 0229-25, Electrotherapy, AMAHHFC.

30. "Electricity: Nature's Chief Restorer," 23.

31. Crystal, "Professor Crystal's Electric Belts and Appliances," 15.

32. Ibid.

33. Mail-order companies often offered to prove to a customer that he suffered from spermatorrhoea by analyzing his urine. A customer would send in a small sample that typically would be found to contain the "leaking" semen. The common diagnosis that this semen revealed, "spinal marrow wasting away," suggests that belt manufacturers believed wholeheartedly in seminal economy. See Haller and Haller, *The Physician and Sexuality*, 214. To compare the similarities between belt companies' descriptions and those in home medical texts, see R. V. Pierce, *Common Sense Medical Adviser* (Buffalo: World's Dispensary Printing, 1909), 772–773.

34. "The Electric Era," 15–16.

35. "Electricity: Nature's Chief Restorer," 22.

36. See Pulvermacher, "Belt and Suspensory Appliance," 27, BLEC, and Dr. A. T. Sanden, "Dr. A. T. Sanden, Originator of the Celebrated Home Treatment for the Cure of All Chronic, Nervous and Wasting Diseases Without Drugs or Medicines" (New York: Prout and Ward Printers, ca. 1910), 30, BLEC.

37. Sanden, "Dr. A. T. Sanden," 16–17.

38. Pulvermacher, "Belt and Suspensory Appliance," 26.

39. Sanden, "Dr. A. T. Sanden," 16–17.

40. Pulvermacher, "Belt and Suspensory Appliance," 26.

41. "The Electric Era."

42. Sanden, "Dr. A. T. Sanden," 9.

43. Ibid., and 36. A testament to the popularity of the image is its longevity: as late as 1915, belt manufacturers like the Vancouver-based Dr. Bell's used almost identical versions.

44. Edison, Jr. in figure 26 is Thomas Edison's son, Thomas, Jr. Much to his father's dismay, Thomas signed a contract with the Edison belt manufacturers agreeing to give his name to the Magno-Electric Vitalizer in exchange for a two-dollar royalty for every device sold. See Paul Israel, *Edison: A Life of Invention* (New York: Wiley & Sons, 1998), 391.

45. For more on these comparisons, see John Kasson, *Houdini, Tarzan, and the Perfect Man: The White Male Body and the Rise of Modernity in America* (New York: Hill & Wang, 2001), and Bederman, *Manliness and Civilization*.

46. The belts' unique combination of diagnoses and treatment may explain why they remained popular over a period of thirty years in spite of their questionable effectiveness. When one considers the high number of "psychically impotent" men seen by regular physicians, it makes sense that many men would

have sought cures in electric belts for illnesses that they did not actually have. In these cases, electric belts may have had a special curative property, given the cultural climate of "electric theology" discussed in chapter 3.

47. For information on the connection between architectural design and domestic feminism, see Dolores Hayden, *The Grand Domestic Revolution: A History of Feminist Designs for American Homes, Neighborhoods, and Cities* (Cambridge: MIT Press, 1981). During the same period that feminists were rethinking domestic architecture, Elsie Clews Parsons rethought the "naturalness" of women's roles inside that living space. See Desley Deacon, *Elsie Clews Parsons: Inventing Modern Life* (Chicago: University of Chicago Press, 1997).

48. For information on the way women were taught to stress abstinence in order to control male sexuality in the nineteenth century, see Haller and Haller, *The Physician and Sexuality*, xii.

49. Karen Lystra, *Searching the Heart: Women, Men and Romantic Love in Nineteenth-Century America* (New York: Oxford University Press, 1989), 81. This sentiment is echoed as well in *The Mosher Survey* on Victorian women's sexual attitudes in which one fifty-year-old female respondent called sex vital to "complete harmony between two people." Clelia Duel Mosher, *The Mosher Survey: Sexual Attitudes of Forty-Five Victorian Women*, ed. James Mahood and Kristine Wenburg (New York: Arno Press, 1980), 328, 254.

50. Davis's survey is discussed in John D'Emilio and Esther Freedman, *Intimate Matters: A History of Sexuality in America* (New York: Perennial Library, 1988), 178.

51. See the introduction to Lystra, *Searching the Heart,* for the idea that love reveals one's ideal self.

52. Stephen Kern, *Anatomy and Destiny: A Cultural History of the Human Body* (Indianapolis: Bobbs-Merrill, 1975), 103.

53. Victor Vecki, *The Pathology and Treatment of Sexual Impotence* (London: 1901), 88, as cited in Kern, *Anatomy and Destiny*, 106.

54. N. F. Cook, *Satan in Society, by a Physician* (Cincinnati: C. F. Vent, 1871), 149. According to Kern, warnings that a lively and sensuous woman could render a man impotent were common in popular advice books, illustrating the belief's significant entrenchment in popular imagination. See Kern, *Anatomy and Destiny*, 108.

55. D'Emilio and Freedman, *Intimate Matters*, 180.

56. Isabelle Rittenhouse Mayne, *Maud*, ed. Richard Lee Strout (New York: Macmillan, 1939). See entry from August 28, 1892, 554, as cited in Rotundo, *American Manhood*, 121.

57. For more information on chippies, see Rotundo, *American Manhood*, 125. D'Emilio and Freedman assert that by the twentieth century, prostitution was an entrenched professional system. See their *Intimate Matters*, 180–182.

58. Quoted in Leslie A. Hall, *Hidden Anxieties: Male Sexuality, 1900–1950* (Cambridge, U.K.: Polity Press, 1991), 122.

59. See *Men's Specialists: Some Quacks and Their Methods* (Chicago: AMA Bureau of Investigation, ca. 1913), 52.

60. William J. Robinson, *Woman Her Sex and Love Life* (New York: Eugenics Publishing Company, 1929; first published in 1917), 286–287. Cited in Michael Gordon, "From an Unfortunate Necessity to a Cult of Mutual Orgasm: Sex in American Marital Education Literature, 1830–1940," in *Studies in the Sociology of Sex*, ed. James Henslin (New York: Appleton-Century Croft, 1971), 61.

61. Bernard S. Talmey, *Woman* (New York: Practitioner's Publishing Company, 1910; first published in 1904), 178. According to Michael Gordon, who quotes this source, the first reference to mutual orgasm in marital advice literature appears in 1900. See Gordon, "From an Unfortunate Necessity," 62.

62. Theodore H. van de Velde, *Sexual Tensions in Marriage: Their Origin, Prevention and Treatment* (New York: Random House, 1931), 104; originally published in German in 1928.

63. Ibid. According to van de Velde, men often concluded that they were impotent after comparing their capacity for orgasm to a female partner's. See ibid., 103.

64. Pulvermacher, "Belt and Suspensory Appliance." Patent medicine purveyors also took this approach. An advertisement for Goldglan, a gland-enhancing pill sold in the 1920s, suggested that it was especially appropriate for the man who "doesn't realize that he is not paying his wife the attention he formerly did." See Arthur Cramp, *Nostrums and Quackery and Pseudo-Medicine*, vol. 3 (Chicago: AMA Press, 1936), 97. The original article is in the *Journal of the American Medical Association* (September 13, 1930). Also see advertisements for Zardon that advertise a gland-enhancing pill as a remedy for the "inability to perform the duties pertaining to married life." See "The Great Nerve Stimulant Zardon" (Toronto, Ohio: Elenita Company, ca. 1901), folder 8, box 9, Patent Medicines, WCBA.

65. Professor Andrew Crystal, "Professor Crystal's Electric Belts and Appliances: Greatest Success of the Nineteenth Century" (Marshall, Mich.: 1898), 11–12, 15. One can find similar themes in belt advertisements by more legitimate vendors. Sears, Roebuck and Co. sold its Heidelberg Electric Belt, most probably a copy of the German Electric Belt, as the Giant Power Electric Belt, complete with suspensory sack. For men who were nervous about their sexual performance, it is likely that the words "giant" and "power" would have appealed. For a copy of the advertisement, see John L. Greenway, "Nervous Disease and Electric Medicine," in *Pseudo-Science and Society in Nineteenth-Century America*, ed. Arthur Wrobel (Lexington: University Press of Kentucky, 1987), 62.

66. German Electric Belt Agency, "The Electric Era," cover, BLEC. The at-

traction worked the other way as well. Advertisements also featured women who were electrically drawn to belt-powered men, such as the advertisement for the Electrovita belt in the *San Francisco Bulletin* in 1913 that featured a woman with electricity emanating from her fingertips toward a muscular man who knows that he has his "restored nerve force" to thank. See "How to Restore Your Nerve Force," *San Francisco Bulletin* (January 22, 1913): 16, folder 0230-03, Electrotherapy, AMAHHFC.

67. See collection abstract 240, Electrothermal Company, 1918–1967, *American Medical Association, Guide to the American Medical Association Historical Health Fraud and Alternative Medicine Collection*, ed. Arthur Hafner, James Carson, and John Zwicky, (Chicago: American Medical Association, 1992), 25.

68. See, for example, "GHR Electric Thermitis Dilator Question Blank," folder 0233-05, Electrotherapy, AMAHHFC.

69. Ibid.

70. John Butler, *Electricity in Surgery* (New York: Boericke & Tafel, 1882), 19–20. Galvanic suppositories had also been in use since the 1880s to cure constipation. Like the GHR and Thermalaid, they were to be used five to ten minutes daily. See *Catalogue and Price List of Electrical Apparatus and Supplies* (Philadelphia: Lyman G. Morey, 1882).

71. Goldglan, sold between 1927 and 1945, was one of the most popular incarnations of the "Keeley Cure," a previous treatment consisting of double bichloride of gold that was given until the 1910s. For information, see "Goldglan: A Superior Gland Treatment for Men and Women," Medical Aid Bureau pamphlet, folder 0205-20, AMAHHFC. For information on how long the company was in business, see *Guide to the American Medical Association Historical Health Fraud and Alternative Medicine Collection*, Diseases of Men folder list, 100.

72. "Goldglan: A Superior Gland Treatment."

73. Ibid.

74. For the quotations, see Tim Armstrong, *Modernism, Technology and the Body: A Cultural Study* (Cambridge: Cambridge University Press, 1998), 145; see 148 for a diagram of the procedure. For more information on Steinach's project as well as precursors such as the Brown-Sequard experiments in the 1880s with injecting animal testicular extract, see Normal Haire, *Rejuvenation: The Work of Steinach, Voronoff, and Others* (London: George Allen & Unwin, 1924), 29. Also useful for information on early experiments is Paul Boernsen, *Radium in the Light of Recent Discovery* (Washington, D.C.: Paul Boernsen, 1915), 4.

75. Fishbein, *The New Medical Follies*, 44–45; for his discussion of the Steinach operation, see 101.

76. See Gerald Stanley Lee, *Rest Working: A Study in Relaxed Concentration* (New York: J. J. Little and Ives Company, 1925), 44.

77. "Just off the Press: Glands of Power and Success," Electro Thermal Company, 1923, folder 0233-19, Electro Thermal Company, AMAHHFC.

78. "Why Many Men Are Old at Forty," Electro Thermal Company, ca. 1926, box 9, folder 7, Patent Medicines, WCBA.

79. Ibid., 4–5.

80. The company had gotten practice with hyperbole as a manufacturer of the Elixir of Youth in the late nineteenth century. See "The GHR Electric Thermitis Dilator," folder 0233-05, Electrotherapy, AMAHHFC.

81. "Are Your Nights Like This," GHR Electric Dilator Company, folder 0233-05, Electrotherapy, AMAHHFC.

82. Ibid.

83. It is difficult to say with certainty who bought this product or what they thought of it. Testimonials are included in the advertising copy, such as the letter from Romulo Pena, owner of the Hotel Pena in Laredo, who claims that he has been cured of prostate gland trouble by the GHR dilator. Yet one must take each of these with an ample grain of salt, given that many patent medicine sellers were notorious for making up such characters. It is safer to rely on the product's persistence on the market, and, in the case with the Thermalaid, on the appearance of imitators, whose existence suggests there was a profit to be made. It is also likely that women and men purchased the device as a dildo, given the restrictions on purchasing explicitly sexual devices or sending them through the mail and the rise of a strong gay subculture by the 1920s. There is no proof for this theory, given the lack of direct evidence. For information on the gay subculture of the period, see George Chauncey, *Gay New York: Gender, Urban Culture, and the Making of the Gay Male World, 1890–1940* (New York: Basic Books, 1994). For the Pena testimonial and others, see "Are Your Nights Like This," and "This Wonderful Treatment," both from the GHR Electric Dilator Company, folder 0233-05, Electrotherapy, AMAHHFC.

84. Today, electrical medicine continues to be held in suspicion by most Western physicians. Two books that discuss why the field remains relegated to "alternative healing" status are Richard Gerber, *Vibrational Medicine: New Choices for Healing Ourselves* (Santa Fe: Bear and Company, 1996), and Robert O. Becker and Gary Selden, *The Body Electric: Electromagnetism and the Foundation of Life* (New York: William Morrow, 1985).

85. For Macfadden's views on prostate massage, see Bernarr Macfadden, *Constipation: Its Cause, Effect and Treatment* (New York: Macfadden Book Company, 1930).

86. Journal of the American Medical Association Bureau of Investigation to Mr. J. F. Price, October 2, 1925, Bureau of Medicine correspondence 1909–1926, folder 0204-03, AMAHHFC.

NOTES TO CHAPTER 5

1. Spencer R. Weart, *Nuclear Fear: A History of Images* (Cambridge: Harvard University Press, 1988), 6.

2. Henry Adams, *The Education of Henry Adams* (New York: Modern Library, 1931; originally published in 1918), 486.

3. Articles often referred to the pain inflicted on subjects during radium treatments. One explained that repeated visits were necessary because the rays could rest on the skin only "as long as the patient could bear it." One physician argued that any attempt to use radium to turn an entire body white was so dangerous that it invited death: "If the entire surface of a negro's body were subjected to X-ray treatments he would probably be fatally burned." See "Burning Out Birthmarks, Blemishes of the Skin and Even Turning a Negro White with the Magic Rays of Radium, the New Mystery of Science," *New York American* (January 10, 1904), box 60, folder 2, William Hammer Collection, National Museum of American History, Smithsonian Institution (hereafter Hammer Collection), and "X-Ray to Turn Black Men White," untitled newspaper (December 28, 1903), box 63, folder 4, Hammer Collection.

4. Wells graphically reported on the practice of southern lynching throughout the 1890s and compiled her evidence into three pamphlets aimed at publicizing and ending the practice. Her "Southern Horrors: Lynch Law in All Its Phases" was published in 1892; "A Red Record," in 1895, and "Mob Rule in New Orleans," in 1900.

5. The very fact that African-Americans turned to science to remove their blackness suggests that scientific knowledge had created a complete circuit of racial inferiority by the end of the nineteenth century. Not only had science proven the "illness" of blackness through racist concepts of "civilization" and "savagery" and schools of thought like social Darwinism, science could also offer the "cure." For information on the characterization of lightened skin as "a beautiful, soft, creamy white color," see "X-Ray to Turn Black Men White."

6. For the southern account, see "Bleaching the Ethopian," *Savannah Press* (February 4, 1904), Hammer Collection, box 61, folder 3. See also "Will Bleach Out the Blacks," untitled Wichita paper (February 2, 1904), Hammer Collection, box 61, folder 1; "X-Ray to Turn Black Men White"; unnamed paper (December 28, 1903), Hammer Collection, box 63, folder 4; untitled article in *North American* (January 10, 1904), Hammer Collection, box 61, folder 2; and "Must Stay Half White," *New York Sun* (April 24, 1904), Hammer Collection, box 61, folder F2. For information on other strategies contemporary African-Americans used to pursue whiteness during the period, see Tom Pendergast, *Creating the Modern Man: American Magazines and Consumer Culture, 1900–1950* (Columbia: University of Missouri Press, 2000), 82–83.

7. Linda Dalrymple Henderson, *Duchamp in Context: Science and Technology in the Large Glass and Related Works* (Princeton: Princeton University Press, 1998), 5. See also Steven Lehner, *Explorers of the Body* (New York: Doubleday & Co., 1979), 407. An excellent source on the history of radium's use remains Lawrence Badash, *Radioactivity in America: Growth and Decay of a Science* (Baltimore: Johns Hopkins University Press, 1979).

8. For more information on the Curies' discovery, see Eve Curie, *Madame Curie: A Biography* (New York: Garden City Publishing Company, 1943). For a more objective account, see Susan Quinn, *Marie Curie: A Life* (New York: Simon & Schuster, 1995). For information on Bequerel, see Lehner, *Explorers of the Body*, 417.

9. William J. Hammer, memo dated approximately 1910, Hammer Collection, box 3, folder 1. See also the biographical outline in box 12, folder 1.

10. Just a few of the towns and cities that hosted radium lectures during this period are Erie, Buffalo, Brooklyn, and Syracuse in New York; Findlay, Ohio; Crawfordsville, Indiana; Pittsburgh, Pennsylvania; Duluth, Minnesota; Denver and Telluride, Colorado. See Hammer Collection, boxes 59 and 63.

11. Hammer Collection, box 59, folder 2.

12. Untitled article from October 23, 1903. Hammer Collection, box 59, folder 2.

13. Letter from Henry A. Lee to W. J. Hammer, March 1, 1904. Hammer Collection, box 59, folder 2. For comment on Hammer's "now famous lectures," see untitled newspaper article from October 16, 1903, Hammer Collection, box 59, folder 2.

14. Henderson, *Duchamp in Context*, 5.

15. Ruth Brecher and Edward Brecher, *The Rays: A History of Radiology in the United States and Canada* (Baltimore: Williams and Wilkins Company, 1969), 23. For more information on Edison, see Paul Israel, *Edison: A Life of Invention* (New York: John Wiley, 1998).

16. Raymond Gagliardi, ed., *A History of the Radiological Sciences*, (Reston, Va.: Radiology Centennial, Inc., 1996) 2.

17. Brecher and Brecher, *The Rays*, 23.

18. Between 1900 and 1910, fifteen U.S. colleges began to teach these subjects. See P. M. Hickey, "Teaching of Röntgenology in America," in *Teaching and Training in Medical Radiology* (Stockholm: Kungl. Bokryckeriet, 1930), 34–40.

19. For information on the founding of the American Radium Society at the Detroit American Medical Association meeting in 1916, see Gagliardi, *A History of the Radiological Sciences*, 16. For information on the beginnings of medical school research, see Claudia Clark, *Radium Girls: Women and Industrial Health Reform, 1910–1935* (Chapel Hill: University of North Carolina Press, 1997), 54–55. Clark also reveals that the major period of research publication on ra-

dium was between 1904 and 1914, after Hammer gained fame for his radium vision on the lecture circuit. See ibid., 54–55.

20. Untitled article in *Syracuse Telegram* (February 25, 1904), Hammer Collection, box 59, folder 2.

21. "Powers of Radium," *Duluth Evening Herald* (March 4, 1904), Hammer Collection, box 63, folder 2.

22. In 1904, the Ouiatenon Club of Crawfordsville, Indiana, heard a lecture on the Louisana Purchase, at the end of which Kent exhibited radium. See the *Crawfordsville Journal* (February 9, 1904), Hammer Collection, box 63, folder 4. Other lecturers also brought their own radium along. Talks at the Commercial Club of New York in 1904 and the Brooklyn Women's Club in 1903 were both followed by radium exhibits. See "Radium and Its Remarkable Properties," *Providence News* (April 13, 1904), Hammer Collection, box 63, folder 2 and the *Brooklyn Eagle* (November 10, 1903), Hammer Collection, box 59, folder 2.

23. See the untitled article describing Hammer's talk before an audience of two hundred in Philadelphia in the *Public Ledger* (October, 17, 1903), Hammer Collection, box 59, folder 2.

24. "Lecture on Radium," Hammer Collection, box 63, folder 2.

25. As Linda Henderson reveals, X rays attracted much interest, but only "the discovery of radioactivity produced a fundamental reorientation of accepted thinking about the natural world." As a result, "the themes of energy and alchemy were prominent elements in the popular literature on radioactivity." See Henderson, *Duchamp in Context*, 23.

26. The era of professional public speakers spans roughly 1870 to 1914 in the United States. According to Robert Oliver, Woodrow Wilson is considered the last great American speaker. See Oliver, *History of Public Speaking in America* (Wesport, Conn.: Greenwood Press, 1977).

27. In 1904, newspaper articles in local papers document discoveries of radium in Wyoming, Connecticut, California, Colorado, Quebec, and London. William Hammer appears to have been involved in authenticating the discovery of radium in Gilpin County, Colorado. The Poughkeepsie, New York, *News* reported on May 6, 1904, that Hammer, "the Edison expert," had examined the first hundred pounds of pitchblende taken from a Gilpin County mine and declared it as "so far ahead of the material" the Curies had gotten in Bohemia that "all demands of science for radium would be supplied in this country." His pronouncement may have accounted for some of the popularity of his Colorado lectures. See Hammer Collection, box 61, folder 3.

28. Hammer Collection, box 59, folder 2. For information on late-nineteenth-century revivals in the United States, see George Thomas, *Revivalism and Cultural Change: Christianity, Nation Building and the Markets in the Nineteenth-Century United States* (Chicago: University of Chicago Press, 1989); William Warren Sweet, *Revivalism in America: Its Origin, Growth and Decline*

(Gloucester, Mass.: Peter Smith, 1965); William G. McLoughlin, Sr., *Modern Revivalism: Charles Grandison Finney to Billy Graham* (New York: Ronald Press, 1959). An account of one of Dwight Moody's revival sermons can be found in McLoughlin, Sr., *Modern Revivalism*, 241–246.

29. "Lecture on Radium," *Erie Daily Times* (March 18, 1904), Hammer Collection, box 63, folder 2.

30. "Cooney Jessap's Overdose of Radium," *Indianapolis Journal* (February 1904), Hammer Collection, box 63, folder 2.

31. *Sacramento Bee* (November 7, 1903), Hammer Collection, box 59, folder 2.

32. Had such a prize actually been awarded, one of the contenders would have been the *New York World*, which, in 1903, reported that radium must be in Connecticut because "curious things" had happened there for five years, including fish clogging a reservoir, fires, mud storms, suicides, and even an infestation of starving cats. See "Is Radium, Which Creates and Kills, Exerting its Marvelous Powers on Every Square Foot of the Nutmeg State?" (1903), Hammer Collection, box 61, folder 2.

33. According to Spencer Weart, journalists believed that radium would revolutionize human evolution by illuminating cities, propelling vehicles, creating new metals, and doing almost "anything else imaginable." Weart, *Nuclear Fear*, 10.

34. "Most Wonderful Thing in the World," unnamed newspaper (February 9, 1904), Hammer Collection, box 59, folder 2.

35. Adams, *The Education*, 381–382.

36. See, for example, "Radium Wonders," *Grand Rapids Herald* (December 13, 1903), Hammer Collection, box 63, folder 2. According to the *Cleveland Plain Dealer*, radium overturned the "so-called law of conservation of energy." The fact that a reporter could refer to a theory that had long been accepted in physics and physiology as now "so-called" shows the dramatic change that radium posed to Americans' thinking. M. A. Bunker, "Radium, Twentieth Century Marvel," *Cleveland Plain Dealer* (April 16, 1904), Hammer Collection, box 63, folder 2.

37. "A Modern Marvel," unnamed paper, Burlington, Iowa, Hammer Collection, box 1, folder 1. For similar reports, see "Radium to the Rescue of an Expiring World," *Boston Herald* (December 20, 1903), Hammer Collection, box 59, folder 1, and C. W. Saleeby, "Radium the Revealer," *Harper's Magazine* (June 1904): 85–88.

38. Weart, *Nuclear Fear*, 6.

39. Story from the *Wichita Eagle*, February 13, 1904, Hammer Collection, box 59, folder 2. See also George Ethelbert Walsh, "A New Light for the World: Radium Light and Heat Rays," untitled magazine article (October 1903): 249–253, Hammer Collection, box 59, folder 2.

40. "What Radium May Do," *Suggestions* (Chicago, June 1903), Hammer Collection, box 59, folder 3. The exact same article appeared in Harrisburg, Pa., paper (April 6, 1904), Hammer Collection, box 63, folder 2. See also *Milwaukee Sentinel* "What We Know of Radium" (December 27, 1903), for predictions that radium will supply heat and light for a building for countless generations, Hammer Collection, box 59, folder 1.

41. "Body Transparent," *New York Press* (December 6, 1903), Hammer Collection, box 59, folder 1. Similar stories on how radium would drive freight trains and automobiles appeared in local papers. See "Radium in Connecticut," *Boston Pilot* (December 19, 1903), Hammer Collection, box 59, folder 1.

42. S. A. Paddock to W. J. Hammer, 1904, Hammer Collection, box 3, folder 1.

43. Cleveland Moffett, "The Sense and the Nonsense about Radium," *Success* (April 1904): 245–248.

44. "A Radium Banquet," *Scientific American* (February 20, 1904), Hammer Collection, box 59, folder 1.

45. See, for example, the *New York Vigilant* (February 18, 1904), Hammer Collection, box 59, folder 2, and "The Radium Cocktail," *Sioux Falls Press* (February 19, 1904), Hammer Collection, box 59, folder 2.

46. "The Radium Cocktail."

47. Untitled article (February 6, 1904), Hammer Collection, box 63, folder 4.

48. "The Radium Cocktail," *Newark News* (Feburary 24, 1904), Hammer Collection, box 63, folder 4.

49. "His Liquid Sunlight," *New York Tribune* (January 15, 1904), Hammer Collection, box 61, folder 3, and "Dr. Morton's Fluorescent Cancer Cure . . . Nature and Blood Should Have Sunshine," *New York Herald* (January 15, 1904), Hammer Collection, box 62, folder 2. Such treatments gained a loyal following in the 1930s. See, for example, Matthew Luckiesh, *Artificial Sunlight: Combining Radiation for Health with Light for Vision* (New York: D. Van Nostrand Company, 1930).

50. "Liquid Sunshine," *New York Sun* (January 12, 1904), Hammer Collection, box 61, folder 2. Though not mentioned directly, "radium cocktails" probably factored in small-town stories of radium's "glow" on the body that appeared around the same time as the cocktail rage. See, for example, in the Austin, Texas, newspaper, *Statesman*, the coverage of radium's projected "glow upon life and its possibilities," which soon would allow life to extend to 150 or 200 years. *Statesman* (January 8, 1904), Hammer Collection, box 61, folder 1.

51. "Radium and Radiomania," *San Francisco Argonaut* (December 28, 1903), Hammer Collection, box 61, folder 3. Other newspapers called it "radiomania" and the "radium craze." See the *Cleveland World* (October 10, 1903),

and an unnamed Wichita paper (October 11, 1903), both in Hammer Collection, box 59, folder 2.

52. For information on the spinthariscope rage, see the *New York Herald* (December 13, 1903), Hammer Collection, box 63, folder 2, and "Fashionable Now to Be Scientific," *New York Herald* (December 13, 1903), Hammer Collection, box 60, folder 1. Saleeby, in "Radium the Revealer," further confirms the device's popularity in commenting that it was something that "most of [his] readers have doubtless seen," 85. For an account of radium roulette, see the *New York Evening Journal* (July 30, 1904), Hammer Collection, box 63, folder 2. For radium punch, see the *Oswego Palladium* (February 16, 1904), Hammer Collection, box 59, folder 2. A general account of the 1904 fad of "radium parties" can be found in the *New York American* (January 17, 1904), Hammer Collection, box 61, folder 2.

53. The *Los Angeles Herald* declared that radium, if touched to the tongue, produced a "wonderful acceleration of the heart," but the practice wouldn't be as popular as drinking a gin rickey because of its prohibitive cost. See the *Herald* (July 20, 1903), Hammer Collection, box 60, folder 3. Other articles agreed that cost was prohibitive. It was $130,000 for only a small particle. The *New London Day* said in 1903 that although many people would like to have radium, "at the present time it is only possible for the very wealthy to possess it." *Day* (July 20, 1903), Hammer Collection, box 60, folder 3. In 1904, the *San Francisco Medical Journal* put the price of radium at $500 to $2,000 a grain. *Medical Journal* (February 1904), Hammer Collection, box 63, folder 2.

54. Regal advertised the sample as originating in Marie and Pierre Curie's laboratory and displayed it in a handsome jewel box for all to see. "Radium in Shop Window," *Wisconsin* (February 22, 1904), Hammer Collection, box 63, folder 2. For information on the lines of people who crowded to see the tiny "radium" tube at the Museum of Natural History in New York City, see "Radium and Crowd," *Magazine* (November 1903), and "Radium Shown in New York," *Lynn Massachusetts Item* (October 8, 1903), both in Hammer Collection, box 59, folder 2. For information on the twice-daily exhibitions of radium in the U.S. Government Building at the 1904 St. Louis World's Fair, see Martha L. Root, "A Week of Wonders," *Pittsburgh Gazette* (June 5, 1904), Hammer Collection, box 59, folder 3. One report asserts that this was actually the sample that had previously been on display at the Museum of Natural History. See untitled newspaper article, St. Louis (October 4, 1903), Hammer Collection, box 59, folder 2. In addition to the U.S. Government Building's display, Columbia University also had a radium exhibit at the fair that occupied 1,100 square feet. See "Columbia's Radium Exhibit," *Harlem Reporter* (June 25, 1904), Hammer Collection, box 60, folder 2.

55. Root, "A Week of Wonders."

56. For more on how department stores created spaces where upper- and

working-class women negotiated power, see Susan Porter Benson, *Counter Cultures: Saleswomen, Managers, and Customers in American Department Stores, 1890–1940* (Urbana: University of Illinois Press, 1986).

57. See Linda Dalrymple Henderson, *Duchamp in Context*, 23. For an account of another "radium dance" performance, see "Radium Dance," an undated, untitled article, Hammer Collection, box 60, folder 1. X rays had also been incorporated into musical performances before radium. Among the many songs written about X rays in the late nineteenth century are "X Rays March Two-Step" (copyright March 31, 1896), "X Rays Will Give It Away" (May 22, 1896), "X Ray Waltzes" (August 6, 1896), and "X Ray March" (January 21, 1897).

58. See Catherine Caufield, *Multiple Exposures: Chronicles of the Radiation Age* (New York: Harper and Row, 1989). For radium cleaners, see "Radium Chemical Company" (Philadelphia) brochure in Hammer Collection, box 59, folder 2. For radium earth, see J. B. King's 1900 scheme discussed in *Health Quackery: Consumers Union's Report on False Health Claims, Worthless Remedies, and Unproved Therapies* (Mount Vernon, N.Y.: Consumers Union, 1980), 226.

59. For more information on the history of American hot springs, see Harvey Green, *Fit for America: Health, Fitness, Sport and American Society* (New York: Johns Hopkins University Press, 1986), and Carolyn Thomas de la Peña, "Recharging at the Fordyce: Machine and Nature in the Modern Bath," *Technology and Culture* 40, no.4 (October 1999): 746–769.

60. I have written elsewhere about how these places taught modern men and women that nature and machine were both necessary for good health: see "Recharging at the Fordyce," 757–769.

61. According to tests by the U.S. Bureau of Standards in 1923, the top radioactive springs in the country were in Massachusetts, New York, Arkansas, Colorado, and Wyoming. See "Directions to Users of Thomas' Radium Ore-Lined Jars," pamphlet, Henry Gaylord Wilshire Collection (hereafter HGWC), box 7, Folder 7, Ionaco 1-2, 1925. A good secondary source on the promotion of radium waters at bathhouses is Jonathan Paul de Vierville, "American Healing Waters: A Chronology (1513–1926) and Historical Survey of America's Major Springs, Spas, and Health Resorts Including a Review of their Medicinal Virtues and Health Care Practices" (Ph.D. diss., University of Texas at Austin, 1992), particularly 447–449.

62. J. J. Moorman, "Montvalle Springs: with the Analysis of its Waters" (Knoxville: John B. G. Kinsloe, 1855), and George Glaze, "The Oak Orchard Acid Springs with Analysis and Testimonials of the Medical Faculty" (New York: Robert Larter, 1864), Warshaw Collection of Business Americana, Spas and Resorts, box 2.

63. Anonymous pamphlet, "Fordyce Bath House" (St. Louis: 1915), 6–7.

64. For more on the construction cost estimate of $230,000, see Thomas de la Peña, "Recharging at the Fordyce," 750.

65. Other resorts also used radium as a central promotional strategy during this same period. For information on Lake Arrowhead, California, which touted the "natural qualities" of its radioactive waters, see David Armstrong, *The Great American Medical Show: Being an Illustrated History of Hucksters, Healers, Health Evangelists, and Heroes from Plymouth Rock to the Present* (New York: Prentice Hall, 1991), 96.

66. Harry Springdale to Gaylord Wilshire, May 20, 1924, 2, HGWC, box 7, folder 1.

67. This connection between radiation and domesticity is discussed in Rebecca Herzig's article on women's use of X rays to remove facial blemishes and unwanted hair in the 1940s. Women pursued this often lethal method of technological beautification more frequently than men, which suggests that gender distinctions in how the technology was used continued in spite of radium water's being offered "for all." It is also telling that popular promoters used X ray technology, like electricity, as an agent to improve women's beauty. See Herzig, "Removing Roots: 'North American Hiroshima Maidens' and the X Ray," *Technology and Culture* 40, no. 4 (October 1999): 723–745.

68. Belgian embassy to Wilshire, June 17, 1924. HGWC, box 7, folder 7.

69. R. P. Sherman to Gaylord Wilshire, June 16, 1924, HGWC, box 7, folder 1.

70. Charles C. Thomas to Gaylord Wilshire, January 12, 1925, HGWC, box 7, folder 7.

71. Wilshire was working on other radium products at the time. He wrote to prospective investors in December 1924 offering an opportunity to fund his radioactive silk pajamas and underjerseys, which would have retailed for twenty-five and ten dollars, respectively. No one seems to have taken him up on the offer. See the letter dated December 17, 1924, in business material, HGWC, box 8, folder 7.

72. *Popular Science Monthly* (June 1923), reprint in HGWC, box 7, folder 1.

73. Pamphlets on these products can be found in American Medical Association Historical Health Fraud Collection (hereafter AMAHHFC), folder 0721-03. Additionally, advertisements for the Radium Ore Revigator and Thomas's Radium Ore-Lined Jars are in Wilshire's personal papers in the HGWC, box 7, folder 7.

74. Pamphlet, Vigoradium Corporation (New York, 1927), AMAHHFC, folder 0721-04.

75. "Put One of These in Your Home." The Revigator brochure carries no publishing information. AMAHHFC, folder 0723-05.

76. Pamphlet, AMAHHFC, folder 0723-05.

77. "Directions to Users of Thomas' Radium Ore-Lined Jars," pamphlet, HGWC, box 7, folder 7.

78. Pamphlet, AMAHHFC, folder 0723-05.

79. "Disease," HGWC, box 7, folder 1.

80. Harry Springdale, president of Hollywood Radium Laboratories, to Gaylord Wilshire, May 20, 1924. HGWC, box 7, folder 1.

81. "The Vitalizer," booklet (The National Radium Corporation, 1925), AMAHHFC, folder 0721-03.

82. Pamphlet, AMAHHFC, folder 0723-05.

83. "Directions to Users," HGWC.

84. Paul Boernsen, *Radium in the Light of Recent Discovery* (Washington, D.C.: The author, 1915), 3–4. The idea that radium's primary benefit was mental was also echoed by Dr. Robert Knox, who declared that "the chief benefit obtained by patients after taking emanation in solution appears to be a feeling of well-being." See Robert Knox, *Radiography, X-Ray Therapeutics and Radium Therapy* (New York: Macmillan, 1915), 357. Other evidence, however, suggests that water jars were actually highly radioactive, and continued to be so eighty years later. The National Park Service continues to warn employees that the jars in their collections are still radioactive. "Conserv-o-Gram," no. 2-19 (Washington, D.C.: August 1998).

85. Weart, *Nuclear Fear*, 53–54.

86. Moffett, "The Sense and the Nonsense," 246. There were some articles that agreed with Moffett that radium had no special medicinal or physiological value. Their voices, however, were overshadowed. See, for example, the York *Gazette* which theorized that radium would be found to have "no more pathological value than other forms of energy, such as light, heat or electricity." See *Gazette* (York, Pa., October 22, 1903), Hammer Collection, box 59, folder 2. Similar doubts are raised in an untitled New York paper from Feburary 11, 1904, Hammer Collection, box 59, folder 2.

87. Eve Curie, *Madame Curie*, 384.

88. Percy Brown, *American Martyrs to Science through Röntgen Rays* (Springfield, Ill.: Charles C. Thomas, 1936), 138. For more on the connection between radium, rays, and self-sacrifice, see Rebecca Herzig, "In the Name of Science: Suffering, Sacrifice, and the Formation of American Roentgenology," *American Quarterly* 53, no. 4 (December 2001): 563–589.

89. "The Vitalizer," AMAHHFC.

90. See "Medical Science Harnesses One of Nature's Rarest Forces for Health," booklet (North American Radium Corporation, 1927), AMAHHFC, folder 0719-02.

91. Roger M. Macklis, "Radiomedical Fraud and Popular Perceptions of Radiation," in Raymond Gagliardi, ed., *A History of the Radiological Sciences* (Reston, Va.: Radiology Centennial, Inc., 1996), 288.

92. Ibid., 288.

93. Ibid.

94. Ibid.

95. Charles Evans Morris, M.D., *Modern Rejuvenation Methods* (New York: Scientific Medical Publishing Co., 1926), 173. The book is stamped as from Radithor Laoratories, a company directed by Dr. William J. A. Bailey and run out of East Orange, N.J.

96. Ibid., 139–141. There are similarities between Bailey's Radithor method and light treatments. Both focused on the importance of the endocrine system in health, and both argued that it needed exposure to radiation to function correctly. Only sunlight therapists argued that that radiation was natural; radium-emanation proponents argued that it was scientifically created. For information on the connection between light therapy and endocrine glands, see M. Luckiesh and A. J. Pacini, *Light and Health: A Discussion of Light and Other Radiations in Relation to Life and Health* (Baltimore: Williams and Wilkins, 1926), 117–134.

97. Morris, *Modern Rejuvenation*, 143.

98. Ibid., 141.

99. Ibid., v.

100. Ibid., 135.

101. Ibid., 143.

102. Ibid., xix.

103. Ibid., 184.

104. Macklis, "Radiomedical Fraud," 286.

105. Caufield, *Multiple Exposures*, 28.

106. Macklis, "Radiomedical Fraud," 289.

107. Ibid.

108. Morris, *Modern Rejuvenation*, 141.

109. Ibid., 182.

110. Quoted, ibid., 165.

111. Henderson, *Duchamp in Context*, 23. Mihran Kassiban, a physician and electrotherapist, was the first to publicize the detrimental effects of X rays by documenting his own gradual amputations and health decline until his death in 1910. Along with the 1904 death of Edison's assistant Clarence Dally, Kassiban's work convinced many that X rays were not primarily benign agents for improved health. See Gagliardi, *A History of the Radiological Sciences*, 14. Even as people were beginning to think X rays were dangerous, they still trusted radium's safety. In 1909, research published by a physician found that radium posed no danger and was almost always preferable to the knife in surgery. See Herbert Robarts, MD, *Practical Radium: The Practical Uses of Radium in the Treatment of Obstinate Forms of Disease* (St. Louis: n.p., 1909), 38–39.

112. Weart, *Nuclear Fear*, 53–55.

113. Hector A. Colwell and Sidney Russ, *X-Ray and Radium Injuries: Prevention and Treatment* (London: Oxford University Press, 1934), 185.

114. Brecher and Brecher, *The Rays*, 420–421.

115. See Langer, "Fast New World," *Colliers* 106, no. 1 (July 6, 1940): 19.

NOTES TO THE CONCLUSION

1. Life Fitness web site, www.lifefitness.com

2. Samuel Fussell claims that most people who take working out seriously are far more concerned with their appearance than with their energy levels. When taken to the extreme, this preference causes them to do physical damage to themselves through steroids and starvation in order to achieve the right "look." See Fussell, *Muscle: Confessions of an Unlikely Bodybuilder* (New York: Poseidon Press, 1991).

3. David Nye, *Consuming Power: A Social History of American Energies* (Cambridge: MIT Press, 1999), 1.

4. www.braintuner.com/braintuner.html. The company also sells Ozonators, which are described as quite similar to the original Electropoise. See also the Health Pax Cranial Electrical Stimulator sold at www.elixa.com/estim/MC400.htm

5. www.redbull.com/product/history/index.html

6. George Lipsitz, *Time Passages: Collective Memory and American Popular Culture* (Minneapolis: University of Minnesota Press, 1990).

7. Strauss quoted in Richard Rhodes, Ed., *Visions of Technology: A Century of Vital Debate About Machines, Systems and the Human World* (New York: Simon & Schuster, 1999), 197.

8. Easterbrook quoted in Rhodes, 358-359. Original quotation is taken from Easterbrook, *Moment On Earth* (Viking, 1995).

9. Anne Balsamo, *Technologies of the Gendered Body: Reading Cyborg Women* (Durham: Duke University Press, 1996), 116.

Bibliography

MANUSCRIPT COLLECTIONS

Austin, Texas
University of Texas at Austin
Todd-McLean Physical Culture Collection [TMPC]

Chicago, Illinois
American Medical Association Headquarters
   Historical Health Fraud Collection [AMAHHFC]

Los Angeles, California
University of California Los Angeles
   Henry Gaylord Wilshire Collection [HGWC]

Minneapolis, Minnesota
Bakken Library and Museum of Electricity in Life [BLEL]
   Ephemera Collection [BLEC]

Reston, Virginia
The History Factory
   American History of Radiology Collection [AHRC]

Washington, D.C.
National Museum of American History, Smithsonian Institution [NMAH]

   Archives Center
      Warshaw Collection of Business Americana [WCBA]
      William Hammer Collection
      Health Spas and Resorts Collection

   Department of Science and Technology
      Division of Medical Sciences, accession memos

INTERVIEWS

Bob Conte, historian, Greenbriar Hotel, White Sulphur Springs, West Virginia, September 1, 1999.
John Hoover, historian, Homestead Resort, Hot Springs, Virginia, August 22, 1999.

NEWSPAPERS

Boston Herald
Boston Pilot
Brooklyn Eagle
Cleveland Plain Dealer
Duluth Evening Herald
Erie Daily Times
Gazette (York, Pennsylvania)
Grand Rapids Herald
Harlem Reporter
Indianapolis Journal
Journal (Crawfordsville, Illinois)
Los Angeles Herald
Lynn, Massachusetts Item
Milwaukee Sentinel
Newark News
New London Day
New York American
New York Evening Journal
New York Herald
New York Press
New York Sun
New York Tribune
New York Vigilant
New York World
News (Providence, Rhode Island)
North American
Oswego Palladium
Pittsburgh Gazette
Public Ledger (Philadelphia)
Sacramento Bee
San Francisco Argonaut
San Francisco Bulletin

Savannah Press
Sioux Falls Press
Statesman (Austin, Texas)
Suggestions (Chicago)
Syracuse Telegram
Wichita Eagle
Wisconsin
World (Cleveland)

TRADE MAGAZINES

Western Electrician
Electric Review
Electric World

CONTEMPORARY SOURCES

Articles, Catalogues, Pamphlets, Reports
Annual Reports of the President and Treasurer of Harvard College, 1883–1884.
"As Wonderful as the Telephone and Electric Light." *Frank Leslie's Illustrated Newspaper* (March 26, 1881).
"Athletics and Gymnastics at Harvard." *The Wheelman* 2 (September 1883), 417–423.
"At Last! An Electric Light for the Necktie." *Ohio Electric Works Illustrated Catalogue* (ca. 1890).
"Awake the Greater Health Within You: A Message of Hope." Chicago: Vit-o-net Corporation, 1928.
Barnett, S. M. "The Gymnasium at Home. Utility and Amusement Combined. Barnett's Patent Parlor Gymnasium and Chest Expander for Schools and Families." New York: J. Becker & Co., 1871.
Beard, George. "American Nervousness: Its Philosophy and Treatment." *Virginia Medical Monthly* 6, no. 4 (July 1879): 253–276.
———. "Nervous Exhaustion (Neurasthenia), with Cases of Sexual Neurasthenia." Undated pamphlet, ca. 1880.
Blaikie, William. "Free Muscular Development." *Harper's Magazine* 56 (May 1878): 915–924.
"The Blood Is Life! An Astonishing Discovery! Accomplished at Last! The Efficacy of Electricity! Nearly All Diseases Effectually Cured by Boyd's Miniature Galvanic Battery." New York: J. C. Boyd, 1879.

Brackett, C. F. "Electricity in the Service of Man: An Introductory Paper." *Scribner's Magazine* 5, no. 6 (June 1889): 643–659.

Bruckner, Samuel. "On the Physical Character of the Pain of Parturition." *Galliard's Medical Journal* (January 1900): 799.

Bryson, Charles Lee. *Health and How to Get It*. Racine, Wis.: Hamilton Beach Manufacturing Company, 1927.

Catalogue and Price List of Electrical Apparatus and Supplies. Philadelphia: Lyman G. Morey, 1882.

Catalogue of the Owen Electric Belts and Appliances. Chicago: Owen Electric Belt and Appliance Company, ca. 1890.

Crystal, Andrew. "Professor Crystal's Electric Belts and Appliances: Greatest Success of the Nineteenth Century." Marshall, Mich.: 1898.

Dana, C. L. "On the Pathology and Treatment of Certain Forms of Nerve Weakness." *Medical Record* 24 (1883): 61.

"A Delightful Road to Health." *Liberty* (January 15, 1927): 82.

Dillings, F. C. "Modern Miracles of the Wonders of Magnetic Healing." New York: Evening Tribune Print, 1882.

Drescher's Illustrated Catalogue and Price List of Electro-Therapeutic Apparatus (New York: self published, 1873).

Dr. Savage Health Studio, n.d. Warshaw Collection of Business Americana.

Duraind, George J. *Gaylord Wilshire and His Amazing Discovery*. Los Angeles: Iona Company, 1927.

"The Electric Boy." *Electrical Review* (October 8, 1887): 7.

"The Electric Era." New York: German Electric Agency, ca. 1901.

Electrical Goods: Everything Electrical for Home, Office, Factory and Shop. Chicago: Sears, Roebuck and Co., 1918.

Electrical Instruments for Physicians and Surgeons. Chicago: R. V. Wagner & Co., 1900.

"Electromagnetism and Your Health." Minneapolis: Thernoid of Minneapolis, ca. 1930.

Electrotherapy in the United States. Minneapolis: Medtronic, 1977.

Figuier, Louis. "The Electrical Girl." *Popular Science Monthly* 6 (March 1875): 588–592.

Fisher, George Jackson. "A Brief Historical Sketch of the Discovery of the Circulation of the Blood." *Popular Science Monthly* 11 (July 1877): 294–306.

"Fordyce Bath House." St. Louis, 1915.

"Future of Electrical Development," Amos Dolbear interview. *Western Electrician* (January 9, 1897).

Glaze, George. "The Oak Orchard Acid Springs with Analysis and Testimonials of the Medical Faculty." New York: Robert Larter, 1864.

"The Great Nerve Stimulant Zardon." Toronto, Ohio: Elenita Company, ca. 1901.

The Greatest Medical Discovery Ever Known: Dr. John Butler's Electro-Massage Machine (or Electric Manipulator) for Curing Disease at Home. 1889.

Gulick, Luther. "Ten Minutes Exercise for Busy Men." New York: American Sports Publishing Company, 1902.

———. "Muscle Building: Practical Points for Practical People." New York: American Sports Publishing Company, 1905.

Hartwell, Edward M. "The Rise of College Gymnastics in the United States." In *Special Report by the Bureau of Education of Educational Exhibits and Conventions at the World's Industrial and Cotton Centennial Exposition at New Orleans, 1884.*

Harvard Catalog. Harvard University (1880–1881).

"Health and Wealth." Chicago: U.S. Insole Company, 1886.

Hickey, P. M. "Teaching of Roentgenology in America." In *Teaching and Training in Medical Radiology.* Stockholm: Kungl. Bokryckeriet, 1930, 34–40.

Higginson, Thomas Wentworth. "Saints and Their Bodies." *Atlantic Monthly* (March 1858): 582–595.

"How to Restore Your Nerve Force." *San Francisco Bulletin* (January 22, 1913): 16.

Huber, John D. "Arrhenius and Electric Children." *Scientific American* (April 13, 1912): 334.

Hutchingson, Woods. "Our Human Misfits." *Everybody's Magazine* 25 (October 1911): 519.

———. "Taking the Waters: The Humbug of Hot Springs." *Everybody's Magazine* (February 1913): 167.

Iles, George. "The Dissipation of Energy." *Popular Science Monthly* 12 (April 1878): 701–705.

Illustrated Catalogue and Price List of the Galvano-Faradic Manufacturing Company. Maine: Schlotterbeck and Co., 1875.

Illustrated Catalogue of Flemming's Electro-Therapeutic Apparatus, Electro-Surgical Apparatus, Electrodes, Etc. Philadelphia: Press of Wm. H. Bartholomew, 1886.

Illustrated, Descriptive List of the McIntosh Galvanic, Faradic and Combined Galvanic and Faradic Batteries. Chicago: McIntosh Galvanic and Faradic Battery Co., ca. 1890.

Kahlo, George. "A European Cure in America, White Sulpher Springs: Climate, Waters, Baths, and other Curatic Resources" (March 1915, reprint May 1916).

Kinesotherapy. New York: The Kny-Scheerer Company, 1914.

Knox, Robert. *Radiography and Radio-Therapeutics.* Macmillan, 1917.

Lake, Henry. "Is Electricity Life?" *Popular Science Monthly* 2 (March 1873): 477–490.

Langer, R. M. "Fast New World." *Colliers* 106, no. 1 (July 6, 1940): 19–20.

Liebig, Justus von. "Century's Progress in Anatomy and Physiology." *Harpers Magazine*, 1898.

The Lift: A Journal Designed to Aid in Showing People How to Lift Themselves up in the World 1, no. 2 (September 1871).

The Lifting Cure: An Original Scientific Application of the Laws of Motion on Mechanical Action to Physical Culture and the Cure of Disease. Boston: D. P. Butler, 1868.

Lungren, Charles. "Electricity at the World's Fair, I." *Popular Science Monthly* 43 (October 1893): 721–740.

———. "Electricity at the World's Fair, II," *Popular Science Monthly* 43 (November 1893): 39–54.

McIntosh Battery and Optical Company: Electro-Therapeutical Catalogue. Chicago: McIntosh, 1881.

McIntosh Combined Galvanic and Faradic Battery. Chicago: McIntosh, 1881.

Narragansett Machine Company: Fine Gymnasium Goods. Providence, R.I.: Narragansett Machine Company, ca. 1887.

Manual for Moorhead's Graduated Magnetic Machine. New York: D. C. Moorhead, 1847.

Men's Specialists: Some Quacks and Their Methods. Chicago: AMA Bureau of Investigation, ca. 1913.

Meyer, Curt. *Illustrated Catalogue and Price List, Physical and Chemical, Electro-Medical, Optical and Scientific Instruments.* New York: Trow's Printing and Bookbinding Co., 1885.

"Modern Miracles or the Wonders of Magnetic Healing," n.d., Warshaw Collection of Americana.

Moffett, Cleveland. "The Wonders of Radium." *McClure's Magazine* 22 (November 1903): 1–15.

———. "The Sense and the Nonsense about Radium." *Success* (April 1904): 245–248.

Moorman, J. J. "Montvalle Springs: With the Analysis of Its Waters." Knoxville: John B. G. Kinsloe, 1855.

Morey, Lyman G. *Catalogue and Price List of Electric Apparatus and Supplies.* Philadelphia, 1882.

Morris, Charles Evans. *Modern Rejuvenation Methods.* New York: Scientific Medical Publishing Co., 1926.

"Moving Display of Electrical Household Appliances." *Western Electrician* (August 3, 1907): 83.

North American Radium Corporation. "Medical Science Harnesses One of Nature's Rarest Forces for Health." New York, n.d.

Official Catalogue of Exhibits and Descriptive Catalogue, World's Columbian Exposition, Department M. Anthropological Building, Midway Plaisance and Isolated Exhibits. Chicago: W. B. Conkey Company, 1893.

Official Catalogue of Exhibits. World's Columbian Exposition, Department of Machinery Hall. Chicago: W.B. Conkey Company, 1893.

Oswald, F. L. "The Age of Gymnastics." *Popular Science Monthly* 13 (June 1878): 129–139.

Oswald, Felix L. "Physical Education." *Popular Science Monthly* 19 (May 1881): 17.

"Our Answer to Numerous Correspondents Pointing Out a Plain Road to Health Without the Use of Medicine." Chicago, ca. 1885.

Owen, A. "Owen Electric Belts." Chicago: The Owen Electric Belt and Appliance Company, ca. 1890.

Paine, Albert Bigelow. "The New Coney Island." *Century* 68 (August 1904): 535.

Papillon, Fernand. "Electricity and Life." *Popular Science Monthly* 2 (March 1873): 526–541.

Partnick, Bunnell & Co. Catalogue and Price List of Telegraphical and Electrical Instruments and Supplies. Philadelphia: Rue & Jones, 1873.

"The Physical Side of College Men." *Illustrated Sporting News* 5 (August 12, 1905): 4.

Pike's Illustrated Catalogue of Scientific Medical Instruments (1856 original). Dracut, Mass.: The Antiquarian Scientist, 1984.

Preece, W. H. "Recent Wonders of Electricity." *Popular Science Monthly* (April 1882): 669–680.

Pulvermacher, J. L. *Galvanic Electricity: Its Pre-Eminent Power and Effects in Preserving and Restoring Health Made Plain and Useful.* London: Galvanic Establishment, 1875.

Pulvermacher Galvanic Company. "Electricity: Nature's Chief Restorer." Cincinnati: Pulvermacher Galvanic Company, 1876.

———. "The Only Rational Means for Self-Cure." Cincinnati: Pulvermacher Galvanic Company, n.d.

"Pure Air and Pure Water by Scientific Methods." New York: Electrozone Corporation of New York, 1927.

"A Radium Banquet." *Scientific American* (February 20, 1904).

"Radium: Its Possibilities as Seen by its Discoverer." Indianapolis Star (December 29, 1903): 4.

Richards, Eugene. "College Athletics and Physical Development." *Popular Science Monthly* 32 (April 1888): 721–732.

"Rogers' Violet Ray." Rogers Electric Labs, ca. 1910.

Saleeby, C. W. "Radium the Revealer." *Harper's Magazine* (June 1904): 85–88.

Sanden, A. T. "Dr. A. T. Sanden, Originator of the Celebrated Home Treatment for the Cure of All Chronic, Nervous and Wasting Diseases Without Drugs or Medicines." New York: Prout and Ward Printers, ca. 1910.

"Sandow Interviewed in America." *Sandow's Magazine* (1902). TMPC.

Sargent, Dudley Allen. "The Apparatus of the Hemenway Gymnasium." *The Harvard Register* 1 (February 1880): 44–45.

———. "Anthropometric Apparatus with Directions for Measuring and Testing the Principal Physical Characteristics of the Human Body." Dudley Allen Sargent, 1887.

———. "The Physical Proportions of the Typical Man." *Scribner's Magazine* 2 (July 1887): 3–17.

———. "The Physical Characteristics of the Athlete." *Scribner's Magazine* 2, no. 5 (November 1887): 540–561.

———. "The Physical Development of Women." *Scribner's Magazine* 5, no. 2 (February 1889): 172–185.

———. "The Inomotor: A Fundamental Mechanism for a New System of Motor Vehicles, Testing Apparatus and Developing Appliances." *American Physical Education Review* 5 (December 1900): 312–323.

———. "Twenty Years' Progress in Efficiency Tests." *American Physical Education Review* 63 (October 1913): 454.

Scrapbook, Alphonso Rockwell, ca. 1865–1900, Bakken Library and Museum of Electricity in Life, Minneapolis, Minnesota.

Sears, Roebuck and Co. *Consumer's Guide* (Fall 1900).

Sidenblah, Elias. *Swedish Catalogue. I. Statistics, International Exhibition, 1876, Philadelphia*. Philadelphia: Hallowell & Company, 1876.

Smith, J. Gardner. "History of Physical Training in New York City and Vicinity in the Young Men's Christian Associations." *American Physical Education Review* 4 (September 1899): 303–308.

Songs for Calisthenics. Springfield, Ill.: Horace S. Taylor, 1849. TMPC.

Songs for Calisthenics. Northhampton, Mass.: Hopkins, Bridgman & Co., 1857. TMPC.

"The Source of Muscular Power." *Popular Science Monthly* 12 (April 1878): 729–736.

Sporting Goods: Sports equipment and clothing, novelties, recreative science, firemen's supplies, magic lanterns and slides, plays and joke books, tricks and magic, badges and ornaments. New York: Peck and Snyder, 1886. Historical reprint from the American Historical Catalog Collection (Princeton: Pine Press, 1976).

Starr, M. Allen. "Electricity in Relation to the Human Body." *Scribner's Magazine* (reprint, ca. 1890): 589–599.

Stevenson, William G. "The Psychological Significance of Vital Force." *Popular Science Monthly* 24 (April 1884): 760–773.

Stillman, J. M. "The Source of Muscular Energy." *Popular Science Monthly* 24 (January 1884): 377–387.

Strong, Josiah. *Expansion*. New York: 1900.

Swedish Catalogue, I. Statistics. Philadelphia: International Exhibition, 1876.

Tesla, Nikola. "The Problem of Increasing Human Energy with Special Reference to Harnessing the Sun's Energy." *The Century Illustrated Monthly Magazine* 60, no. 2 (June 1900): 175–211.

Thompson, Sir William (Lord Kelvin). "The Available Energy of Nature." *Popular Science Monthly* 20 (November 1881): 87–95.

U.S. Senate. Report of Immigration Commission on Changes in Bodily Form from Descendants of Immigrants. 61st Cong., 2d sess., 1910. S. Doc. 208.

"The Use of Illuminated Girls." *Electrical World* (February 6, 1886).

"Violet Rays: The Master Violet Ray." Chicago: The Master Electric Company, ca. 1925.

Walling, H. F. "Dissipation of Energy." *Popular Science Monthly* 4 (February 1874): 430–433.

Wells, Ida B. "Mob Rule in New Orleans," "A Red Record," and "Southern Lynch Law in All Its Phases." Reprinted in *Southern Horrors and Other Writings*, ed. Jacqueline Jones Royster (Boston: Bedford Books, 1997).

Wendell, Barrett. "Social Life at Harvard." *Lippincott's Monthly Magazine* 39 (January 1887): 157.

"What to Do with Radium." *Literary Digest* (May 7, 1921): 21.

"Why Not Try Our Home Spas?" *Journal of the Arkansas Medical Society* 11 (1914): 144.

Williams, Henry Smith. "The Century's Progress in Anatomy and Physiology." *Harpers* 96 (1898): 621–632.

Williams, Mattieu. "Electromania." *Popular Science Monthly* 21 (September 1882): 650–655.

Windship, George Barker. "Autobiographical Sketches of a Strength-Seeker." *Atlantic Monthly* (January 1862): 102–115.

Worcester, Alfred. "Gymnastics." *Popular Science Monthly* 23 (May 1883): 77–85.

World's Columbian Exposition, 1893, Official Catalogue, part 9, Electricity Building. Chicago: W. B. Conkey Company, 1893.

Books

Adam, G. Mercer. *Sandow's System of Physical Training.* New York: J. Selwin Tait & Sons, 1894.

Adams, Henry. *The Education of Henry Adams.* New York: Modern Library, 1931.

Althaus, Julius. *Cases Treated by Faradisation.* London: Truebner and Co., 1861.

Bagg, J. H. *Bagg on Magnetism or the Doctrine of Equilibrium.* Detroit: Bagg and Harmon, 1845.

Baum, L. Frank. *The Master Key: An Electrical Fairy Tale.* Indianapolis: Bowen-Merrill Company, 1901.

Beard, George M. *American Nervousness: Its Causes and Consequences*. New York: G. Putnam's, 1881.

———. *The Study of Trance, Muscle Reading and Allied Nervous Phenomena in Europe and America, with a Letter on the Moral Character of Trance Subjects and a Defense of Dr. Charcot*. New York, 1882.

———, and A. D. Rockwell. *Practical Treatise on Nervous Exhaustion*. New York: E. B. Treat, 1869.

———. *A Practical Treatise on Nervous Exhaustion*. 3d ed. New York: E. B. Treat, 1894.

Beecher, Catharine. *Physiology and Calisthenics for Schools and Families*. New York: Harper & Bros., 1856.

Bernard, Barnard. *Sex Weaknesses: Their Cause and Remedy*. Sausalito: Physical Culture Consultants, 1929.

Blaikie, William. *How to Get Strong and How to Stay So*. New York: Harper & Brothers, 1879.

Boernsen, Paul. *Radium in the Light of Recent Discovery*. Washington, D.C.: 1915.

Bowen, Wilbur Pardon. *Applied Anatomy and Kinesiology: The Mechanism of Muscular Movement*. Philadelphia: Lea and Febiger, 1917.

Brackett, Cyrus, et al. *Electricity in Daily Life: A Popular Account of the Applications of Electricity to Every Day Uses*. New York: Charles Scribner's Sons, 1891.

Brittan, S. *Man and His Relations: Illustrating the Influence of the Mind on the Body*. New York: W. A. Townsend, 1864.

Britten, Emma Harding. *The Electric Physician: Self Cure through Electricity*. New York: William Britten, 1875.

Brown, Percy. *American Martyrs to Science through Roentgen Rays*. Springfield, Ill.: Charles C. Thomas, 1936.

Butler, D. P. *The Lifting Cure: An Original Scientific Application of the Laws of Motion on Mechanical Action to Physical Culture and the Cure of Disease*. Boston: D. P. Butler, 1868.

Butler, John. *Electricity in Surgery*. New York: Boericke & Tafel, 1882.

Caldwell, John J. *Report of Cases Treated by Electricity, Being a Reprint from the Transactions of the Medical and Surgical Faculty of the State of Maryland at its Seventy-Forth Annual Session Held at Baltimore*. Baltimore: William K. Boyle and Son, 1873.

Call, Annie Payson. *Power Through Repose*. Boston: Roberts Brothers, 1891.

Channing, William. *The Medical Application of Electricity*. Boston: Thomas Hall, 1865.

Chaplin, J. *The Origin and Use of the Electro-Chemical Bath for the Extraction of Mercury and Other Metallic Substances from the Human Body and its Curative Agency in Other Diseases*. London: William Freeman, 1856.

Chase, Stuart. *Men and Machines.* New York: Macmillan, 1929.

Chavannes, Albert. *Magnetation.* Knoxville: Albert Chavannes, 1899.

Chiosso, Captain James. *The Gymnastic Polymachinon: Instructions for Performing a Systematic Series of Exercises on the Gymnastic & Calisthenic Polymachinon.* London: Walton & Maberly, 1855.

Colwell, Hector A., and Sidney Russ. *X-Ray and Radium Injuries: Prevention and Treatment.* London: Oxford University Press, 1934.

Comstock, J. L. *Outlines of Physiology, Both Comparative and Human.* New York: Robinson, Pratt & Co., 1836.

Cook, N. F. *Satan in Society, by a Physician.* Cincinnati: C. F. Vent, 1871.

Cramp, Arthur. *Nostrums and Quackery.* Vol. 1. Chicago: American Medical Association Press, 1912.

———. *Nostrums and Quackery: Articles on the Nostrum Evil, Quackery and Allied Matters Affecting the Public Health.* Vol. 2. Chicago: AMA Press, 1921.

———. *Miscellaneous Nostrums.* Chicago: Propaganda Department of the Journal of the American Medical Association, 1923.

———. *Nostrums and Quackery and Pseudo-Medicine.* Vol. 3. Chicago: AMA Press, 1936.

Curie, Eve. *Madame Curie: A Biography.* New York: Garden City Publishing Company, 1943.

Davis's Manual of Magnetism, Including Galvanism, Magnetism, Electro-Magnetism, Electro-Dynamics, Magneto-Electricity, and Thermo-Electricity. Boston: Palmer and Hall, Magnetical and Telegraphic Instrument Makers, 1857.

Directory of Deceased American Physicians, 1804–1929. Chicago: American Medical Association, 1993.

The Doctor's Story: A Treatise on Electricity and Electro Magnetism. New York: Pall Mall Electric Company, 1888.

Dowse, Thomas Stretch. *Lectures on Massage and Electricity in the Treatment of Disease.* New York: E. B. Treat & Co., 1906.

Eastman, Mary. *Biography of Dio Lewis, M.D.* New York: Fowler and Wells, Co., 1890.

Eberhart, Noble. *A Brief Guide to Vibratory Technique.* Chicago: New Medicine Publishing Co., 1908.

———. *Physicians' Directions for Renulife Treatments.* Detroit: Renulife Electric Company, 1926.

"Electrotherapy." In *A System of Electrotherapeutics as Taught by the International Correspondence Schools.* Vol. 4. Scranton: International Textbook Co., 1902.

Engelmann, George. *Labor Among Primitive Peoples.* St. Louis: J. H. Chambers & Co., 1882.

Fishbein, Morris. *The New Medical Follies: An Encyclopedia of Cultism and Quackery in these United States*. New York: Boni and Liverright, 1927.

Flint, Austin. *The Physiology of Man*. New York: D. Appleton and Company, 1868.

Fournier, Marian. *The Medico-Mechanical Equipment of Dr. Zander*. Leiden: Museum Boerhaave, 1989.

Fowler, Orson. *The Practical Phrenologist; and Recorder and Delineator of the Character and Talents*. New York: Mrs. O. S. Fowler, 1869.

Fraser, E. J. *Medical Electricity: A Treatise on the Nature of Vital Electricity in Health and Disease with Plain Instructions in the Uses of Artificial Electricity as a Curative Agent*. Chicago: C. S. Halsey, 1863.

Galvani, Luigi. *Effects of Electricity on Muscular Motion*. Translated from 1791 original. Norwalk, Conn.: Burndy Library, 1953.

Garratt, Alfred. *Electro-Physiology and Electro-Therapeutics: Showing the Best Methods of the Medical Uses of Electricity*. Boston: Ticknor and Fields, 1860.

General Faradism, A System of Electrotherapeutics as Taught by the International Correspondence Schools. Vol. 4. Scranton: International Textbook Company, 1902.

Gottschalk, Franklin B. *Static Electricity, X-Ray and Electro-Vibration, Their Therapeutic Application*. Chicago: T. Eisele, 1903.

Grier, M. J. *The Treatment of Some Forms of Sexual Debility by Electricity*. Philadelphia: Medical Press Company, 1891.

Grover, Burton Baker. *Electro-Therapy in the Abstract for the Busy Practitioner*. New York: Thompson-Plaster Co., 1922.

Gulick, Luther. *Manual of Physical Measurements in Connection with the Association Gymnasium Records*. New York: International Committee of Young Men's Christian Association, 1892.

Haire, Norman. *Rejuvenation: The Work of Steinach, Voronoff, and Others*. London: George Allen & Unwin, 1924.

Hamilton, Alan McLane. *Clinical Electro-Therapeutics, Medical and Surgical: A Hand-Book for Physicians in the Treatment of Nervous and Other Diseases*. New York: D. Appleton and Company, 1873.

Hancock, Irving. *Physical Training for Business Men: Basic Rules and Simple Exercises for Gaining Assured Control of the Physical Self*. New York: G. P. Putnam's Sons, 1917.

Haynes, C. M. *Elementary Principles of Electro-Therapeutics for the Use of Physicians and Students*. Chicago: McIntosh Galvanic and Faradic Battery Co., 1884.

The Health Lift: Reduced to a Science, Cumulative Exercise, a Thorough Gymnastic System in Ten Minutes Once a Day. New York: Health-Lift Company, 1876.

Hedley, W. S. *The Hydro-Electric Methods in Medicine*. London: H. K. Lewis, 1892.

——. *Therapeutic Electricity and Practical Muscle Testing*. Philadelphia: P. Blakiston's Son and Co., 1900.

The History and Philosophy of Animal Magnetism with Practical Instructions for the Exercise of this Power. Boston: J. N. Bradley & Co., 1843.

Herrick, Robert. *Together*. New York: Macmillan, 1908.

Hollick, Frederick. *Popular Treatise on Venereal Disease*. New York, 1852.

Houston, Edwin. *Electricity in Everyday Life in Three Volumes*. New York: P. F. Collier & Son, 1905.

——, and A. E. Kennelly. *Electricity in Electro-Therapeutics*. New York: W. J. Johnston Company, 1896.

Idone, Frank. *US Army Exercises: Rearranged for General Use*. New York: Richard K. Fox, 1904.

Inch, J. S. *Centennial Exposition, Described and Illustrated, Being a Concise and Graphic Description of this Grand Enterprise*. Philadelphia: Hubbard Brothers, 1876.

Ives, John. *Electricity as a Medicine and Its Mode of Application*. New York: John T. Ives, 1879.

James, George Wharton. *Indians' Secrets of Health*. Pasadena: Radiant Life Press, 1908.

Jouston, Edwin, and A. E. Kennelly. *Electricity in Electro-Therapeutics*. New York: W. J. Johnston Company, 1896.

Kellogg, John Harvey. *The Art of Massage: Its Physiological Effects and Therapeutic Applications*. Battle Creek, Mich.: Modern Medicine Publishing Co., 1895.

——. *The Battle Creek Sanitarium Book*. Battle Creek, Mich.: n.p., ca. 1906.

——. *Light Therapeutics: A Practical Manual of Phototherapy for the Student and the Practitioner*. Battle Creek, Mich.: Good Health Publishing Company, 1910.

Kidder, Jerome. *Electro-Allotropo-Physiology Uses of Different Qualities of Electricity to Cure Disease*. New York: Jerome Kidder, 1873.

Knox, Robert. *Radiography, X-Ray Therapeutics and Radium Therapy*. New York: Macmillan, 1915.

Lawrance, Richard Moore. *On Localized Galvanism Applied to the Treatment of Paralysis and Muscular Contractions*. London: Henry Renshaw, 1858.

Leavitt, John W. *Exercise a Medicine; or Muscular Action as Related to Organic Life*. New York: J. W. Leavitt, 1870.

Lee, Gerald Stanley. *Crowds, A Moving Picture of Democracy*. New York: Page & Co., 1913.

——. *Rest Working: A Study in Relaxed Concentration*. New York: J. J. Little and Ives Company, 1925.

Levertin, A. *Dr. G. Zander's Medico-Mechanische Gymnastik.* Stockholm: P. A. Norstedt, 1892.

———. "A Short Review of Dr. G. Zander's Medico-Mechanical Gymnastics Method." In A. Levertin, F. Heiligenthal, G. Schuetz, and G. Zander, *The Leading Features of Dr. G. Zander's Medico-Mechanical Gymnastic Method and Its Use.* Wiesbaden: Rossel, Schwartz & Co., 1906.

Lewis, Dio. *New Gymnastics for Men, Women, and Children.* Boston: James R. Osgood and Company, 1873.

Lindquist, Jerome. *Approach to Electrotherapeutics.* Los Angeles: Ward Richie Press, 1939.

London, Jack. *Call of the Wild.* New York: Macmillan, 1903.

———. *White Fang.* New York: Macmillan, 1906.

Luckiesh, Matthew. *Artificial Sunlight: Combining Radiation for Health with Light for Vision.* New York: D. Van Nostrand Company, 1930.

Luckiesh, M., and A. J. Pacini. *Light and Health: A Discussion of Light and other Radiations in Relation to Life and Health.* Baltimore: Williams and Wilkins, 1926.

Lyman, Henry. *Artificial Anesthesia and Anesthetics.* New York: William Wood & Company, 1881.

Macfadden, Bernarr. *Constipation: Its Cause, Effect and Treatment.* New York: Macfadden Book Company, 1930.

Maclaren, Archibald. *A System of Physical Education: Theoretical and Practical.* Oxford: Clarendon Press, 1869.

The Magicians Own Book. New York: Dick & Fitzgerald, 1857.

Marey, Etienne-Jules. *Animal Mechanism: A Treatise on Terrestrial and Aerial Locomotion.* New York, 1874.

Martin, Franklin. *Electricity in Diseases of Women and Obstetrics.* Chicago: W. T. Keener, 1892.

Massey, G. Betton. *Electricity in the Diseases of Women, with Special Reference to the Application of Strong Currents.* Philadelphia: F. A. Davis, 1889.

Mayne, Isabelle Rittenhouse. *Maud.* Ed. Richard Lee Strout. New York: Macmillan, 1939.

Mitchell, John. *A System of Physiologic Therapeutics: A Practical Exposition of the Methods, other than Drug-Giving, Useful for the Prevention of Disease and in the Treatment of the Sick.* Philadelphia: P. Blakiston's Son & Co., 1904.

Morrill, S. E. *A Treatise of Practical Instructions in the Medical and Surgical Uses of Electricity.* Kalamazoo: Kalamazoo Publishing Company, 1882.

Morris, Charles Evans. *Modern Rejuvenation Methods.* New York: Scientific Medical Publishing Co., 1926.

Mumford, Lewis. *Sketches from Life: The Autobiography of Lewis Mumford: The Early Years.* New York: Dial Press, reprint, 1982.

Neiswanger, Charles S. *Electro-Therapeutical Practice: A Ready Reference Guide for Physicians in the Use of Electricity and X-Rays*. 21st ed. Chicago: Ritchie & Co., 1920.

Norton, Frank, ed. *Frank Leslie's Historical Register of the United States Centennial Exposition, 1876*. New York: Frank Leslie, 1877.

O'Brien, J. Emmett. *The Identity of Nerve Force and Electricity*. Chicago: AMA Press, 1903.

Owen, J. *"Our Little Doctor": Helen Craib-Beighle and the Magic Power of Her Electric Hand*. San Francisco: The Hicks-Judd Co., 1893.

Paige, A. *The Electropathic Guide Devoted to Electricity and Its Medical Applications*. Boston: Damrell & Moore, 1849.

———. *Mental and Physical Electropathy, or Electricity; Its Physiological Relations and Medical Applications*. Philadelphia: Browns' Steam Power Book and Job Printing Office, 1852.

Petinak, Marko J. *Knowledge for Correct Living*. Los Angeles: Marko Petinak, 1926.

Philbrook, H. B. *Cause and Cure of Disease: Offices of Electricity in the Origin and Removal of the Disorders and Injuries of the Organization of the Human Body*. New York: Office of Problems of Nature, 1886.

Pierce, R. V. *Common Sense Medical Adviser*. Buffalo: World's Dispensary Printing, 1909.

Pilgrim, Maurice F. *Mechanical Vibratory Stimulation: Its Theory and Application in the Treatment of Disease*. New York: Metropolitan Publishing Co., 1903.

Pitzer, George C. *Electricity as a Remedial Agent*. St. Louis, 1885.

Poyen, Charles. *Progress of Animal Magnetism in New England*. Boston: Weeks & Jordan, 1837.

The Reactionary Lifter: Its Use in the System of Cumulative Exercise. New York: Health Lift Company, 1872.

Reynolds, J. Russell. *Lectures on the Clinical Uses of Electricity, Delivered in University College Hospital*. Philadelphia: Lindsay and Blakiston, 1872.

Ries, W. F. *Perfect Health Based on Science and Experience*. Toledo: W. F. Ries, 1927.

Robarts, Herbert. *Practical Radium: The Practical Uses of Radium in the Treatment of Obstinate Forms of Disease*. St. Louis, 1909.

Robinson, William J. *Woman, Her Sex and Love Life*. New York: Eugenics Publishing Company, 1929.

Rockwell, Alphonso. *Electrotherapeutics of the Male Genital Organs*. New York: William Wood & Co., 1874.

———. *The Medical and Surgical Uses of Electricity*. New York: W. Wood, 1896.

Rohland, Robert. *Od, or Odo-Magnetic Force: And Explanation of Its Influence on Homeopathic Medicines*. New York: Robert Rohland, 1871.

Sandow, Eugen. *Physical Development for Men*. London: published by author, n.d.

Sargent, Dudley Allen. *Handbook of Developing Exercises*. Boston: Franklin Press, 1886.

———. "The System of Physical Training at the Hemenway Gymnasium." In *Physical Training: A Full Report of the Papers and Discussions of the Conference Held in Boston in November, 1889*, ed. Isabel C. Barrows. Boston: Press of George H. Ellis, 1890, 62–77.

———. *Universal Test for Health, Speed and Endurance of the Human Body*. Cambridge: Dudley Allen Sargent, 1902.

Sargent, Ledyard, ed. *Dudley Allen Sargent: An Autobiography*. Philadelphia: Lea & Febiger, 1927.

Schmidt, F. A., and Eustace H. Miles. *The Training of the Body for Games*. New York: E. P. Dutton & Co., 1901.

Schneider, Edward. *Physiology of Muscular Activity*. Philadelphia: W. B. Saunders Company, 1940.

Schütz, M. "On Medico-Mechanical Treatment of Injuries." In A. Levertin et al., *The Leading Features of Dr. G. Zander's Medico-Mechanical Gymnastic Method and Its Use*. Wiesbaden: Rossel, Schwartz & Co., 1906.

Schweig, George M. *The Electric Bath: Its Medical Uses, Effects and Appliance*. New York: G. P. Putnam's Sons, 1877.

Scoresby, Rev. W. *Zoistic Magnetism: Being the Substance of Two Lectures, Descriptive of Original Views and Investigations Respecting This Mysterious Agency*. London: Longman, Brown, Green, and Longmans, 1849.

Scott, George. *The Doctor's Story: A Treatise on Electricity and Electro Magnetism*. New York: Pall Mall Electric Company, 1888.

Shaftesbury, Edmund. *Instantaneous Personal Magnetism*. Meriden, Conn.: Ralston University Press, 1926.

———. *Private Lessons in the Cultivation of Magnetism of the Sexes*. Cleveland: Ralston Society, 1934.

Sherwood, H. H. *The Motive Power of the Human System, with the Symptoms and Treatment of Chronic Diseases*. New York: Jared W. Bell, 1840.

Snow, Arnold. *Mechanical Vibration and Its Therapeutic Application*. New York: Scientific Author's Publishing Co., 1904.

Steele, Albert J. *Theory and Practice of Electrical Therapeutics, or Electricity as a Curative Agent*. New York: American News Company, 1871.

Talmey, B. S. *Woman*. New York: Practitioner's Publishing Company, 1910.

———. *Male Impotence and Sterility in Marriage*. New York: A. R. Elliott Publishing, 1917.

Taylor, Frederick Winslow. *Principles of Scientific Management*. New York: Harper and Brothers, 1911.

Tibbits, Herbert. *How to Use a Galvanic Battery in Medicine and Surgery*. London: J. & A. Churchill, 1879.

Tipton, A. W. *A Revised and Enlarged Edition of Clark's New System of Electrical Medication*. Chicago: Chas. J. Johnson, 1882.

Tousey, Sinclair. *Medical Electricity, Röntgen Rays and Radium*. Philadelphia: W. B. Saunders Co., 1921.

Trowbridge, John. *The Electrical Boy or the Career of Greatmen and Greatthings*. Boston: Roberts Brothers, 1891.

Turner, Dawson. *Radium: Its Physics and Therapeutics*. New York: William Wood & Co., 1911.

van de Velde, Theodore H. *Sexual Tensions in Marriage: Their Origin, Prevention and Treatment*. New York: Random House, 1931.

Vaughan, John. *Observations on Animal Electricity in Explanation of the Metallic Operation of Doctor Perkins*. Wilmington, Del.: W. C. Smyth, 1787.

Vecki, Victor. *The Pathology and Treatment of Sexual Impotence*. London, 1901.

von Humbolt, Alexander. *Views of Nature: Or Contemplations on the Sublime Phenomena of Creation*. London: Henry G. Bohn, 1850.

Waterman, L. E. *A Manual of the Exercise Known as the Butler Health Lift*. New York: Lewis G. Janes & Co., 1871.

Watson, J. Madison. *Watson's Manual of Calisthenics: A Systematic Drill-Book Without Apparatus for Schools, Families, and Gymnasiums*. New York: E. Steiger & Co., 1882.

Wells, S. M. *The Electropathic Guide: Prepared with Particular Reference to Home Practice*. Chicago: S. M. Wells, 1888.

Wells, W. R. *A New Theory of Disease; Based Upon the Principle that Man is a Compound Electrical Magnet*. Rochester, N.Y.: Steam Press, 1862.

Winjum, A. R. T. *Manual of Physical Exercise: "A Health Hand-Book."* Battle Creek, Mich.: A. R. T. Winjum, 1909.

Winslow, Kalem. *The Home Medical Adviser*. New York: D. Appleton & Co., 1927.

Wolf, Heinrich F. *The Practice of Physical Medicine*. Chicago: Wilcox & Follett Co., 1947.

Zachos, J. C. *The Butler Health Lift: Its Reasons and Its Facts*. New York: Lewis G. Janes & Co., 1871.

Zander, Gustav, and L. Wischnewetzky. "Mechanical-Electrotherapeutics and Orthopedics by Means of Apparatus." In Alfred Levertin, *Dr. Zander's Medico-Mechanische Gymnastik, ihre Methode, Bedeutung und Anwendung*. Stockholm: Königl. Buchdruckerei, P. A. Norstedt & Söner, 1892.

Zettel, H. A. *Life—Its Origin, Health and Diseases*. Herbert A. Zettel, 1918.

SECONDARY SOURCES

Articles and Reports

Alaimo, Stacy. "Cyborgs and Ecofeminist Interventions: Challenges for an Environmental Feminism." *Feminist Studies* 20, no. 1 (April 1994): 133–145.

Betts, John. "The Technological Revolution and the Rise of Sports, 1850–1900." In *The Sporting Image: Readings in American Sport History*, ed. Paul Zingg. Lanham, Md.: University Press of America, 1988.

Chiu, J. A., et al. "Transcutaneous Electrical Nerve Stimulation (TENS) Helps Manage Pain." *Essential Information on Alternative Health Care* 5, no. 7 (November 1999): 16.

Cohen, Michael. "The Homestead Zander Collection." Unpublished report in the accession files of the Homestead, Hot Springs, Virginia.

Davis, Donald Jr. "The Ionaco of Gaylord Wilshire." *Southern California Quarterly* (December 1967): 425–453.

Enserink, Martin. "Can the Placebo Be the Cure?" *Science* 284, no. 5412 (April 9, 1999): 238.

Gordon, Michael. "From an Unfortunate Necessity to a Cult of Mutual Orgasm: Sex in American Marital Education Literature." In *Studies in the Sociology of Sex*, ed. James Henslin. New York: Appleton-Century Croft, 1971, 53–77.

Haraway, Donna. "A Manifesto for Cyborgs: Science, Technology, and Socialist Feminism in the 1980s." In *Coming to Terms: Feminism, Theory, Politics*, ed. Elizabeth Weed. New York: Routledge, 1989.

Harris, Nigel, et al. "The Microvascular Effects of Electrical Spinal Cord Stimulation in Painful Diabetic Neuropathy and Other Painful Conditions." *Diabetes* 49, no. 5 (May 2000): A:164.

Herzig, Rebecca. "In the Name of Science: Suffering, Sacrifice, and the Formation of American Rotentgenology." *American Quarterly* 53, no. 4 (December 2001): 563–589.

———. "Removing Roots: 'North American Hiroshima Maidens' and the X Ray." *Technology and Culture* 40, no. 4 (October 1999): 723–745.

Kopytoff, Verne. "A Fitness Coach with a Muscular Memory." *New York Times* (May 6, 1999): D1.

Krull, Anne. "The Cyborg as an Interpretation of Culture-Nature." *Zygon* 36, no. 1 (March 2001): 49–56.

Lewchuck, Wayne. "Men and Monotony: Fraternalism as a Management Strategy at the Ford Motor Company." *Journal of Economic History* 5, no. 4 (December 1993): 824–856.

Morus, Iwan Rhys. "Marketing the Machine: The Construction of Electrotherapeutics as Viable Medicine in Early Victorian England." *Medical History* 36 (1992): 34–52.

Motluk, Alison. "Some of the Best Medicines Are All in the Mind." *New Scientist* 171, no. 2304 (August 18, 2001): 19.

Neustadter, Roger. "The 'Deadly Current': The Death Penalty in the Industrial Age." *Journal of American Culture* 12 (1989): 79–87.

Noon, Mitchell J. "Placebo to Credebo: The Missing Link in the Healing Process." *Pain Reviews* 6, no. 2 (July 1999): 133–142.

Paul, Joan. "The Health Reformers: George Barker Windship and Boston's Strength Seekers." *Journal of Sport History* 10, no. 3 (Winter 1983): 41–57.

Talbot, Margaret. "The Placebo Effect," *New York Times Sunday Magazine* (January 9, 2000): 34–39, 44, 58–60.

Thomas de la Peña, Carolyn. "Recharging at the Fordyce: Machine and Nature in the Modern Bath." *Technology and Culture* 40, no. 4 (October 1999): 746–769.

Todd, Janice. "Strength Is Health: George Barker Windship and the First American Weight Training Boom." *Iron Game History* (September 1993): 3–14.

———. "From Milo to Milo: A History of Barbells, Dumbbells and Indian Clubs." *Iron Game History* (April 1995): 4–16.

Young, Dwight. "To Form a More Perfect Human." *The Wilson Quarterly* (Spring 1990): 120–128.

Books

Ames, Kenneth. *Death in the Dining Room and Other Tales of Victorian Culture*. Philadelphia: Temple University Press, 1992.

Armstrong, David. *The Great American Medical Show: Being an Illustrated History of Hucksters, Healers, Health Evangelists, and Heroes from Plymouth Rock to the Present*. New York: Prentice Hall, 1991.

Armstrong, Tim. *Modernism, Technology and the Body: A Cultural Study*. Cambridge: Cambridge University Press, 1998.

Badash, Lawrence. *Radioactivity in America: Growth and Decay of a Science*. Baltimore: Johns Hopkins University Press, 1979.

Balsamo, Anne. *Technologies of the Gendered Body: Reading Cyborg Women*. Durham: Duke University Press, 1996.

Banta, Martha. *Taylored Lives: Narrative Productions in the Age of Taylor, Veblen, and Ford*. Chicago: University of Chicago Press, 1993.

Barber, Benjamin. *Jihad vs. McWorld*. New York: Times Books, 1995.

Barker-Benfield, G. J. *The Horrors of the Half-Known Life: Male Attitudes towards Women and Sexuality in the Nineteenth Century*. New York: Routledge, 1974; 2000.

Barney, Robert K. "German Turners in America: Their Role in Nineteenth Century Exercise Expression and Physical Education Legislation." In *A History of Physical Education and Sport in the United States and Canada*, ed. Earle F. Ziegler, 111–120. Champaign, Ill.: Stipes Publishing, 1975.

Becker, Robert, and Gary Selden. *The Body Electric: Electromagnetism and the Foundation of Life*. New York: William Morrow, 1985.

Bederman, Gail. *Manliness and Civilization: A Cultural History of Gender and Race in the United States, 1880–1917*. Chicago: University of Chicago Press, 1995.

Belfer, Lauren. *City of Light*. New York: Dial Press, 1999.

Bennett, Bruce. *Contributions of Dr. Sargent to Physical Education*. Minot, N.D.: State Teachers College, 1948.

———. "The Life of Dudley Allen Sargent and His Contributions to Physical Education." Ph.D. diss., University of Michigan, 1947.

Bennett, Paula, and Vernon A. Rosario. *Solitary Pleasures: The Historical, Literary and Artistic Discourses of Autoeroticism*. New York: Routledge, 1995.

Benson, Susan Porter. *Counter Cultures: Saleswomen, Managers, and Customers in American Department Stores, 1890–1940*. Urbana: University of Illinois Press, 1986.

Benthall, Jonathan. *The Body Electric: Patterns of Western Industrial Culture*. London: Thames and Hudson, 1976.

Berryman, Jack W. "Exercise and the Medical Tradition from Hippocrates through Antebellum America: A Review Essay." In *Sport and Exercise Science: Essays in the History of Sports Medicine*, ed. Jack W. Berryman and Roberta J. Park. Urbana: University of Illinois Press, 1992.

Bett, John R. "The Technological Revolution and the Rise of Sport, 1850–1900." In *The Sporting Image: Readings in American Sport History*, ed. Paul Zingg. Lanham, Md.: University Press of America, 1988.

Bledstein, Burton, and Robert D. Johnston, eds. *The Middling Sorts: Explorations in the History of the American Middle Class*. New York: Routledge, 2001.

Blocker, Jack. *"Give to the Wind Thy Fears": The Women's Temperance Crusade, 1873–1874*. Westport, Conn.: Greenwood Press, 1985.

Bordeau, Sanford. *Volts to Hertz: The Rise of Electricity: From the Compass to the Radio through the Works of Sixteen Great Men of Science Whose Names are Used in Measuring Electricity and Magnetism*. Minneapolis: Burgess Publishing Co., 1982.

Braun, Marta. *Picturing Time: The Work of Etienne-Jules Marey*. Chicago: University of Chicago Press, 1992.

Brecher, Ruth, and Edward Brecher. *The Rays: A History of Radiology in the United States and Canada*. Baltimore: Williams and Wilkins Company, 1969.

Brock, William. *Justus von Liebig: The Chemical Gatekeepers*. New York: Cambridge University Press, 1997.

Brush, Stephen. *The Temperature of History: Phases of Science and Culture in the Nineteenth Century*. New York: Burt Franklin & Co., 1978.

Budd, Michael. *The Sculpture Machine: Physical Culture and Body Politics in the Age of Empire.* Houndsmills: Macmillan, 1997.

Cardwell, Donald S. *From Watt to Clausius: The Rise of Thermodynamics in the Early Industrial Age.* Ithaca: Cornell University Press, 1971.

Caufield, Catherine. *Multiple Exposures: Chronicles of the Radiation Age.* New York: Harper and Row, 1989.

Chapman, David. *Sandow the Magnificent: Eugen Sandow and the Beginnings of Bodybuilding.* Urbana: University of Illinois Press, 1994.

Chauncey, George. *Gay New York: Gender, Urban Culture, and the Making of the Gay Male World, 1890–1940.* New York: Basic Books, 1994.

Clark, Claudia. *Radium Girls: Women and Industrial Health Reform, 1910–1935.* Chapel Hill: University of North Carolina Press, 1997.

Coffman, Elizabeth. "Women in Motion: Dance, Gesture and Spectacle in Film, 1900–1935." Ph.D. diss., University of Florida, 1995.

Cogan, Frances. *All American Girl: The Ideal of Real Woman-Hood in Mid-Nineteenth-Century America.* Athens: University of Georgia Press, 1989.

Cogdell, Christina. "Reconsidering the Streamline Style: Evolutionary Thought, Eugenics, and U.S. Industrial Design, 1925–1940." Ph.D. diss., University of Texas, Austin, 2001.

Colbert, Charles. *Phrenology and the Fine Arts in America.* Chapel Hill: University of North Carolina Press, 1997.

Corbusier, Le. *Towards a New Architecture.* New York: Payson & Clarke, 1927.

Cottrell, Deborah Lynn. "Women's Minds, Women's Bodies: The Influence of the Sargent School for Physical Education." Ph.D. diss., University of Texas at Austin, 1993.

Davis, Audrey, and Mark Dreyfuss. *The Finest Instruments Ever Made: A Bibliography of Medical, Dental, Optical, and Pharmaceutical Company Trade Literature, 1700–1939.* Arlington, Mass.: Medical History Publishing Associates, 1986.

Davis, Mike. *City of Quartz: Excavating the Future in Los Angeles.* New York: Verso, 1990.

Deacon, Desley. *Elsie Clews Parsons: Inventing Modern Life.* Chicago: University of Chicago Press, 1997.

Debre, Patrice. *Louis Pasteur.* Translated by Elborg Forster. Baltimore: Johns Hopkins University Press, 1998.

D'Emilio, John, and Esther Freedman. *Intimate Matters: A History of Sexuality in America.* New York: Perennial Library, 1988.

Drinka, George. *The Birth of Neurosis: Myth, Malady, and the Victorians.* New York: Simon & Schuster, 1984.

Duffy, John. *The Healers: A History of American Medicine.* Urbana: University of Illinois Press, 1979.

Dutton, Kenneth R. *The Perfectible Body: The Western Ideal of Male Physical Development.* New York: Continuum Publishing Company, 1995.

Earnest, Earnest. S. *Weir Mitchell, Novelist and Physician.* Philadelphia: University of Pennsylvania Press, 1950.

Easterbrook, Gregg. *Moment on Earth.* New York: Viking, 1995.

Ernst, Robert. *Weakness Is a Crime: The Life of Bernarr Macfadden.* Syracuse: Syracuse University Press, 1991.

Fox, Renée, and Judith Swazey. *Spare Parts: Organ Replacement in American Society.* New York: Oxford University Press, 1992.

Fox, Richard Wightman. *Trials of Intimacy: Love and Loss in the Beecher-Tilton Scandal.* Chicago: University of Chicago Press, 1999.

Fussell, Samuel. *Muscle: Confessions of an Unlikely Bodybuilder.* New York: Poseidon Press, 1991.

Gagliardi, Raymond, ed. *A History of the Radiological Sciences.* Reston, Va.: Radiology Centennial Inc., 1996.

Gauld, Alan. *Electrotherapy in the United States.* Minneapolis: Medtronic, 1977.

———. *A History of Hypnotism.* Cambridge: Cambridge University Press, 1992.

Gay, Peter. *The Tender Passion.* New York: Oxford University Press, 1986.

Gerber, Richard. *Vibrational Medicine: New Choices for Healing Ourselves.* Santa Fe: Bear and Company, 1996.

Ginger, Ray. *The Age of Excess: The United States from 1877 to 1914.* New York, 1965.

Gorn, Elliott. *The Manly Art: Bare-Knuckle Prize Fighting in America.* Ithaca: Cornell University Press, 1986.

Gosling, F. G. *Before Freud: Neurasthenia and the Medical Community.* Urbana: University of Illinois Press, 1987.

Green, Harvey. *Fit for America: Health, Fitness, Sport and American Society.* Baltimore: Johns Hopkins University Press, 1986.

Greenway, John. "Nervous Disease and Electric Medicine." In *Pseudo-Science and Society in Nineteenth-Century America,* ed. Arthur Wrobel. Lexington: University Press of Kentucky, 1987.

Grover, Kathryn, ed. *Hard at Play: Leisure in America, 1840–1940.* Amherst: University of Massachusetts Press, 1992.

———. *Fitness in American Culture: Images of Health, Sport, and the Body, 1830–1940.* New York: Margaret Woodbury Strong Museum, 1989.

Hafner, Arthur, et al. American Medical Association, *Guide to the American Medical Association Historical Health Fraud and Alternative Medicine Collection.* Chicago: American Medical Association, 1992.

Haggard, Howard. *Devils, Drugs, and Doctors: The Story of the Science of*

Healing from Medicine-Man to Doctor. New York: Blue Ribbon Books, 1929.

Hall, Lesley. *Hidden Anxieties: Male Sexuality, 1900–1950.* Cambridge, U.K.: Polity Press, 1991.

Haller, John S. *Outcasts from Evolution: Scientific Attitudes of Racial Inferiority, 1859–1900.* Urbana: University of Illinois Press, 1971.

———, and Robin Haller. *The Physician and Sexuality in Victorian America.* Urbana: University of Illinois Press, 1974.

Harris, Leon. *Upton Sinclair, American Rebel.* New York: Crowell, 1975.

Harris, Michael R. "Iron Therapy and Tonics." In *Fitness in American Culture: Images of Health, Sport, and the Body, 1830–1940,* ed. Kathryn Grover, 67–85. New York: Margaret Woodbury Strong Museum, 1989.

Hayden, Dolores. *The Grand Domestic Revolution: A History of Feminist Designs for American Homes, Neighborhoods, and Cities.* Cambridge: MIT Press, 1981.

Health Quackery: Consumers Union's Report on False Health Claims, Worthless Remedies, and Unproved Therapies. Mount Vernon, N.Y.: Consumers Union, 1980.

Hemphill, C. Dallett. *Bowing to Necessities: A History of Manners in America, 1620–1860.* New York: Oxford University Press, 1999.

Henderson, Linda Dalrymple. *Duchamp in Context: Science and Technology in the Large Glass and Related Works.* Princeton: Princeton University Press, 1998.

Henning, Michelle. "Don't Touch Me (I'm Electric): On Gender and Sensation in Modernity." In *Women's Bodies: Discipline and Transgression,* ed. Jane Arthurs and Jean Grimshaw. London: Cassell, 1999.

Himrich, Brenda, and Stew Thornley. *Electrifying Medicine: How Electricity Sparked a Medical Revolution.* Minneapolis: Lerner Publications Company, 1995.

Holbrook, Stewart, and Eric Jameson. *The Golden Age of Quackery.* New York: Macmillan, 1959.

Hopkins, C. Howard. *History of the YMCA in North America.* New York: Association Press, 1951.

Horowitz, Helen Lefkowitz. *Alma Mater: Design and Experience in the Women's Colleges from Their Nineteenth-Century Beginnings to the 1930s.* New York: Knopf, 1984.

Hoy, Suellen. *Chasing Dirt: The American Pursuit of Cleanliness.* Oxford: Oxford University Press, 1995.

Hughes, Thomas. *American Genesis: A Century of Invention and Technological Enthusiasm, 1870–1970.* New York: Viking, 1989.

Hughes, Thomas, ed. *Changing Attitudes Towards American Technology.* New York: Harper & Row, 1975.

Israel, Paul. *Edison: A Life of Invention.* New York: John Wiley, 1998.

Ives, John. *Electricity as a Medicine and Its Mode of Application.* New York: John T. Ives, 1879.

Jameson, Eric. *The Natural History of Quackery.* Springfield, Ill.: Charles C. Thomas, 1961.

Kasson, John. *Amusing the Million: Coney Island at the Turn of the Century.* New York: Hill and Wang, 1978.

———. *Civilizing the Machine: Technology and Republican Values in America, 1776–1900.* New York: Grossman, 1976.

———. *Houdini, Tarzan and the Perfect Man: The White Male Body and the Challenge of Modernity.* New York: Hill & Wang, 2001.

Kern, Stephen. *Anatomy and Destiny: A Cultural History of the Human Body.* Indianapolis: Bobbs-Merrill, 1975.

———. *The Culture of Time and Space, 1880–1918.* Cambridge: Harvard University Press, 1983.

Kett, Joseph. *Rites of Passage: Adolescence in America, 1790 to the Present.* New York: Basic Books, 1977.

Kevles, Daniel. *In the Name of Eugenics: Genetics and the Uses of Human Heredity.* New York: Knopf, 1985.

Kimmel, Michael. *Manhood in America: A Cultural History.* New York: Free Press, 1996.

Klaw, Spencer. *Without Sin: The Life and Death of the Oneida Community.* New York: Penguin Press, 1993.

Kneeland, Timothy. "The Use of Electricity to Treat Mental Illness in the United States, 1870 to the Present." Ph.D. diss., University of Oklahoma, 1996.

Koolhaas, Rem. *Delirious New York: A Retroactive Manifesto for Manhattan.* New York: Monacelli Press, 1994. (orig. pub 1973).

Kostof, Spiro. *A History of Architecture, Settings, and Rituals.* New York: Oxford University Press, 1985.

Lears, T. J. Jackson. *Fables of Abundance: A Cultural History of Advertising in America.* New York: Basic Books, 1994.

———. *No Place of Grace: Antimodernism and the Transformation of American Culture, 1880–1920.* Chicago: University of Chicago, 1994.

Leavitt, Judith Waltzer. *Brought to Bed: Childbearing in America, 1750–1950.* New York: Oxford University Press, 1986.

Lehner, Steven. *Explorers of the Body.* New York: Doubleday & Co., 1979.

Lipsitz, George. *Time Passages: Collective Memory and American Popular Culture.* Minneapolis: University of Minnesota Press, 1990.

Lutz, Tom. *American Nervousness, 1903: An Anecdotal History.* Ithaca: Cornell University Press, 1991.

Lystra, Karen. *Searching the Heart: Women, Men and Romantic Love in Nineteenth-Century America.* New York: Oxford University Press, 1989.

Macklis, Roger. "Radiomedical Fraud and Popular Perceptions of Radiation." In *A History of the Radiological Sciences*, ed. Raymond Gagliardi. Reston, Va.: Radiology Centennial Inc., 1996.

Maines, Rachel. *Technology of Orgasm: Hysteria, the Vibrator, and Women's Sexual Satisfaction*. Baltimore: Johns Hopkins University Press, 1994.

Martin, Ronald. *American Literature and the Universe of Force*. Durham: Duke University Press, 1981.

Marvin, Carolyn. *When Old Technologies Were New: Thinking about Electric Communication in the Late Nineteenth Century*. New York: Oxford University Press, 1988.

McLoughlin, William, Sr. *Modern Revivalism: Charles Grandison Finney to Billy Graham*. New York: Ronald Press, 1959.

Meyer, Donald. *The Positive Thinkers: A Study of the American Quest for Health, Wealth and Personal Power from Mary Baker Eddy to Norman Vincent Peale*. Garden City, N.Y.: Doubleday, 1965.

Mosher, Clelia Duel. *The Mosher Survey: Sexual Attitudes of Forty-Five Victorian Women*, ed. James Mahood and Kristine Wenberg. New York: Arno Press, 1980.

Mrozek, Donald. *Sport and American Mentality, 1880–1910*. Knoxville: University of Tennessee Press, 1983.

Nash, Roderick. *Wilderness and the American Mind*. New Haven: Yale University Press, 1967.

Nye, David. *Electrifying America: Social Meanings of a New Technology*. Cambridge: MIT Press, 1990.

———. *American Technological Sublime*. Cambridge: MIT Press, 1994.

———. *Consuming Power: A Social History of American Energies*. Cambridge: MIT Press, 1998.

Oliver, Robert T. *History of Public Speaking in America*. Westport, Conn.: Greenwood Press, 1977.

Oppenheim, Janet. *"Shattered Nerves": Doctors, Patients, and Depression in Victorian England*. New York: Oxford University Press, 1991.

Ott, Katherine. *Fevered Lives: Tuberculosis in American Culture Since 1870*. Cambridge: Harvard University Press, 1996.

Park, Roberta. "Healthy, Moral, and Strong: Educational Views of Exercise and Athletics in Nineteenth-Century America." In *Fitness in American Culture: Images of Health, Sport, and the Body, 1830–1940*, ed. Kathryn Grover, 123–168. New York: Margaret Woodbury Strong Museum, 1989.

———. "Physiologists, Physicians and Physical Educators." In *Sport and Exercise Science: Essays in the History of Sports Medicine*, ed. Jack Berryman. Urbana: University of Illinois Press, 1992.

Pendergast, Tom. *Creating the Modern Man: American Magazines and Consumer Culture, 1900–1950*. Columbia: University of Missouri Press, 2000.

Pera, Marcello. *The Ambiguous Frog: The Galvani-Volta Controversy on Animal Electricity.* Translated by Jonathan Mandelbaum. Princeton: Princeton University Press, 1992.

Petravage, Carol. *The Fordyce Bathhouse, Hot Springs National Park, Arkansas.* Harpers Ferry, W.V., 1988.

Porter, Roy. *Health for Sale: Quackery in England, 1660–1850.* Manchester: Manchester University Press, 1989.

Pursell, Carroll. *The Machine in America: A Social History of Technology.* Baltimore: Johns Hopkins University Press, 1995.

Quinn, Susan. *Marie Curie: A Life.* New York: Simon & Schuster, 1995.

Rabinbach, Anson. *The Human Motor: Energy, Fatigue and the Origins of Modernity.* New York: Basic Books, 1990.

Rhodes, Richard, ed. *Visions of Technology: A Century of Vital Debate about Machines, Systems, and the Human World.* New York: Simon & Schuster, 1999.

Rosenberg, Charles. *No Other Gods: On Science and American Social Thought.* Baltimore: Johns Hopkins University Press, 1978.

Rothman, Sheila. *Living in the Shadow of Death: Tuberculosis and the Social Experience of Illness in America.* New York: Basic Books, 1994.

Rotundo, Anthony. *American Manhood: Transformations in Masculinity from the Revolution to the Modern Era.* New York: Basic Books, 1993.

Rowbottom, Margaret, and Charles Susskind. *Electricity and Medicine: History of Their Interaction.* San Francisco: San Francisco Press, 1984.

Russett, Cynthia. *Sexual Science: The Victorian Construction of Womanhood.* Cambridge: Harvard University Press, 1989.

Rylance, Rick. *Victorian Psychology and British Culture, 1850–1880.* New York: Oxford University Press, 2000.

Sandelowski, Margarete. *Pain, Pleasure and American Childbirth: From the Twilight Sleep to the Read Method, 1914–1960.* Westport, Conn.: Greenwood Press, 1984.

Schaller, Warren, and Charles Carroll. *Health, Quackery and the Consumer.* Philadelphia: W. B. Saunders Co., 1976.

Schwartz, Hillel. "Torque: The New Kinaesthetic of the Twentieth Century." In *Incorporations: Zone 6,* ed. Jonathan Cray and Sanford Kwinter. New York: Urzone, 1992.

Sears, John. *Sacred Places: American Tourist Attractions in the Nineteenth Century.* New York: Oxford University Press, 1989.

Shorter, Edward. *From Paralysis to Fatigue: A History of Psychosomatic Illness in the Modern Era.* New York: Free Press, 1992.

Siler, Brooke. *The Pilates Body: The Ultimate At-Home Guide to Strengthening, Lengthening, and Toning Your Body Without Machines.* New York: Bantam Doubleday, 2000.

Smith, Terry. *Making the Modern: Industry, Art, and Design in America.* Chicago: University of Chicago Press, 1993.

Stage, Sarah. *Female Complaints: Lydia Pinkham and the Business of Women's Medicine.* New York: Norton, 1979.

Stengers, Jean, and Anne Van Neck. *Masturbation: The History of a Great Terror,* trans. Kathryn Hoffman. New York: Palgrave, 2001.

Swanson, Richard, and Betsy Spears. *History of Sport and Physical Education in the United States.* 4th ed. New York: McGraw-Hill, 1995.

Swazey, Judith. *Spare Parts: Organ Replacement in American Society.* New York: Oxford University Press, 1992.

Sweet, William Warren. *Revivalism in America: Its Origin, Growth, and Decline.* Gloucester, Mass.: Peter Smith, 1965.

Thomas, George M. *Revivalism and Cultural Change: Christianity, Nation-Building, and the Market in the Nineteenth-Century United States.* Chicago: University of Chicago Press, 1989.

Tichi, Cecelia. *Shifting Gears: Technology, Literature and Culture in Modernist America.* Chapel Hill: University of North Carolina Press, 1987.

Todd, Janice. *Physical Culture and the Body Beautiful: Purposive Exercise in the Lives of American Women, 1800–1870.* Macon: Mercer University Press, 1998.

Tomes, Nancy. *The Gospel of Germs: Men, Women and the Microbe in American Life.* Cambridge: Harvard University Press, 1998.

Vertinsky, Patricia. *The Eternally Wounded Woman: Women, Doctors, and Exercise in the Late Nineteenth Century.* New York: St. Martin's Press, 1990.

Vierrille, Jonathan Paul. "American Healing Waters: A Chronology (1513–1926) and Historical Survey of America's Major Springs, Spas, and Health Resorts, Including a Review of Their Medicinal Virtues and Health Care Practices." Ph.D. diss., University of Texas, Austin, 1992.

Weart, Spencer. *Nuclear Fear: A History of Images.* Cambridge: Harvard University Press, 1988.

Wertz, Dorothy, and Richard Wertz. *Lying-In: A History of Childbirth in America.* New Haven: Yale University Press, 1989.

Whorton, James. *Crusaders for Fitness: The History of American Health Reform.* Princeton: Princeton University Press, 1982.

Williams, Brett. *John Henry: A Bio-Bibliography.* Westport, Conn.: Greenwood Press, 1983.

Young, Katharine, ed. *Bodylore.* Knoxville: University of Tennessee Press, 1993.

Zunz, Olivier. *Making America Corporate, 1870–1920.* Chicago: University of Chicago Press, 1990.

Index

About the Author

Carolyn Thomas de la Peña is Assistant Professor of American Studies at the University of California at Davis. Her research interests include material culture, consumer culture, gender, technology, and design. Her current projects explore the meanings of consumer spaces and American business culture of the early twentieth century.